Contents

Assessment of Motor Speech Disorders

Edited by

Anja Lowit, Ph.D. and Raymond D. Kent, Ph.D.

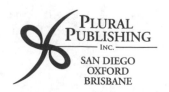

PLURAL
PUBLISHING
INC.

SAN DIEGO
OXFORD
BRISBANE

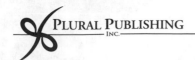

5521 Ruffin Road
San Diego, CA 92123

e-mail: info@pluralpublishing.com
Web site: http://www.pluralpublishing.com

49 Bath Street
Abingdon, Oxfordshire OX14 1EA
United Kingdom

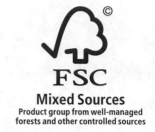

FSC
Mixed Sources
Product group from well-managed
forests and other controlled sources

Cert no. SW-COC-002283
www.fsc.org
© 1996 Forest Stewardship Council

Library of Congress Cataloging-in-Publication Data

Assessment of motor speech disorders / [edited by] Anja Lowit and Raymond D.
Kent.
        p. ; cm.
  Includes bibliographical references and index.
  ISBN-13: 978-1-59756-367-3 (alk. paper)
  ISBN-10: 1-59756-367-6 (alk. paper)
  1. Articulation disorders—Diagnosis. I. Lowit, Anja. II. Kent, Raymond D.
  [DNLM: 1. Dysarthria—diagnosis. 2. Speech Disorders—diagnosis. WL 340.2]
  RC424.7.A87 2010
  616.85'5—dc22

                                                                2010033933

Preface

Motor speech disorders (MSD) are a complex set of disorders. Although the resulting communication disturbances are largely phonetic by nature, the underlying causes for the speech disorder often result in deficits in associated areas, such as physiologic, linguistic, cognitive, or psychosocial functioning. Clinical assessment thus requires a holistic approach that encompasses a range of variables to arrive at a full understanding of how various aspects of communication are affected by the disorder. Historically, assessment of MSD focused on phonetic speech aspects and their presumed underlying physiological functioning, as initially suggested by Darley, Aronson, and Brown's (1975) seminal work, and later adapted by other assessment batteries, such as the recently updated Frenchay Dysarthria Assessment (Enderby & Palmer, 2008). In addition, a number of intelligibility tests have been developed to complement these assessments (Kent, Weismer, Kent, & Rosenbek, 1989; Yorkston & Beukelman, 1981).

The adoption of the ICF framework, which recognizes the importance not just of the underlying speech deficits, but also of their impact on the individual's activities and participation, has spurned a rethinking of the way speech disorders should be assessed nowadays. The focus of assessment thus has moved away from the impairment-based analysis of the speech deficit to the more holistic evaluation of the person's ability to function with their impairment.

Although an increasing number of research publications are becoming available on methods designed to assess clients more holistically, this information is currently not readily available in a form that supports informed clinical decisions to be made by practitioners. Clinicians lack a definitive text that critically reviews existing and newly developed evaluation techniques and provides guidance for the most suitable assessment resource or method for the MSD client group.

In parallel to devising more holistic clinical assessments methods, new techniques for the evaluation of phonetic and physiological aspects have been developed to further our understanding of the underlying motor control processes that lead to the observed speech deficits. Although these techniques are well established in other fields such as theoretical phonetics, physics, and kinesiology, they have not been used extensively in the clinical study of speech disorders. There thus exists a need to identify relevant techniques and to discuss their clinical application to MSD.

This book brings together a wide range of researchers to present an up-to-date summary of assessment and evaluation techniques for disordered speech, both with a clinical focus as well as for research purposes. After setting the scene with an introduction to the ICF framework (chapter 1), chapters 2 to 9 review research evidence pertaining to best practice in the assessment of established areas such as intelligibility and physiological functioning, as well as introducing recently developed topics such as conversation analysis, impact, and telehealth. In chapters 10 to 16, established and new research methods in the areas of phonetics/phonology, kinematics, imaging, and neural modeling are reviewed in relation to their applicability and value for the study of disordered speech.

It is the hope of the editors of this book that this comprehensive look at the assessment of motor speech disorders will help to stimulate progress in the clinical and research arenas. The chapters offer both a record of accom-plishment and suggestions for the future of assessment. We thank the authors for making our vision of this book a reality.

Anja Lowit, Ph.D.
Raymond D. Kent, Ph.D.

References

Darley, F. L., Aronson, A. E., & Brown, J. R. (1975). *Motor speech disorders*. Philadelphia, PA: W. B. Saunders.

Enderby, P., & Palmer, R. (2008). *Frenchay dysarthria assessment* (2nd ed.). Austin, TX: Pro-Ed.

Kent, R. D., Weismer, G., Kent, J. F., & Rosenbek, J. C. (1989). Toward phonetic intelligibility testing in dysarthria. *Journal of Speech and Hearing Disorders, 54*, 482–499.

Yorkston, K. M., & Beukelman, D. R. (1981). *Assessment of intelligibility of dysarthric speech*. Tigard, OR: CC Publications.

Contributors

Andrew Anderson, Ph.D.
Research Fellow
Cognitive Perceptual and Brain Sciences
University College London
London
United Kingdom
Chapter 13

Steven M. Barlow, Ph.D.
Professor
Speech-Language-Hearing,
    Neuroscience, Human Biology and
    Bioengineering
University of Kansas
Lawrence, Kansas
United States
Chapter 10

Carolyn R. Baylor, Ph.D.
Assistant Professor
Rehabilitation Medicine
University of Washington
Seattle, Washington
United States
Chapter 6

Steven Bloch, Ph.D., MRCSLT
National Institute for Health Research
    Fellow
Psychology and Language Sciences
University College London
London
United Kingdom
Chapter 8

Shin Ying Chu, M.A.
Doctoral Candidate in Speech Physiology

Department of Speech-Language-
    Hearing
Communication Neuroscience
    Laboratories
The University of Kansas
Lawrence, Kansas
United States
Chapter 10

Volker Dellwo, Ph.D., M.A.
Assistant Professor in
    Phonetics/Phonology
Department of General Linguistics
University of Zürich
Zürich
Switzerland
Chapter 11

Lena Hartelius, Ph.D.
Professor
Division of Speech and Language
    Pathology
Institute of Neuroscience and
    Physiology
University of Gothenburg
Gothenburg
Sweden
Chapter 1

Peter Howell, Ph.D.
Professor
Psychology and Language
    Sciences
University College London
London
United Kingdom
Chapter 13

Raymond D. Kent, Ph.D.
Professor Emeritus of Communicative
    Disorders
University of Wisconsin-Madison
Madison, Wisconsin
United States
Chapter 2

Yunjung Kim, Ph.D.
Assistant Professor
Department of Communication
    Sciences and Disorders
Louisiana State University
Baton Rouge, Louisiana
United States
Chapter 2

Bernd J. Kröger, Ph.D.
Professor
Department of Phoniatrics,
    Pedaudiology, and Communication
    Disorders
RWTH and University Hospital
    Aachen (UKA)
Aachen
Germany
Chapter 16

Anja Kuschmann, M.A.
Doctoral Candidate in Clinical
    Linguistics and Speech Pathology
Speech and Language Therapy
    Division
University of Strathclyde
Glasgow
United Kingdom
Chapter 12

Julie M. Liss, Ph.D.
Associate Professor
Department of Speech and Hearing
    Science
Arizona State University
Scottsdale, Arizona
United States
Chapter 11

Anja Lowit, PhD., MRCSLT
Reader
Speech and Language Therapy Division
University of Strathclyde
Glasgow
United Kingdom
Chapters 12, 13 and 16

**Catherine Mackenzie, Ph.D., M.Ed.,
FRCSLT**
Professor
Speech and Language Therapy Division
School of Psychological Sciences and
    Health
University of Strathclyde
Glasgow
United Kingdom
Chapter 7

Ineke Mennen, Ph.D.
Professor
Centre for Research on Bilingualism
Bangor University
Bangor,
United Kingdom
Chapter 12

Nick Miller, Ph.D., MRCSLT
Professor
Speech and Language Sciences
Institute of Health and Society
University of Newcastle
Newcastle upon Tyne
United Kingdom
Chapters 1, 12, and 16

Bruce E. Murdoch, Ph.D., D.Sc.
Professor
Centre for Neurogenic
    Communications Research,
School of Health and Rehabilitation
    Sciences
The University of Queensland
Queensland
Australia
Chapter 3

Christiane Neuschäfer-Rube, Ph.D.
Professor
Department of Phoniatrics,
    Pedaudiology, and Communication
    Disorders
RWTH and University Hospital
    Aachen (UKA)
Aachen
Germany
Chapter 16

Rupal Patel, Ph.D.
Associate Professor
Northeastern University and
Affiliated Faculty Harvard-MIT
    Health Science and Technology
    Program
Boston, Massachusetts
United States
Chapter 4

Serge Pinto, Ph.D.
CNRS Researcher (National Scientific
    Research Centre)
Laboratoire Parole et Langage
    (Aix-en-Provence, France)
CNRS/Aix-Marseille University
Aix-en Provence
France
Chapter 14

Meredith Poore, M.A.
Doctoral Candidate in Speech Physiology
Department of Speech-Language-
    Hearing
Communication Neuroscience
    Laboratories
The University of Kansas
Lawrence, Kansas
United States
Chapter 10

Deborah Theodoros, Ph.D.
Professor
Division of Speech Pathology
School of Health and Rehabilitation
    Sciences

The University of Queensland
Brisbane
Australia
Chapter 9

Margaret Walshe, Ph.D., M.Sc.
Lecturer
Department of Clinical Speech and
    Language Studies
Trinity College Dublin
Ireland
Chapter 5

Laurence White, Ph.D.
Research Fellow
International School for Advanced
    Studies (SISSA)
Trieste
Italy
Chapter 11

Ray Wilkinson, Ph.D., MRCSLT
Reader
Neuroscience and Aphasia Unit
School of Psychological Sciences
University of Manchester
Manchester
United Kingdom
Chapter 8

Kathryn M. Yorkston, Ph.D., BC-NCD
Professor
Rehabilitation Medicine
University of Washington
Seattle, Washington
United States
Chapter 6

Wolfram Ziegler, Ph.D.
Professor of Neurophonetics
Head of Clinical Neuropsychology
    Research Group
Department of Neuropsychology
City Hospital Munich
Munich
Germany
Chapter 15

1

The ICF Framework and Its Relevance to the Assessment of People with Motor Speech Disorders

LENA HARTELIUS, PH.D.
NICK MILLER, PH.D.

I knocked on Alexander's door several times and finally had to open without having heard him say "come in!" The sparsely furnished room in the nursing home contained most of what he feels he needs to get him through the day—a large TV set, audio books, a refrigerator filled with fruit, juice, chocolate bars, and beer. Although he has been a nursing home resident for the last two years, he spends a lot of time at home with his wife. He begins our conversation by telling me about his birthday party a couple of months earlier. He turned 70, and his wife and three children had arranged a "photo and film party" for him, featuring visual memories from a life full of activities, including travelling around the world. None of the five grandchildren were invited. "Only people who were actually there when it happened were allowed to take part," he said without my asking. "And it also makes it easier for me to talk, less

noise. I feel very self-conscious about my speech problems. My wife tries to help; every time I inhaled, she exclaimed, Hush —he is going to say something! Which makes me even more self-conscious, and I can't think anymore. It is difficult to get started and difficult to be heard. But once I get started, it helps a lot that she is very active, more of a verbal coach than a listener, really."

Alexander was diagnosed with Parkinson's disease in the 1970s. After 20 years of carefully balanced treatment, he still suffered from pronounced on–off variability and was treated surgically in the late 1990s. Since then, he has received bilateral deep brain stimulation in his subthalamic nuclei. The procedure has been very helpful to him generally, although it created speech problems that he did not have initially. He, himself, discovered that it was the electrostimulation that produced the speech

1

problem. A year after his operation, he was having an electrocardiogram, and the stimulation had to be turned off. As the stimulators were turned off, he immediately began to speak fluently without any problems in terms of voice or articulation. He sounded like his old self. After that, he and his neurologist have spent numerous hours trying to find the right combination of voltage for him so that he doesn't have to "choose whether to walk or talk."

After a while, I come to the reason for my visit—I want to ask him about measurement. Alexander has been an architect, a builder, and an artist, and my impression is that he has spent a lot of time thinking about how to measure things, works of use as well as works of art. "Do you think speech problems can be measured? And if so, how would you go about measuring them?" Alexander pondered for a long time and answered, "First of all, I would measure the strength of the voice; if you are not loud enough, you can't be heard. Secondly, I would measure how clear the speech is. That might not be easy to measure, but I'm sure it can be done. And, finally, if you want a measure of effect, I would measure how many times each utterance had to be repeated. I think that covers it; the rest of the effects can be inferred from that information." I promised to pass on his insights.

Alexander has more than 30 years of experience of living with his neurologic disease, as opposed to another person visiting the clinic the same week, Anna. She is 31 years old and has spinocerebellar ataxia, SCA3, as do one of her older sisters and her mother, who is now deceased. Anna lives in an apartment on the ground floor with her boyfriend. She uses a walking frame on wheels indoors and a wheelchair when she goes shopping. She has a personal assistant all through the day, and her boyfriend helps out evenings and mornings. Although she

wants to do as much as possible herself, she is often very tired. She trained as an engineer but has never had a job. She also had to give up her church choir singing because it was too difficult for her to hold the tune. Because she worries a lot about what is going to happen to her communication, she wants to come in for a "speech check-up" in the clinic every six months to keep track of any changes for the worse. She has a mild ataxic dysarthria and is 100% intelligible. What affects Anna's communication the most is not her respiratory or phonatory function and not her articulatory precision and prosody, although there is slight audible speech impairment. Environmental conditions also are close to optimal in terms of support and relationships although she finds that her circle of friends and acquaintances is narrowing. The fact that the disease is known and understandable to her family makes it easier in some ways but creates a lot of worry in others, since older family members "represent versions of the future," as Anna puts it. Her communication mostly is affected by influencing personal factors, both unchangeable ones, such as her general health condition and earlier experience, and potentially changeable personal factors such as coping style and current psychological assets. Our regular clinic meetings often center around confirming that the speech difficulties are very mild, reviewing helpful strategies, and talking through her communicative concerns. A questionnaire is helpful in bringing out and formulating these concerns.

These vignettes neatly encapsulate many of the issues broached in this chapter, and we will return to them regularly. The authors' aim is to provide readers with a brief overview of the International Classification of Functioning, Disability and Health (ICF) framework and its application and relevance to the assessment of individuals with motor speech disorders. After a short introduction, this chapter outlines the aims and the main constructs of the ICF model and classification. This model makes an important contribution to thinking about motor speech disorders and provides us with a way to manage the complex clinical and research challenges of this diverse and multifaceted client group. However, how the model, and particularly the classification should be applied to the area of speech and language pathology in general and motor speech disorders in particular, is not immediately transparent or evident. In this chapter, the authors draw out some issues in the interpretation of a number of concepts and items of measurement and through this raise a number of questions to deal with in the work ahead. Finally, we review earlier use of ICF in motor speech disorders research and other places in this book, concluding with possible areas of further research.

Introduction

Alexander's Parkinson's Disease and Anna's spinocerebellar ataxia, like many other neurological disorders, are associated with prominent changes in motor control and/or neuromuscular status. The movement disorder associated with these conditions rests largely on alterations to motor control, muscle tone, power, and coordination. Speech and voice changes associated with these conditions also are linked to these alterations in that they may influence velocity, force, and coordination of movements of the articulators. Degradation of these variables in turn affects the range, rate, precision, and sustainability of movements for producing speech sounds.

The logical step in describing the type and severity of speech disorder therefore would appear to be a speech motor assessment to precisely measure these parameters—rate, range, force, precision, sustainability, and so on. Thus, one might conduct diadochokinetic tasks to look at speed and coordination of lip, tongue tip, or tongue dorsum performance or infer intactness of velar movement through e.g. alternating repetition of syllables me-bee. Vocal fold and respiratory function might be gauged from maximum sustainability of /a:/, maximum loudness for /a/, maximum inspiratory capacity and expiratory force, and so forth. In some clinics or settings, these perceptual measures might be supplemented by instrumental measures.

Not so long ago, the recommendations in textbooks were that, having identified the speech motor deficit, one sought therapeutic activities that directly targeted them—for instance, increase diadochokinetic rate, increase precision of tongue tip control, or oral gymnastics to maintain or increase sustainability of movements. The implication was that gains in rate, range, force, precision, and sustainability of movement would be reflected in benefits for speech performance and intelligibility and amelioration of other negative consequences of the underlying movement disorder for speech and communication.

The rationale appears sound enough. But, several issues exist here when it comes to understanding the nature of the speech or broader communication disorder and issues concerning whether therapy directed at these variables really would bring about successes in communication gains. These issues include, for instance, that many assessments of motor speech status actually are assessments of nonverbal movements of the articulators very distant from the kinds of movements required for speech (Clark, 2003; Weismer, 2006). Added to that, the assumption of a direct link between outcomes of motor speech examinations and speech performance and intelligibility status is not strongly supported in the literature, or at least the interpretation of relationships is fraught with many complexities (McHenry & Minton, 1994; Hustad, 2008; Solomon, 2004; Weismer, Yeng, Laures, Kent, & Kent, 2001; Whitehill & Tsang, 2002; Ziegler, 2003). Furthermore, although the disorders introduced previously traditionally are associated with acquired motor *speech* disorders, they now are firmly recognized to have appreciable cognitive and language change components that also can have a significant bearing on communication.

The major issue, though, in relation to the topic of this chapter and an overall rationale for understanding, describing, measuring, and rehabilitating communication disorders is that an impairment perspective narrowly focused on the underlying movement disorder provides very restricted insights into the nature of a disorder and its consequences. At a minimum, one would wish to know whether and how, for example, slowed diadochokinetic rates, reduced maximum expiratory force, and similar underlying changes to the speech mechanism affect intelligibility, and in turn the impact that altered intelligibility or changed speech natu-

ralness might exercise on the person, the family, and social circle. Crucially, focusing on the underlying motor speech fails to disclose how any real or perceived (on the part of the speaker or the listener) change impacts on the person as a communicator. For instance, it tells nothing of their view of themselves as communicators, their moods, motivations, and aims in life in relation to communication. It indicates nothing about the family's view of them in relation to how they used to be and now are. It provides no insights into or understanding of the individual's ability to (continue to) engage in the activities they enjoyed previously or new ones they may wish to take up. It ignores the ways in which their participation in society may have been curtailed or modified and the impact this change has on their lives.

It is well known, and not just in the domain of speech, that there is not necessarily a one-to-one correspondence between underlying motor or neuropathological status and the changes that pervade the life of the person with neurological diseases or stroke (Chiara, Martin, & Sapienza, 2007; Hartelius, Elmberg, Holm, Lövberg, & Nikolaidis, 2008; Klasner & Yorkston, 2005; Miller, Allcock, Jones, Noble, Hildreth, & Burn, 2007; Walshe, Peach, & Miller, 2008). It is quite possible to find individuals who, on formal motor speech articulatory testing, present what appears to be a severe impairment profile, yet they do not perceive themselves to be severely impaired; they continue to enjoy life as they did previously, and their families may see no significant change regarding communication. Conversely, one can find others who, in the opinion of the speech-language pathologist or other professionals sound as if no speech or communication change is present. They score within normal ranges on motor speech examination. Yet, when asked, they tell of severe impacts on their lives—they have had to give up work and curtail their social activities; they are no longer the person they were; their families view them as different people (Hartelius, Jonsson, Rickeberg, & Laakso, 2010; Miller, Noble, Jones, Allcock, & Burn, 2008; Yorkston, Baylor, Klasner, Deitz, Dudgeon, Eadie, Miller, & Amtmann, 2007). They sense themselves as no longer in control when communicating; speaking is no longer the pleasant, easy, natural task it once was; the way people appear to judge them and the character others assign to them is not one they recognize as being their old selves. The general implication is that there is much more to neuromuscular disorders than can be disclosed in a speech motor examination.

Alexander's and Anna's stories bring into focus several of these issues, especially in terms of personal adjustments and the relationship between underlying pathology and behavioral consequences. To thoroughly understand this wider perspective requires a revised mindset in conceptualizing what constitutes illness or disability and how these impact people's lives.

The ICF was developed to address just this necessity. It sought to give a rationale and framework for understanding illness and the illness process, not within the narrow confines of a focus on underlying pathology, but within the broader experiential, psychosocial context in which any change occurred and had to be accommodated. The emphasis in understanding change associated with underlying pathology was not to understand the basic neuropathology, but to take up the challenge of understanding the impact of changes on individuals as thinking, feeling beings who live in real-life social and emotional contexts, with a past and with aims for the future.

ICF: A Conceptual Framework and a Classification Tool of Health Conditions

The current edition of the International Classification of Functioning, Disability, and Health, commonly known as ICF, was endorsed by the World Health Assembly of the WHO in May, 2001. It replaced the earlier International Classification of Impairments, Disabilities, and Handicap (ICIDH), which had undergone several field trials and systematic revisions since its first publication in 1980. The main differences between ICF as compared to ICIDH are that (1) it focuses on *health* rather than diseases and disorders and can, thus, be used to characterize the health conditions of *all* individuals and not just individuals with disabilities; (2) it has an increased level of complexity and multidimensionality; and (3) contextual factors are included. These notions are expanded in the following paragraphs.

ICF is meant to complement the existing classifications of diseases and interventions. The WHO Family of International Classifications (WHO-FIC) consists of the International Statistical Classification of Diseases and Related Health Problems (ICD-10), the

ICF and the International Classification of Health Interventions (ICHI, under development). ICD-10 gives an etiological framework for classification, by diagnosis of diseases and disorders, whereas ICF classifies function and disability associated with health conditions. In short, ICD-10 provides a disease perspective and ICF a functioning and disability perspective. The two classifications are, therefore, complementary and used together. They can give a more comprehensive and meaningful picture both of the health condition and of the experience of health of individuals and populations. In focusing on health and disability rather than disease, ICF acknowledges that every person can experience impaired health and some (temporary or long-term) disability. Consequently, there has been an important paradigm shift, from a focus on *cause* to a focus on *impact*, and the classification acknowledges that disability is a universal human experience. Sooner or later, we will all, to various degrees and durations, experience impaired health and disability.

The chief aims of the ICF classification are as follows:

- To provide a scientific basis for consequences of health conditions
- To establish a common language to improve communications
- To permit comparison of data across countries, health care disciplines, services, and time
- To provide a systematic coding scheme for health information systems

The ICF was developed because diagnosis alone does not provide information on service needs or functional outcomes. The use of a medical classification of diagnoses alone does not give us the information we need for health planning and management purposes.

The contrast between medical and functional classification is revealed readily when we attempt to determine the prevalence of different types of communication disorders. This is notoriously difficult, because we need to take into account a double or even triple prevalence. First, there is the prevalence of the different underlying causes, for example, that Parkinson's Disease (PD) occurs in approximately 150/100,000 of the population. But not everyone with a given neurological disorder necessarily presents with a voice or speech disorder. Hence, one needs to consider the prevalence of voice and speech disorders in a particular group. The third dimension, however, is that, even though we might diagnose the presence of a motor speech disorder in 90% of people with PD, this fails to indicate how many of those individuals are likely to be perceived by themselves or by others to have a disabling disorder, to experience different levels of difficulty in communicative situations. So, it is certainly useful to establish how common different types of communication disorders are, not only the number of individuals with an ICD-10 diagnosis of dysarthria or apraxia of speech, but more pertinently in terms of the consequences of disability (i.e., the burden of a motor speech disorder). The ICF allows us to go beyond the primary diagnosis and also beyond broad communication disorder diagnoses, to arrive at descriptions of populations with speech impairments in terms that are more relevant to personal experiences and personal daily living goals in rehabilitation as well as being comparable across countries and languages.

As indicated in this section's heading, the ICF can be viewed, described, and used in two different ways. First, it is a conceptual framework, a model combining different health-related constructs. Second, it is a classification tool comprising items used for the description of health conditions. Put simply, the ICF model is the theory, and the ICF classification is the theory put into practice. The model and the classification obviously share several characteristics, but also have their differences. In the following sections, we describe the ICF as a model and as a classification, before moving into its relevance for people with motor speech disorders.

The ICF Model and Its Concepts

The conceptual model of disability proposed by ICF is a *biopsychosocial* model stressing a threefold perspective: biological, individual, and societal. The well-known structure of the model including key concepts is presented in Figure 1–1. This model integrates the two common earlier models of disability, the medical model and the social model. The medical model views disability as something caused by a disease or trauma, making it a personal feature requiring medical, individual care provided by professionals to rectify or repair the problem. By contrast, the social model views disability as created in the encounter between the individual and the society in which he or she lives; the problem being created through a dissonance between the individual's needs and the social and physical environment. In terms of intervention, the social model proposes a political response to mitigate the environmental effects, and thereby support the individual. Of course, the notion of disability is more

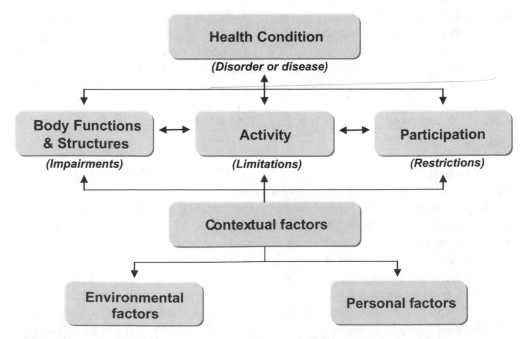

Figure 1–1. The ICF biopsychosocial model of disability.

complex than these two inadequate models allow. The more complex bio-psychosocial model acknowledges the fact that some disability aspects are internal to the person, and others are more external, and both medical and social responses are appropriate to the problems associated with disability.

Increased complexity leads to a need for an increased number of concepts and terms to permit a comprehensive description of the complexity. To be able to use the model as flexibly and in an as detailed and complete a way as was intended, the agreement on definitions of terminology is crucial. Detailed information about terminology and use, including an online version of the classification itself is provided at WHO's Web site (http://www.who.int/classifications/icf/en/).

ICF is a classification of *health* and *health-related domains* intended to facilitate the description of changes in *body function* and *structure*, what a person with a health condition can do in a standard environment (i.e., their level of *capacity*) as well as what they actually do in their usual environment (i.e., their level of *performance*) in terms of *activities* and *participation*. According to WHO terminology, *health* is defined as a state of complete physical, mental, and social well-being and not merely the absence of disease or infirmity. *Disability* is defined as any restriction or lack of ability to perform an activity in the manner or within the range considered normal for a human being. Disability may be physical, intellectual, sensory, permanent, or transitory. In ICF, *functioning* refers to all body functions, activities, and participation, whereas *disability* is a catchall term for *impairments*, *activity limitations,* and *participation restric-*

tions. Activity limitations are problems an individual may have in executing activities (*tasks* or *actions*). Participation restrictions are problems an individual may experience in *involvement in life situations*. In ICF, functioning and disability are viewed as outcomes of interactions between health conditions (diseases, disorders, and injuries) and contextual factors. These contextual factors comprise *environmental factors* (such as social attitudes, architectural conditions, and social and legal structures) and *personal factors* (including gender, age, social background, profession, coping styles, character and so forth).

The hierarchical structure of ICF is shown in Table 1–1. The two *parts* consist of *components* (e.g., in Part 1, body function, structures, activity/participation). These in turn consist of *chapters*, numbered from 1–9, and chapters comprise several *domains*. For example, one domain within Chapter 3 (voice and speech functions) is voice functions (including, for example, quality of voice), another is fluency and rhythm of speech functions (including, for example, speed of speech). Each of the domains is given an alphanumeric code consisting of one letter, indicating the relevant component and 3 or 4 additional digits indicating level of detail in the domain.

The ICF Classification

The model and the list of chapters becomes a classification when the qualifiers are used. The qualifiers indicate the presence and severity of a problem regarding *body* (*structure* and/or *function*), *activity*, or *participation*).

For the classifications of *body function* and *structure*, the primary qualifier

Table 1–1. The ICF Chapters

Part 1. Functioning and Disability			Part 2. Contextual Factors	
Body Function	Body Structures	Activity and Participation	Environmental Factors	Personal Factors
1. Mental functions	1. Structures of the nervous system	1. Learning and applying knowledge	1. Products and technology	(not coded)
2. Sensory functions and pain	2. The eye, ear, and related structures	2. General tasks and demands	2. Natural environment and human-made changes to environment	Gender Age Coping styles
3. Voice and speech functions	3. Structures involved in voice an speech	3. Communication	3. Support and relationships	Social background
4. Functions of the cardiovascular, haematological, immunological, and respiratory systems	4. Structures of the cardiovascular, haematological, immunological, and respiratory systems	4. Mobility	4. Attitudes	Education Profession Past and current experience
5. Functions of the digestive, metabolic, and endocrine systems	5. Structures related to the digestive, metabolic, and endocrine systems	5. Self care	5. Services, systems, and policies	Overall behaviour pattern Character
6. Genitourinary and reproductive functions	6. Structures related to the genitourinary and reproductive systems	6. Domestic life		
7. Neuromusculoskeletal and movement-related functions	7. Structures related to movement	7. Interpersonal interactions and relationships		
8. Functions of the skin and related structures	8. Skin and related structures	8. Major life areas		
		9. Community, social, and civic life		

indicates the presence of an impairment and the degree of the impairment of function or structure, on a five-point scale (*no problem*, *mild/small*, *moderate*, *severe/extreme/difficult*, and *profound/ complete*). An example of how Alexander's and Anna's speech problems could be classified as a functional impairment is presented in Table 1–2. Note that this is only a characterization in terms of voice and speech function, another relevant domain to use in the description of Alexander's problem would be s3400 "classifying structural changes of the vocal folds." Also, note that language functions are found in Chapter 1 "Mental Functions," and are not classified here. However, as an example, in both cases the domain b1672 "integrative language functions" (described as "mental functions that organize seman-

tic and symbolic meaning, grammatical structure, and ideas for the production of messages in spoken, written, or other forms of language") could be used.

For the classifications of *activity* and *participation*, two types of qualifiers and the same five-point scale are used. The *performance* qualifier describes what an individual does in his or her *current environment*. The current environment is a person's actual context including assistive devices or personal assistance. The *capacity* qualifier describes an individual's ability to execute a task or an action. This construct indicates the highest probable level of functioning of a person. To assess this full ability of the individual, one needs to have a *standardized environment* to equalize the varying impact of different environments on the ability of the individual.

Table 1–2. Examples of How Alexander's and Anna's Speech Problems Could Be Classified As a Functional Impairment

Part	Component	Chapter	Domain	Qualifier	
				Alexander	Anna
Functioning and disability	Body functions	3. Voice and speech functions	b3100 Production of voice	b3100.4	b3100.1
			b3108 Quality of voice	b3108.3	b3108.3
			b320 Articulation function	b3200.2	b3200.1
			b3302 Speed of speech	b3302.2	b3302.1
			b3303 Melody of speech	b3303.4	b3303.3

The standardized environment often is an actual environment commonly used for capacity assessment in test settings, that is, the clinic room, a laboratory, or an environment with precisely defined parameters based on extensive scientific research. The capacity construct usually reflects the person's capacity without personal assistance or the use of assistive devices. For assessment purposes, this environmental adjustment has to be the same for all persons in all countries to allow for international comparisons. For precision and international comparability, features of the uniform or standard environment can be coded using the environmental factors classification.

Having both performance and capacity data enables the clinician or researcher to determine the gap between capacity and performance. If capacity is less than performance, the person's current environment has *en*abled him or her to perform better than what data about capacity would predict. If capacity is greater than performance, then some aspect of the environment has *dis*abled, that is, is a barrier to performance. For example, Alexander's wife uses very active strategies as a conversation partner to help him make himself understood. In these situations, he communicates better than his percentage intelligibility, as measured in the therapy room, would predict. His performance rises above his capacity. On the other hand, Anna likes to give direct comments when she goes to a movie with her boyfriend, but he can never understand her and prefers to discuss the movie afterward. In a quiet setting, she is completely intelligible. In the movie situation, her performance falls below her capacity.

As mentioned previously, both capacity and performance qualifiers can be used with and without assistive devices or personal assistance. The use of these facilitators does not alter the impairments, but may reduce activity limitation. It is particularly useful to define how far the functioning of the individual would be limited without the assistive devices.

Applying ICF

Given its complexity, the classification has the potential to answer a wide range of questions, including clinical, research, and policy development questions. Regarding research, ICF can assist in scientific research by providing a framework or structure for interdisciplinary research in disability and for making results of research comparable. The concern in modern day health care is more on assessment of functioning at the level of the whole human being in day-to-day life, and ICF has great potential as a universally applicable classification and assessment tool for both different types of activities and overall levels of participation in basic areas and roles of social life. In addition, ICF can facilitate the coding of outcomes in intervention studies by clearly distinguishing interventions (and coding outcomes) in light of the aspect of disability addressed by the intervention in question. Some interventions focus primarily on the body structure or function, in the case of motor speech disorders, for example, a palatal lift, phonatory strengthening exercises, or articulation drills. Some interventions focus on the activity or participation—

for example, practicing reading out loud, having a conversation with a neighbor, ordering a meal at a restaurant without verbal assistance. Or, interventions can focus on the contextual facilitators or barriers aiming to improve capacity or modify the environment, for example, by introducing a voice amplifier or training facilitative strategies in a conversational partner.

ICF also allows a comparison of outcomes of different types of interventions on similar populations. In particular, the introduction of environmental factors is a major innovation in ICF and contributes considerably to the flexibility and possibilities in terms of choice of treatment target. The classification makes it possible to identify environmental barriers and facilitators for both capacity and performance of actions and tasks in daily living. Accumulated knowledge of barriers and strategies allows guidelines and advice to extend the functioning levels of persons with disabilities across a wide range of life activities rather than focus on descriptions of limitations. As a consequence, ICF classification data also can be used in analyses of the economic impact of functional limitations as compared to the costs of modifying the environment. The disability burden of different diseases and health conditions also needs to be investigated and compared. Health economic analyses then can be used in disability-related social policy development.

Having gone through the rationale, aims, model, structure, and terminology of ICF and stressing its complexity, it becomes evident that the magnitude of ICF is both an advantage and a limitation for its users. Indeed, a criticism raised regarding its use is that it does not provide sufficient information on how professionals in these fields could apply it in their work. The conceptual model is easy enough to embrace, but the classification is so detailed it might seem unwieldy. It has been described as a Swiss army knife—it has the potential to carry out a great number of tasks, but you have to choose the right (and the right number of) tools for the tasks. One particular problem is that an exact correspondence rarely exists between instruments for measurement and the ICF codes. Core sets of codes and assessments suitable for different diseases, disorders, and conditions (e.g., stroke, multiple sclerosis) currently are being developed to facilitate international comparisons of data and other adaptations that might be called for. These are a few of the issues that currently prevent full clinical and research use of the ICF. The dissemination of the manual, the *Procedural Manual and Guide for the Standardized Use of the ICF: A Manual for Health Professionals*, hopefully will clarify some of these issues.

ICF and Its Relevance and Application to Assessment of People with Motor Speech Disorders

Communication as an activity is at the heart of participation, and a number of body structures and functions need to be intact in order for communication to be optimal. Communication (from the Latin, "to make common") is also per definition an interaction, a joint effort that gives contextual factors a key role as potential facilitators. One of the earliest attempts to apply ICF—or even ICIDH—was undertaken in the area of motor speech disorders (Yorkston, Beukelman, & Bell, 1988) and several special issues have been dedicated to the application of ICF to the speech-language pathology area (*Advances in Speech-Language Pathology 6*(1) 2004; *Seminars in Speech and Language 28*(4) 2007; *International Journal of Speech-Language Pathology 10*(1–2) 2008). Also, a number of speech-language pathology organizations worldwide have endorsed use of the ICF to guide standards of practice.

Based on the work by Yorkston, et al. (1988) and Yorkston, Beukelman, Strand, & Hakel, 2010), Table 1–3 describes a tentative application of ICF to the area of motor speech disorders. The defining characteristics of motor speech disorders as structural/functional impairments are, of course, loss or abnormality of psychological, physiological, or anatomical structure or function that results in slow, weak, imprecise, and/or uncoordinated movements of the speech musculature (dysarthria) or inability to plan speech movements (apraxia of speech). The resulting activity limitation is a negative effect on speech intelligibility, naturalness, prosody, speaking rate, and articulatory adequacy. These limitations, in turn, restrict communicative participation in different life situations. Several contextual factors, both barriers and facilitators in the environment, as well as personal factors, are thought to influence the effects of this health condition.

At least two points in this table could be questioned: (1) Whether or not communication, and in this case communication in persons with motor speech disorders, can be differentiated and characterized both as activity and participation, and (2) whether or not decreased intelligibility should be referred to as an activity limitation or a functional impairment. These points are discussed in the following paragraph.

In the list of chapters in the *activity and participation component, communication* is Chapter 3 of the nine chapters (see Tables 1–1 and 1–2). In handling the nine chapters used to describe activity and participation, ICF suggests differentiating chapters (Chapters 1–3 as activity, Chapters 6–9 as participation), overlapping chapters (Chapters 1–5 as activity, Chapters 3–9 as participation), or merging chapters (all chapters potentially activity *and* participation). Because communication-related activities are included in other chapters of the activities and participation component (such as *learning and applying knowledge, interpersonal interactions and relationships* and *community, social and civic life*), one could argue in favor of merging chapters. This is also the default approach used in ICF, and it is suggested that the qualifiers should be used to distinguish the information acquired. The qualifiers in this case are as we know *capacity* and *performance*, which suggests that one could assess intelligibility, naturalness, prosody, rate, and so on, as *capacity* (what a person is able to do under ideal conditions, assisted or unassisted) in the lab or in the clinic and assess the same variables as *performance* (what a person actually does, assisted or unassisted, in her current environment) directly or indirectly (using subjective reports) in live situations. Another approach, which seems to have some support in the classification itself, is to bear in mind that the literal definition of activity limitation in ICF is "problems an individual may *have*" and the full description of participation restriction is "problems an individual may *experience.*" Consequently, one can choose to assess chosen variables as *activity* when they are assessed by the clinician or researcher, and as

Table 1–3. Assessment of People with Motor Speech Disorders within the ICF Framework

Motor speech disorders as . . .	. . . structural/functional impairment	. . . activity limitation	. . . participation restriction	Influencing environmental factors	Influencing personal factors
Defining **characteristics**	Loss or abnormality of psychological, physiologic, or anatomical structure or function, which results in slow, weak, imprecise, and/ or uncoordinated movements of the speech musculature or inability to plan sequence of speech movements	Impairments affecting: Intelligibility Naturalness Prosody Speaking rate Articulatory adequacy	Impairments affecting: Participation in life situations using communication	Environmental conditions Support and relationships Attitudes Services and technology, etc.	Gender Age Coping styles Background Education Profession Experience Character etc.
Descriptive **qualifiers**	Functions and Structures	Capacity and Performance (with or without assistance)		Barriers and Facilitators	
Types of **assessments**	Instrumental and perceptual assessments of respiration, phonation, oral motor and velopharyngeal function, articulation	Intelligibility measures Instrumental and perceptual assessments of naturalness, prosody, speaking rate, and articulatory adequacy	Interviews Self-report questionnaires	? ↑	? ↑

Modified from Yorkston, Beukelman, Strand, and Hakel (2010).

participation when they are assessed by the person with a motor speech disorders or a close other. For Anna, for example, a self-report questionnaire used as a starting point for discussions of difficulties and strategies reveals that the participation restrictions perceived by her do not mirror the activity limitations perceived by the clinician using her clinical judgment and clinical measures. An in-depth discussion of how activity and participation relate to each other and how they have been operationalized in research with adults with acquired communicative disability is provided by O'Halloran and Larkins (2008).

Intelligibility is another problematic concept that is not readily defined within the ICF structure. A thorough analysis of how reduced speech intelligibility in dysarthria relates to the ICF structure is presented in Dykstra, Hakel, and Adams (2007). Intelligibility is defined in its most simplistic way as the extent to which an acoustic signal, generated by a speaker, can be recovered correctly by a listener. The acoustic signal carrying a spoken message to be understood can be viewed as a number of functions (respiration, phonation, oral motor function, etc.) coordinated in an activity that has a purpose. As such it seems reasonable to classify it as an *activity*, and it has most often been associated with the activity level of functioning, although the components that compromise intelligibility are all linked with the construct of *body functions and structures*.

The assessment of intelligibility has been considered a primary measure of disability and an index of severity. However, because traditional measurements of speech intelligibility typically are undertaken under decontextualized environments and do not reveal functional limitations and restrictions, the ICF manual states that intelligibility be considered under body functions rather than an activity level code. (Some recent developments have sought to bridge this divide by, for instance, assessing intelligibility against standard background noise or while the person is involved in a competing task, Bunton & Keintz, 2008) Intelligibility also is linked closely to *participation* and related to the concepts enhanced intelligibility (or comprehensibility, using the qualifiers unassisted or assisted performance). The extent to which intelligibility correlates with functional performance in real communicative contexts is relatively unknown, but it has been considered likely that intelligibility scores underestimate communicative success (Hustad & Weismer, 2007). In ICF terms, the performance exceeds the capacity. On the other hand, the reason for this presupposition is that intelligibility testing may focus on single minimal pair context words without any contextual clues, which does not resemble any natural conversational situations. However, many speakers with dysarthria are restricted to single words, with very degraded signal, and at times are unable to signal context/change of topic, that is, to give contextual clues. In addition, intelligibility testing usually takes place in ideal clinic situations, but real-life communication usually is in noisy, rushed multitalker real-life situations. Finally, in many disorders when speakers have to think and speak, the dual/competing task nature of communication causes deterioration in speech. Consequently, one might argue that clinical intelligibility tests may actually overestimate success.

Regardless of where in the ICF structure one places key concepts, there is a need to develop new techniques of description and quantification of the effects that motor speech disorders have in terms of limiting and restricting communication and communicative interaction.

Assessments of the structural/functional aspects of motor speech disorders typically are perceptual and instrumental assessments of respiration, phonation, oral motor, and velopharyngeal function and articulation. We listen, and we try to quantify the deviations we perceive. Or we measure and try to hear the deviations the instrumental assessments indicate. Quantification of the impaired function underlying motor speech disorders typified the earliest research and clinical efforts of speech disorder pioneers, including the seminal work of Darley, Aronson, and Brown in the late 1960s. Almost in tandem with the development of perceptual measures was an interest in physiologic and other types of instrumental measures and a continued interest in this area has delivered a cumulative increase in our knowledge. In this book, this approach is discussed in Chapter 3, "Physiological Assessment", by Bruce Mudoch, and also, reflecting the extensive development of instrumental techniques in recent years, Chapters 10–16.

By the 1980s, the focus was widened and came to include the listener as a relevant part and assessments of intelligibility were developed (see Chapter 2, "The Assessment of Intelligibility in Motor Speech Disorders," by Ray Kent and Yunjung Kim, in this book). Also, the characteristics of prosody, including speaking rate, received increased attention, and the use of different assess-

ment options are reviewed in the chapter by Rupal Patel.

Successively, the beam of our searchlight has increased its range, and we are now devoting time and energy to learn more about the effects of motor speech disorders in terms of restricted communicative participation. So far, this has mostly been done conducting qualitative interviews and using self-report questionnaires. Quantifying the impact of dysarthria on the individual (Chapter 5 by Margaret Walshe) and in particular, developing measures of communicative participation (Chapter 6, "Measurement of Communicative Participation," by Kathryn Yorkston and Carolyn Baylor), are research efforts in this direction. Furthermore, exploring the effect of contextual variables, such as other concomitant disease factors (e.g., cognitive impairment, Chapter 7, "Dysarthria: The Cognitive Dimension," by Catherine Mackenzie) and investigating how assessment and intervention can be conducted with the patient in their current environment rather than in the clinic (via telehealth, Chapter 9 by Deborah Theodoros) and looking at everyday interaction (Chapter 8 by Steven Bloch and Ray Wilkinson) all represent our increasing awareness that the assessment of the patient's speech without considering environmental or personal factors is insufficient for clinical purposes.

Future Directions of Development and Challenges

Clearly, we need to continue the path set out and develop measures that cover different aspects of activity and participation, measures of intelligibility, enhanced intelligibility, listener comprehension, and communicative participation but also measures that can quantify environmental factors and personal factors (Howe, 2008). Contextual elements can impact intelligibility and participation considerably in individuals with motor speech disorders, and if we shift our attention away from measuring the severity of speech impairment to barriers and strategies in the environment that will allow us to establish new targets of intervention (e.g., environmental adjustments, partner training).

It is also important to remember that the ICF codes and qualifiers do not in any way replace other types of detailed assessments. Note, for instance, that Alexander and Anna both were described as severe (3 or 4) regarding b.3108 *quality of voice* and b3303 *melody of voice*. However, their difficulties in speech motor control as well as their perceptual symptoms are completely different, Alexander having a breathy monotonous voice and Anna a harsh voice quality with difficulties to control pitch level.

Also, agreeing on the number of codes necessary to describe our client populations, which tools in the Swiss army knife to use, is an urgent and important challenge. We need to develop a core set of codes and measures for motor speech disorders. In its most detailed use, ICF has more than 1400 codes, and unless there is agreement on the use of the relevant ones for speech-language pathologists, comparison between countries and across languages will be virtually impossible.

One interesting development is the use of graphic models to illustrate the intricate relationships between data generated by ICF codes. Generalized linear models were used by Strobl, Stucki, Grill, Muller, and Mansmann (2009) to identify dependencies between ICF categories. This procedure is a way to reduce complex information and visualize interactions and associations, similar to the way Darley, Aronson, and Brown used cluster analysis of co-occurring dimensions to illustrate complex perceptual impressions. These graphic models might aid in the selection of a parsimonious set of variables for description and are considered a potential basis for identification of suitable targets for rehabilitation interventions.

In 1965, at a conference regarding brain mechanisms underlying speech and language, Fredric Darley asked *"What shall we let the term dysarthria encompass?"* (Darley 1967; Duffy, 2007). He defined it primarily as a function of nervous system level of involvement (cerebellum, lower motor neuron, etc.) and speech system level of involvement (phonation, articulation). Together with Aronson and Brown, he provided a conceptual framework for perceptual and instrumental studies that have increased our understanding of motor speech disorders immensely. Forty-five years later, we are definitely ready to extend the framework and let the term dysarthria, and apraxia of speech, encompass the nervous system level and the speech system level, but also the behavioral consequences for intelligibility, social interaction, individual opportunities, self-concept, and the like. In doing so, we hopefully will be able to see more of the entire picture and serve our clients better.

References

Advances in Speech-Language Pathology. (2004). *Classifying communication disability using the ICF, 6*(1).

Bunton, K., & Keintz, C. (2008). Use of dual task paradigm for assessing speech intelligibility in clients with Parkinson's disease. *Journal of Medical Speech-Language Pathology, 16*(3), 141–155.

Chiara, T. D., Martin, D., Sapienza, C. (2007). Expiratory muscle strength training: Speech production outcomes in patients with multiple sclerosis. *Neurorehabilitation and Neural Repair, 21*(39), 239–249.

Clark, H. M. (2003). Neuromuscular treatments for speech and swallowing: A tutorial. *American Journal of Speech-Language Pathology, 12,* 400–415.

Darley, F. L. (1967). Lacunae and research approaches to them. In C. Milliken & F. L. Darley (Eds.), *Brain mechanisms underlying speech and language* (pp. 236–240). New York, NY: Grune & Stratton.

Duffy, J. R. (2007). History, current practice, and future trends and goals. In G. Weismer (Ed.), *Motor speech disorders: Essays for Ray Kent* (pp. 7–56). San Diego, CA: Plural Publishing.

Dykstra, A. D., Hakel, M. E., & Adams, S. G. (2007). Application of the ICF in reduced speech intelligibility in dysarthria. *Seminars in Speech and Language, 28*(4), 301–311.

Hartelius, L., Elmberg, M., Holm, R., Lövberg, A-S., & Nikolaidis, S. (2008). Living with dysarthria: Evaluation of a self-report questionnaire. *Folia Phoniatrica et Logopaedica, 60,* 11–19.

Hartelius, L., Jonsson, M., Rickeberg, A., & Laakso, K.(2010. Communication and Huntington's disease: Qualitative interviews and focus groups with persons with Huntington's disease, family members, and caregivers. *International Journal of Language and Communication Disorders, 45*(3), 381–393.

Howe, T. J. (2008). The ICF Contextual Factors related to speech-language pathology. *International Journal of Speech-Language Pathology, 10*(1–2), 27–37.

Hustad, K. C. (2008). The relationship between listener comprehension and intelligibility scores for speakers with dysarthria. *Journal and Speech Language and Hearing Research, 51*(3), 562–573.

Hustad, K. C., & Weismer, G. (2007). A continuum of interventions for individuals with dysarthria. In G. Weismer (Ed.), *Motor speech disorders: Essays for Ray Kent* (pp. 261–303). San Diego, CA: Plural Publishing.

International Journal of Speech-Language Pathology. (2008). *Contribution of the ICF to speech-language pathology, 10*(1–2).

Klasner, E., & Yorkston, K. M. (2005). Speech intelligibility in ALS and HD dysarthria: The everyday listener's perspective. *Journal of Medical Speech-Language Pathology, 13*(2), 127–139.

McHenry, M., & Minton, J. (1994). Intelligibility and nonspeech oral strength and force control following traumatic brain injury. *Journal of Speech and Hearing Research, 37,* 1271–1283.

Miller, N., Allcock, L., Jones, D., Noble, E., Hildreth, A. J., & Burn, D. J. (2007). Prevalence and pattern of perceived intelligibility changes in Parkinson's disease. *Journal of Neurology, Neurosurgery and Psychiatry, 78*(11), 1188–1190.

Miller, N., Noble, E., Jones, D., Allcock, L., & Burn, D. J. (2008). "How do I sound to me?" Perceived changes in communication in Parkinson's disease. *Clinical Rehabilitation, 22*(1), 14–22.

O'Halloran, R., & Larkins, B. (2008). The ICF Activities and Participation related to speech-language pathology. *International Journal of Speech-Language Pathology, 10*(1–2), 18–26.

Seminars in Speech and Language. (2007). *The international classification of functioning, disability and health (ICF) in clinical practice, 28*(4).

Solomon, N. P. (2004). Assessment of tongue weakness and fatigue. *International Journal of Orofacial Myology, 30*, 8–19.

Strobl, R., Stucki, G., Grill, E., Müller, M., & Mansmann, U. (2009). Graphical models illustrated complex associations between variables describing human functioning. *Journal of Clinical Epidemiology, 62*(9), 922–933.

Walshe, M., Peach, R. K., & Miller, N. (2008). Dysarthria impact profile: Development of a scale to measure psychosocial effects. *International Journal of Language and Communication Disorders, 25*, 1–23.

Weismer, G. (2006). Philosophy of research in motor speech disorders. *Clinical Linguistics & Phonetics, 20*(5), 315–349.

Weismer, G., Yeng, J. Y., Laures, J. S., Kent, R. D., & Kent, J. F. (2001). Acoustic and intelligibility characteristics of sentence production in neurogenic speech disorders. *Folia Phoniatrica et Logopaedica, 53*(1), 1–18.

Whitehill, T. L., & Tsang E.S.L. (2002). Relationship between diadochokinetic and speech measures in hypokinetic speakers. *Journal of Medical Speech-Language Pathology, 10*(4), 333–338.

Yorkston, K. M., Beukelman, D. R., Strand, E. A., & Hakel, M. (2010). *Management of motor speech disorders in children and adults* (3rd ed.). Austin, TX: Pro-Ed.

Yorkston, K. M., Baylor, C. R., Klasner, E. R., Deitz, J., Dudgeon, B. J., Eadie, T., Miller, R. M., & Amtmann, D. (2007). Satisfaction with communicative participation as defined by adults with multiple sclerosis; a qualitative study. *Journal of Communication Disorders, 40*(6), 433–451.

Yorkston, K. M., Beukelman, D. R., & Bell, K. R. (1988). *Clinical management of dysarthric speakers*. Austin, TX: Pro-Ed.

Ziegler, W. (2003). Speech motor control is task-specific: Evidence from dysarthria and apraxia of speech. *Aphasiology, 17*(1), 3–36.

2

The Assessment of Intelligibility in Motor Speech Disorders

RAYMOND D. KENT, PH.D.
YUNJUNG KIM, PH.D.

Introduction

Reduced speech intelligibility is a common consequence of motor speech disorders (dysarthria and apraxia of speech) and can be a significant component of the burden of neurological disease. As Confucius said, we speak to be understood. But how do we measure the failed understanding of another person's message? This central and longstanding problem in speech-language pathology has been addressed with a variety of methods, all of which yield useful information, but none of which suffices for all speakers and all listeners under all communicative situations. Discussion of this issue considers variables arising from the different components of the communication process: listener, message, medium, and speaker.

Speech intelligibility is the joint product of a speaker who transmits a message, the message itself, the medium over which the message is transmitted, and a listener who decodes the message. Variables associated with each link in this chain ultimately determine the success of a communicative event. Although the aim of clinical intelligibility assessment is to be able to say something like, "the individual was 85% intelligible," such a statement really should be understood to mean that "the individual was 85% intelligible (putting aside for a moment the problems of quantification) for a particular kind of message (e.g., a single word, a phrase, a reading passage) transmitted over a particular medium (e.g., face-to-face, a telephone, a high-quality sound system, or a video system with sound) and interpreted by a particular listener or group of listeners (e.g., a clinician, a family member, or a panel of listeners unfamiliar with the speaker)."

Constructs and Definitions

It is important to recognize and distinguish several terms that are used to label various facets of communication. In one recent definition, *intelligibility* "refers to how well a speaker's acoustic signal can be accurately recovered by a listener" (Hustad, 2008). We suggest that this definition should be amended to read that intelligibility "refers to how well a speaker's message, transmitted acoustically (or visually and acoustically as the case may be), can be accurately recovered by a listener." That is, intelligibility does not so much focus on recovery of the acoustic signal but, rather, almost always on recovery of the intended message carried by that signal. The focus on the intended message is evident in the procedures that commonly are used to measure intelligibility and the terminology used in measurement. The recovery is indexed either in linguistic units (such as phonemes or words) accurately transmitted or on a listener's global understanding of the speaker's thoughts or intent (the gist), neither of which are expressed at the acoustic level per se. It also should be noted that these two alternatives (linguistic units transmitted versus gist) are not equivalent because they focus on different aspects of the speaker's message. Acoustic information in the form of time-varying spectral details is of value only as it enables the recovery of the encoded linguistic message. The original definition given earlier restricts the medium to the acoustic signal, but this need not be the case in all circumstances.

Several other constructs are complementary to, and sometimes conflated with, intelligibility. *Comprehensibility* has been defined as "contextual intelligibility," or intelligibility when contextual information is present in different forms, such as semantic cues, syntactic cues, orthographic cues, and gestures (Yorkston, Strand, & Kennedy, 1996). But the literature on intelligibility studies in fields such as psychology, audiology, and communication engineering often refers to the effect of most of these variables on intelligibility. Comprehensibility has been contrasted with transcription methods of intelligibility testing (Hustad, 2008), but this distinction is restricted to one particular way of assessing intelligibility and does not pertain to other methods such as perceptual scaling of intelligibility. Another term is *listener comprehension*, defined as a listener's ability to interpret the meaning of messages without regard for accuracy of phonetic and lexical parsing (Hustad & Beukelman, 2002). And, finally, *communicative participation* is defined as communication in social contexts (Eadie et al., 2006; Yorkston & Baylor, Chapter 6, "Measurement of Communicative Participation," in this book).

Intelligibility and related constructs also have been defined in the field of linguistics, where intelligibility often is invoked to define languages and dialects. Smith and Nelson (1985) distinguished the terms intelligibility, comprehensibility, and interpretability using categories in speech act theory. Specifically, they define *intelligibility* as pertaining to the recognition of words and utterances (that is, linguistic units of some kind). *Comprehensibility* is the recognition of the meaning of a word or utterance (*locutionary* force in speech act terms). *Interpretability* is the meaning behind the word or utterance (the *illocutionary* force). The main points to be made are that (1) intelligibility typically is defined at the level of linguistic units, however these units may be understood; and (2) intelligibility is one aspect of a communicative transaction that potentially is deep and far-ranging.

The conceptual overlap for the terminology used to denote intelligibility and related constructs in communication complicates a review and interpretation of the literature. Some important differences come into relief when these constructs are considered in terms of the ICF framework (World Health Organization, 2001). Intelligibility, comprehensibility and listener comprehension generally would be categorized as "Activities" measures in the ICF framework. (Dykstra, Hakel, & Adams, 2007; Hartelius & Miller, Chapter 1, "The ICF Framework and Its Relevance to the Assessment of People with Motor Speech Disorders," in this book). These constructs have physiological and acoustic correlates in the act of speech production, and these correlates would fall in the "Structure and Function" category of the ICF. It bears repeating that intelligibility per se nearly always is measured as an "Activity" and not as a "Function." Communicative participation—as its name suggests—would be classified as a "Participation" measure. Intelligibility may help to determine a speaker's participation, but it is not, in itself, a participation measure.

Intelligibility tests have several clinical uses. Hodge and Whitehill (2010) comment that these uses include determining the need for intervention, planning the nature of intervention, determining the effectiveness of intervention, and understanding intelligibil-

ity deficits. These uses are harmonious with the principles of evidence-based practice. Ideally, an intelligibility test will yield a reliable quantitative result (an intelligibility score) along with sufficient analytical detail to justify and design treatment and to demonstrate treatment outcome. The following discussion summarizes the assessment of intelligibility as it relates to methods for the measurement of intelligibility, characteristics of listeners, effect of the medium, properties of the message to be communicated, and the speakers themselves. For additional reviews of these issues, see Barreto and Ortiz (2008); Hodge and Whitehill (2010); Kent, Weismer, Kent, and Rosenbek (1989); Weismer (2008); and Yorkston and Beukelman (1978).

Intelligibility Measures

Table 2–1 lists the procedures that most commonly are used to assess intelligibility of individuals with motor speech disorders (or any communication disorder). Intelligibility measures differ in two primary dimensions—the speech material (message) and the listener response. The most frequently used materials for assessing intelligibility in dysarthria are words, phrases, or sentences and conversation. These are discussed in more detail in a following section, "The Message." The most commonly used listener responses are scaling judgments and item identification (primarily transcription and word identification). A common and long-standing scaling method is to rate a speaker's intelligibility on an equal-appearing interval scale, such as those used by

Table 2–1. Characteristics of Procedures Commonly Used in Assessing the Intelligibility of Individuals with Motor Speech Disorders

	Measure	Advantages	Disadvantages
Equal Appearing Interval Scale	Numerical value on a predetermined scale	Ease of use in both stimulus presentation and obtaining listener judgments	Questionable psychometric validity for intelligibility (a prothetic dimension)
Direct Magnitude Estimation	Numerical ratio assigned to stimuli	Psychometric suitability to intelligibility	Requires preparation of stimuli suited to task; assumes listeners can make ratio judgments
Visual Analog Scale	Point on a line that represents the perceptual dimension	Ease of use; avoids numerical response; continuum of possible responses	Possible differences in how different raters interpret the scale
Percentage Estimate of Speech Understood	Numerical percentage	Ease of use; large number of values available to rater	Raters' criteria may differ
Item Intelligibility from Structured Materials	Number of items (usually words) correctly identified by a listener or panel of listeners	Quantification of intelligibility for isolated words; in some cases, phonetic interpretation of errors can be achieved through item analysis	Results may not be representative of connected speech
Transcription	Number of words or syllables correctly identified by transcribers	Can be used with conversational samples	Analysis can be difficult, especially for speakers with severe intelligibility deficits

Darley, Aronson, and Brown (1969a) and in rating systems used in Parkinson's disease (Zraick et al., 2003) and Huntington's disease (Zraick et al., 2004). An alternative scaling method is direct magnitude estimation (DME). Schiavetti (1992) comments that DME is preferable to EAIS for intelligibility scaling because the former is better suited to prothetic dimensions (dimen-

sions that are additive, such as stimulus intensity and intelligibility). EAIS is suitable for metathetic dimensions (nonadditive dimensions such as pitch or hue). Schiavetti explains that when an EAIS scale is applied to a dimension such as intelligibility, (a) listeners do not divide interval scales equally, so that the scale becomes ordinal rather than interval, and (b) confidence intervals around ratings can be large, especially in the middle part of the scale (as shown by Bunton, Kent, Duffy, Rosenbek, & Kent, 2007, for the perceptual dimensions used in the classic study of Darley et al., 1969a). Intelligibility also has been scaled with percentage estimates; that is, listeners are asked to estimate the percentage of the message that they understood. This judgment requires that listeners have a reliable and valid internal standard that is shared by others. DME with a standard stimulus (modulus) has the advantage of giving listeners a common referent for making their ratio judgments. Weismer and Laures (2002) discuss the importance of careful selection of a standard in DME of intelligibility.

The Listener

No such person as a standard human listener exists. Listeners vary in their life experiences, sensory and cognitive abilities, familiarity with a given topic and a given talker, and even their disposition to understand a message. Attempts to measure a speaker's intelligibility in clinical circumstances often rely on judgments made by clinicians, but other listeners, such as family members or strangers, may be more relevant to the predicament of reduced

intelligibility. Comprehension of a spoken message is itself a complicated process that draws on various sensory and cognitive resources. These resources may be deployed to advantage in listening to degraded messages, whether the degradation affects the source (as in motor speech disorders) or the transmission (as in masking or other signal interference).

Listeners have manifold resources that can be exploited to understand speech, and research on neural processing of degraded speech is opening new doors to understanding the nature of these resources. Neural adaptation to signal degradation of speech is based to a large degree on the acoustic properties of the speech signal. The auditory cortex of the right hemisphere is advantaged for coding syllable patterns (Abrams, Nichol, Zecker, & Kraus, 2008), which helps to explain the participation of this cortical region in speech processing. Both facial movements and vocal envelopes are modulated in the 2 to 7 Hz frequency range, which is the basic tempo of speech syllabicity (Chandrasekaran, Trubanova, Stillittano, Capier, & Ghazanfar, 2009). Activation of right dorso-lateral prefrontal cortex has been observed for degraded speech (Sharp, Scott, & Wise, 2004), and activation of various regions in both hemispheres may be a strategy for dealing with degraded speech, whatever the source of the degradation (source or medium). It is becoming clear that listeners can deploy neural strategies to deal with speech signals that are contaminated or otherwise lacking in clarity.

Intelligibility of dysarthric speech is improved when listeners are familiar with a listener (DePaul & Kent, 2000; D'innocenzo, Tjaden, & Greenman, 2006; Hustad & Cahill, 2003) or even with the type of dysarthria that a speaker has (Liss, Spitzer, Caviness, & Adler, 2002). Variation also exists among listeners who are unfamiliar with a speaker. DePaul and Kent (2000) used the term *listener proficiency* to refer to these intrinsic (and sometimes large) differences among listeners. Although no standard human listener exists, it may be possible to design a standard machine listener through the use of speech-processing technology (Carmichael, 2007; Doyle et al., 1997; Van Nuffelen, Middag, De Bodt, & Martens, 2008). One advantage of this approach is that it affords a degree of control and stability that is not accomplished easily with human listeners, who may shift their criteria as the result of familiarization, context, and expectations. Van Nuffelen et al. (2008) reported high correlations between perceptual and objective intelligibility scores (as high as 0.943 when both phonemic and phonological features were used in the objective analysis). The high correlations were based on a selected set of features in six categories: (1) vowel-related phonemic and phonological features, (2) lateral-related features, (3) silence-related features, (4) fricative-related features, (5) velar-related features and (6) plosive-related features.

The Message

As mentioned earlier, the message can take a variety of forms. The selection of a particular message depends on the purpose of the intelligibility assessment, the population of speakers, and the resources available for analysis of the results. The most common types of message are single words, sentences, a reading passage, and conversation. Table 2–2 lists some of the tools that have been developed for intelligibility testing. Some of the tests are commercially available, while others are free for use. Some were developed for research purposes, others for immediate clinical application.

Single Words

These tests require the speaker to produce lists of single words that may be designed to meet certain design criteria, such as phonetic analysis of items not transmitted correctly. Tests of this kind accommodate a range of speech production capabilities, from talkers who can produce little more than monosyllabic utterances to talkers with nearly normal speech. Generally, these tests allow quantification of intelligibility in terms of the percentage of words correctly identified by listeners, and, if the words are selected carefully, they can be used to determine the phonetic contrast errors underlying an intelligibility deficit (Kent, et al., 1989, and other sources listed in Table 2–2). A systematic analysis of phonetic contrasts requires a lengthy list of words, ideally balanced with respect to the appearance of different values for a phonetic contrast (e.g., target words representing both voiced and voiceless initial consonants to evaluate the contrast of voicing). A notable limitation of single words is that they obviously cannot be used to assess the kinds of prosodic and sequencing complexities that characterize multi-word utterances. Some breakdowns in intelligibility become apparent only with longer utterances.

Table 2–2. Tests and Materials Developed for the Assessment of Intelligibility in Children or Adults

Test and Source	Population/ Language	Description
The Preschool Speech Intelligibility Measure (PSIM) (Morris, Wilcox, & Schooling, 1995)	Children/English	Single-word test with closed set responses
Test of Children's Speech Plus (TOCS+) (Hodge & Daniels, 2005)	Children/English	Intelligibility scored for isolated words (open or closed response set) and sentences (open response only)
Word intelligibility lists (Tikofsky & Tikofsky, 1964)	Adults/English	Three word lists: 50 consonant-vowel-consonant words, 50 randomly selected spondees, and 60 monosyllabic words containing a number of initial and final consonant clusters
Single word intelligibility test (Tikofsky, 1970)	Adolescents to adults/English	Intelligibility scored for 50 monosyllabic or bisyllabic words
Frenchay Dysarthria Assessment (FDA) (Enderby, 1980, 2008)	12 years to adults/ English	Intelligibility rated for three tasks: isolated words, short sentences, and five-minute conversational sample
Phonetically balanced single-word test (Platt, Andrews, Young & Quinn, 1980)	Adults/English	List of 50 phonetically balanced words
Single-word intelligibility test (Kent, Weismer, Kent, & Rosenbek, 1989)	Adults/English	List of 52 words from which 19 phonetic contrast errors can be determined
Phonetic intelligibility test (Gentil, 1992)	Adults/French	72-word list with closed response sets to examine 17 phonetic contrasts; an additional paired-word test for severe dysarthria examines 12 phonetic contrasts

continues

Table 2–2. *continued*

Test and Source	Population/ Language	Description
Test af Fonetisk Forståelighed (Petersen, 1997a, 1997b)	Adults/Danish	Word list from which phonetic contrast errors can be identified
Münchner Verständlichkeits-Profil (MVP) (Ziegler, Hartmann & Wiesner, 1992)	Adults/German	Word lists from which phonetic contrast errors can be identified; available in an on-line version (Ziegler & Zierdt, 2008)
Cantonese Single-Word Intelligibility Test (CSIT) (Whitehill & Ciocca, 2000)	Adults/Cantonese	List of 75 words allowing examination of 17 phonetic contrasts
Single word intelligibility test (Ozawa et al., 2003)	Adults/Japanese	List of 80 words, with analysis of 24 phonetic contrasts
Mandarin Single-Word Intelligibility (Jeng, Weismer, & Kent, 2006)	Adults/Mandarin	List of 78 words including contrasts for 4 mandarin tones
Nederlandstalig SpraakVerstaanbaarheids-Onderzoek (NSV0) (De Bodt, Guns, & Van Nuffelen, 2006)	Adults/Dutch	50 consonant-vowel consonant words divided into 3 subtests for initial consonants, final consonants, and medial vowels and diphthongs; analysis by segmental errors
Speech Intelligibility Test (SIT) (Yorkston, Beukelman, & Hakel, 1996)	Adults/English	Intelligibility tests for isolated words and sentences
Unpredictable sentences for intelligibility testing (McHenry & Parle, 2006)	Adults/English	A set of 50 7-word sentences designed so that each word is relatively unpredictable (e.g., "Some creative authors try inventing exotic styles")
Le Test Phonétique d'Intelligibilité (TPI) (available as part of BEDC, Auzou, 2007) (Crochemore & Vannier, 2001)	Adults/French	List of words allowing examination of 14 phonetic contrasts

Sentences

The individuals being tested can read sentences from printed materials or a computer monitor, or they can repeat sentences produced by the examiner or a recording. Sentences provide control over linguistic variables and can be designed to offer various degrees of complexity (length, phonetic variation, predictability, and other variables). An advantage of sentences over isolated words is the inclusion of prosody and the opportunity to ask the speaker to modify features such as speaking rate and stress pattern. The usefulness of sentences can be limited by the listener's ability to predict words in a sentence based on factors such as syntax and semantics. Therefore, sentences with low predictability have been devised (McHenry & Parle, 2006). Intelligibility data usually are obtained either by transcription of the sentences, which allows word-level scoring, or by scaling methods such as EAIS or DME.

Reading Passages

Passages that are read orally offer control over lexical, syntactic, and phonetic properties of the test materials. But reading can introduce complications, particularly if the reading level is not suited to the abilities of the person taking the test. Although this task presumably incorporates prosodic variation, the prosodic patterns may not be wholly representative of those in extemporaneous speech. Some passages have been used frequently enough to qualify as standardized. Several of these (The Rainbow Passage, Comma Gets a Cure, The North Wind and the Sun, Arthur the Rat, The Grandfather Passage) are found on the following Web site: (http://www.abdn.ac.uk/langling/re sources/Standardised%20reading%20 passages.doc).

Reading passages also may be designed to be conversational in nature, thereby increasing the likelihood that they will be produced with prosodic variation (Lowit, Brendel, Dobinson, & Howell, 2006). As in the case of sentences, intelligibility can be gauged by transcription or by scaling methods.

Conversation

This task has face value as the most authentic communicative act. But it has disadvantages in that there may limited control over cognitive, syntactic, semantic, and phonological aspects. With some severely involved individuals, it may be difficult to understand some or all of the speech. Because the speaker's intent may not be clear, it can be impossible to gauge the accuracy of speech production. One approach to restricting vocabulary in conversation is to ask the person being examined to describe a picture or an event, so that at least some vocabulary items are predictable. As appealing as conversation may be for its naturalness as a communicative message, it presents formidable challenges in quantification and analysis of intelligibility failures. The former has been addressed in studies of children's speech using calculations of an intelligibility index (Flipsen, 2006; Shriberg, Austin, Lewis, McSweeny, & Wilson, 1997).

The Medium

Most studies of the intelligibility of dysarthric speech strive to optimize the medium by ensuring little or no interference by noise or other distractions. Although an optimal medium is assumed in most of the discussion in this chapter, it is an interesting question if disordered speech is more susceptible to interference because of reduced redundancy. Few studies have been reported on this issue. It has been shown that even highly proficient accented speech (native Chinese speakers using English as a second language) was reduced more significantly in intelligibility than native speech when noise was added to the signal (Rogers, Dalby, & Nishi, 2004). If the same result applies to disordered speech, then it is logical to hypothesize that dysarthric speech would be more susceptible than healthy speech to environmental interference such as noise background. But research to date does not give much support to this hypothesis. Schiltz (1994) observed a surprisingly small effect of multi-talker babble on the speech intelligibility of women with amyotrophic lateral sclerosis. Turner, Martin, and de Jonge (2008), in another study of dysarthric speakers with amyotrophic lateral sclerosis, found little change in both word intelligibility and phonetic contrast errors across different presentation levels (35 dB to 75 dB HL). A similar conclusion was reached in a study showing limited improvement of speech intelligibility when dysarthric speech was presented at a higher level (Kim, Weismer, Kuo, Kent, and Duffy, 2007). Interestingly, in the Kim et al., 2007, study, presentation level seemed to affect the scaling of normal utterances to a greater degree than it did dysarthric utterances.

The Speaker

The ultimate goal in clinical practice is to assess the intelligibility of an individual with a motor speech disorder. A major challenge to understanding intelligibility reduction is that these disorders are heterogeneous, and it is likely that the intelligibility deficits in any given individual are associated with the type and severity of the disorder, along with accompanying factors, such as compensatory adjustments and co-existing sensory or cognitive problems. In a study of normally speaking adult and child talkers, Hazan and Markham (2004) reported that high levels of intelligibility can be achieved through a combination of different acoustic-phonetic characteristics. The inverse is probably true as well: Low levels of intelligibility can be related to different combinations of acoustic-phonetic or physiological characteristics. Nonetheless, certain acoustic and physiological correlates may have a general value in indexing the functional limitations associated with reduced intelligibility. For example, in the acoustic realm, the common (but not universal) correlates appear to be reduced acoustic vowel space (i.e., a smaller area of the vowel quadrilateral depicted in the F1–F2 space), reduced slope of formant transitions, particularly the F2 transition, vocal dysfunction, and irregularities in speech timing. (Kim, Weismer, Kent, & Duffy, 2009; Liu, Tsao,

& Kuhl, 2005; Weismer, 2008; Weismer & Martin, 1992).

Enhancing Intelligibility: Clear Speech

Intelligibility can vary circumstantially, and it's helpful to understand variations in intelligibility observed in intra-speaker and interspeaker comparisons. When asked to enhance their intelligibility, individual talkers can systematically adjust their speech patterns to increase the likelihood that they will be understood. The relevant research pertains especially to distinguishing "clear speech" (hyperarticulated speech) from "conversational speech" (Picheny, Durlach, & Braida, 1985, 1986, 1989). Acoustic analyses of the two forms of speech have shown consistent differences, thereby laying a foundation for a general understanding of the acoustic correlates of intelligibility. Moreover, the adjustments that speakers make are not only a matter of speaking more slowly, because enhancements of intelligibility can be achieved even at rapid speaking rates (Krause & Braida, 1995). Interestingly, the acoustic differences between "clear" and "conversational" speech appear to explain intrinsic intelligibility differences among individual speakers (Bond & Moore, 1994; Bradlow, Torretta, & Pisoni, 1996). Bradlow et al., concluded that global characteristics (e.g., speaking rate and mean f_0 level) are not correlated strongly with intelligibility, but fine-grained characteristics (f_0 and F1 variation, formant frequency range for vowels, and intersegmental timing) are correlated. The acoustic profile of a highly intelligible speaker for a sentence task included a relatively wide range of f_0, a relatively expanded vowel space with a substantial F1 variation, precise articulation of the point vowels, and a high precision of intersegmental timing.

Studies of dysarthria also have established fine-grained acoustic characteristics relating to differences in speaker intelligibility (Kent et al., 1989; Kim et al., 2009; Turner, Tjaden, & Weismer, 1995; Weismer, 1997; Weismer & Martin, 1992). The results from dysarthric speech generally are congruent with the results for neurologically healthy speech. That is, the differences in intelligibility appear to be rooted in a common set of fine-grained acoustic measures including vowel formant frequencies and intersegmental timing. The question then arises whether individuals with dysarthria can capitalize on clear speech modifications to improve their own intelligibility. The answer is affirmative, at least for some individuals. Benefits of clear speech in dysarthria are shown by (1) a mean increase of 8% in intelligibility scores when speakers with dysarthria implemented clear speech (Beukelman, Fager, Ullman, Hanson, & Logemann, 2002); (2) improved intelligibility when dysarthric speakers used clear speech in verbal repairs (Kennedy, Strand, & Yorkston, 1994); and (3) acoustic analyses confirming that individuals with Parkinson's disease produced clear speech with some of the same acoustic properties that characterize clear speech in healthy individuals (decreased articulation rate, increased mean vocal fundamental frequency, and increased variability of vocal fundamental frequency) (Goberman & Elmer, 2005). Note that not all speakers with dysarthria demonstrate improved intelligibility with reduced speaking rate, and some even show the inverse (Van Nuffelen, De Bodt, Wuyts, & Van de Heyning, 2009).

These considerations have relevance to the specification of the speaker's task and the concept of intelligibility measurement. That is, exactly what instructions should be given to a person whose intelligibility is being tested? If individuals with dysarthria retain some capability to enhance their intelligibility, should we be interested not only in typical performance (however that would be defined) but also in the range of intelligibility performance under various conditions of speaking rate and attempted "clear speech" adjustments? A measure of capacity for change may be more useful than a single estimate, especially given that any single estimate can never be absolute.

The Analysis of Factors Causing Reduced Intelligibility in Dysarthria

It is one thing to measure intelligibility, but another to analyze or interpret the reasons for reduced intelligibility. Discovery of the factors underlying failed intelligibility adds value to the assessment and can be useful in treatment planning. It would be helpful to know (1) whether the reasons for reduced intelligibility vary systematically across types of dysarthria; (2) how individuals with the same dysarthria type vary from one another; and (3) how the severity of dysarthria affects the factors underlying reduced intelligibility.

One of the most common taxonomies used for the classification of motor speech disorders, especially the dysarthrias, was introduced by Darley, Aronson, and Brown (1969a, 1969b). Each type of dysarthria (ataxic, flaccid, hyperkinetic, hypokinetic, and spastic) had characteristics that are consistent with standard descriptions of the underlying neurologic disease or damage. But even within a given perceptually determined type of dysarthria, large variations may exist in the severity of the disorder and the manifestation of the neuropathology across the muscular systems underlying speech production. A full examination of intelligibility deficit, therefore, involves the measurement of the intelligibility loss and an assessment of the factors contributing to this loss. Historically, most of the effort has been given to the former and much less to the latter.

What aspects of speech disturbance determine an intelligibility deficit? De Bodt, Hernandez-Diaz, and Van De Heyning (2002) studied 76 speakers with various types of dysarthria who were rated by two judges on intelligibility and four primary dimensions of speech production: voice quality, articulation, nasality, and prosody. A multiple regression model showed that intelligibility can be expressed as a linear combination of the individual dimensions, with articulation being the strongest contributor. This result confirms the expectation that features of supraglottal function are most important in determining speech intelligibility. But a remaining question is whether reduced intelligibility takes different forms, depending on the type of dysarthria. Although much more research is needed to provide a complete answer, available evidence points to intelligibility profiles that are sensitive to dysarthria type (Blaney &

Hewlett, 2007; Kent et.al, 1989; Klasner & Yorkston, 2005; Liss, Spitzer, Caviness, & Adler, 2002). Another aspect of reduced intelligibility is that in addition to the distortion or absence of acoustic cues that characterize healthy speech, dysarthria can have abnormally inserted cues that potentially mislead or confuse listeners (DiCicco & Patel, 2008). Abnormal prosody can make a further contribution to reduced intelligibility; aspects of disturbed prosody are discussed in other chapters in this book (Chapter 4, "Assessment of Prosody," Patel; Chapter 11, "Assessment of Rhythm," White, Liss, & Dellwo; Chapter 12, "Assessment of Intonation," Kuschmann, Miller, Lowit, & Mennen).

Elaborated profiles for different types of dysarthria would be a major contribution to the study of intelligibility deficits in motor speech disorders. Information of this kind also may be highly useful to the design of treatments to enhance intelligibility.

Conclusion

The assessment of speech intelligibility in motor speech disorders has been marked by progress in the development of test materials to quantify reduced intelligibility and, to a lesser degree, by the design of methods to explain intelligibility failures. The steady increase in knowledge about the effects of listener, medium, and message on determinations of intelligibility is helpful when accounting for intelligibility failures in terms of individual patterns of motor impairment and planning treatments based partly on this information.

References

Abrams, D. A., Nichol, T., Zecker, S., & Kraus, N. (2008). Right-hemisphere cortex is dominant for coding syllable patterns in speech. *Journal of Neuroscience, 28*, 3958–3965.

Auzou, P. (2007). *BECD*. Isbergues, France: Ortho Edition.

Barreto, S. dos Santos, & Ortiz, K. Z. (2008). Intelligibility measurements in speech disorders: a critical review of the literature. (Original title: Medidas de inteligibilidade nos distúrbios da fala: revisão crítica da literatura). *Pro-Fono Revista de Atualizacao Cientifica, 20*, 201–206.

Beukelman, D., Fager, S., Ullman, C., Hanson, E. K., & Logemann, J. (2002). The impact of speech supplementation on the intelligibility of persons with traumatic brain injury. *Journal of Medical Speech Language Pathology, 10*, 237–242.

Blaney, B., & Hewlett, N. (2007). Dysarthria and Friedreich's ataxia: What can intelligibility assessment tell us? International *Journal of Language & Communication Disorders, 42*, 19–37.

Bond, Z. S., & Moore, T. J. (1994). A note on the acoustic-phonetic characteristics of inadvertently clear speech. *Speech Communication, 14*, 325–337.

Bradlow, A. R., Toretta, G. M., & Pisoni, D. B. (1996). Intelligibility of normal speech. I. Global and fine-grained acoustic-phonetic talker characteristics. *Speech Communication, 20*, 255–272.

Bunton, K., Kent, R. D., Duffy, J. R., Rosenbek, J. C., & Kent, J. F. (2007). Listener agreement for auditory-perceptual ratings of dysarthria. *Journal of Speech, Language, and Hearing Research, 50*, 1481–1495.

Carmichael, J. N. (2007). Introducing objective acoustic metrics for the Frenchay Dysarthria Assessment procedure. Ph.D. dissertation, University of Sheffield, UK.

Chandrasekaran, C., Trubanova, A., Stillittano, S., Capier, A., & Ghazanfar, A. A. (2009). The natural statistics of audiovisual speech. *PLoS Computational Biology, 5*, e1000436. doi:10.1371/journal.pcbi.10 00436.

Crochemore, E., & Vannier, F. (2001). Phonetic analysis of dysarthric speech. In P. Auzou & C. Ozsancak (Eds.), *Les Dysarthries* (pp. 71–82). Paris, France: Masson.

Darley, F. L., Aronson, A. E., & Brown, J. R. (1969a). Differential diagnostic patterns of dysarthria. *Journal of Speech Hearing Research, 12*, 246–269.

Darley, F. L., Aronson, A. E., & Brown, J. R. (1969b). Clusters of deviant speech dimensions in the dysarthrias. *Journal of Speech and Hearing Research, 12*, 462–496.

De Bodt, M. S., Guns, C., & Van Nuffelen, G. (2006). *NSVO: Nederlandstalig Spraak-VerstaanbaarheidsOnderzoek [DIA: Dutch Intelligibility Assessment]*. Herentals, The Netherlands: Viaamse Vereniging voor Logopedisten.

De Bodt, M. S., Hernandez-Diaz, H. M., & Van De Heyning, P. H. (2002). Intelligibility as a linear combination of dimensions in dysarthric speech. *Journal of Communication Disorders, 35*, 283–292.

DePaul, R., & Kent, R. D. (2000). A longitudinal case study of ALS: Effects of listener familiarity and proficiency on intelligibility judgments. *American Journal of Speech Language Pathology, 9*, 230–240.

DiCicco, T. M., & Patel, R. (2008). Automatic landmark analysis of dysarthric speech. *Journal of Medical Speech-Language Pathology, 16*, 213–220.

D'innocenzo, J., Tjaden, K., & Greenman, G. (2006). Intelligibility in dysarthria: Effects of listener familiarity and speaking condition. *Clinical Linguistics & Phonetics, 20*, 659–675.

Doyle, P. C., Leeper, H. A., Kotler, A. L., Thomas-Stonell, N., O'Neil, C., Dylke, M. C., & Rolls, K. (1997). Dysarthric speech: A comparison of computerized recognition and listener intelligibility. *Journal of Rehabilitation Research & Development, 34*, 309–316.

Dykstra, A. D., Hakel, M. E., & Adams, S. G. (2007). Application of the ICF in reduced speech intelligibility in dysarthria. *Seminars in Speech and Language, 28*, 301–311.

Eadie, T. L., Yorkston, K. M., Klasner, E. R., Dudgeion, B. J., Deitz, J. C., Baylor, . . . Amtmann, D. (2006). Measuring communicative participation: A review of self report instruments in speech-language pathology. *American Journal of Speech Language Pathology, 15*, 307–320.

Enderby, P. M. (1980). Frenchay dysarthria assessment. *British Journal of Disorders of Communication, 15*, 165–173.

Enderby, P. M. (2008). *Frenchay dysarthria assessment-2nd edition (FDA-2)*. Austin, TX: ProEd.

Flipsen, P., Jr. (2006). Measuring the intelligibility of conversational speech in children. *Clinical Linguistics & Phonetics, 20*, 303–312.

Gentil, M. (1992). Phonetic intelligibility testing in dysarthria for the use of French language clinicians. *Clinical Linguistics & Phonetics, 6*, 179–189.

Goberman, A. M., & Elmer, L. W. (2005). Acoustic analysis of clear versus conversational speech in individuals with Parkinson disease. *Journal of Communication Disorders, 38*, 215–230.

Hazan, V., & Markham, D. (2004). Acoustic-phonetic correlates of talker intelligibility for adults and children. *Journal of the Acoustical Society of America, 116*, 3108–3118.

Hodge, M. & Daniels, J. (2005). Test of Children's Speech and Spelling—TOCS+ version 4.1. [Software]. University of Alberta, Edmonton, AB.

Hodge, M., & Whitehill, T. (2010). Intelligibility impairments. In J. S. Damico, N. Muller, & M. J. Ball (Eds.), *The handbook of language and speech disorders* (pp. 99–114). Oxford, UK: Wiley-Blackwell.

Hustad, K. C. (2008). The relationship between listener comprehension and intelligibility scores for speakers with dysarthria. *Journal of Speech, Language, and Hearing Research, 51*, 562–573.

Hustad, K. C., & Beukelman, D. R. (2002). Listener comprehension of severely dysarthric speech: Effects of linguistic cues and stimulus cohesion. *Journal of Speech, Language, and Hearing Research, 45*, 545–558.

Hustad, K. C., & Cahill, M. A. (2003). Effects of presentation mode and repeated familiarization on intelligibility of dysarthric speech. *American Journal of Speech-Language Pathology, 12*, 198–208.

Jeng, J.-Y., Weismer, G., & Kent, R. D. (2006). Production and perception of mandarin tone in adults with cerebral palsy. *Clinical Linguistics & Phonetics, 20*, 67–87.

Kennedy, M. R. T., Strand, E. A., & Yorkston, K. M. (1994). Selected acoustic changes in the verbal repairs of dysarthric speakers. *Journal of Medical Speech-Language Pathology, 2*, 263–279.

Kent, R. D., Weismer, G., Kent, J. F., & Rosenbek, J. C. (1989). Toward phonetic intelligibility testing in dysarthria. *Journal of Speech, Language, and Hearing Disorders, 54*, 482–499.

Kim, Y-J., Weismer, G., Kent, R. D., & Duffy, J. R. (2009). Statistical models of F2 slope in relation to severity of dysarthria. *Folia Phoniatrica et Logopaedica, 61*, 329–335.

Kim, Y-J., Weismer, G., Kuo, C., Kent, R. D., & Duffy, J. R. (2007). Effect of level of presentation to listeners on scaled speech intelligibility of speakers with dysarthria. [Abstract] *Journal of the Acoustical Society of America, 122*, 3028.

Klasner, E. R., & Yorkston, K. M. (2005). Speech intelligibility in ALS and HD dysarthria: the everyday listener's perspective. *Journal of Medical Speech-Language Pathology, 13*, 127–139.

Krause, J. C., & Braida, L. D. (1995). The effects of speaking rate on the intelligibility of speech for various speaking modes. [Abstract]. *Journal of Acoustical Society of America, 98*, 2982.

Liss, J. M., Spitzer, S. M., Caviness, J. N., & Adler, C. (2002). The effect of familiar-ization on intelligibility and lexical segmentation in hypokinetic and ataxic dysarthria. *Journal of the Acoustical Society of America, 112*, 3022–3030.

Liu, H. M., Tsao, F. M., & Kuhl, P. K. (2005). The effect of reduced vowel working space on speech intelligibility in Mandarin-speaking young adults with cerebral palsy. *Journal of the Acoustical Society of America, 117*, 3879–3789.

Lowit, A., Brendel, B., Dobinson, C., & Howell, P. (2006). An investigation into the influences of age, pathology, and cognition on speech production. *Journal of Medical Speech Language Pathology, 14*, 253–262.

McHenry, M., & Parle, A. M. (2006). Construction of a set of unpredictable sentences for intelligibility testing. *Journal of Medical Speech-Language Pathology, 14*, 269–271.

Morris, S. R., Wilcox, K. A., & Schooling, T. L. (1995). The preschool speech intelligibility measure. *American Journal of Speech-Language Pathology, 4*, 22–28.

Ozawa, Y., Shiromoto, O., Ishizaki, F., Hasegawa, J., Nishimura, H., & Watamori, T. (2003). Word intelligibility testing using phonetic contrasts for Japanese speakers with articulation disorders. *Japan Journal of Logopedics and Phoniatrics, 44*, 119–130.

Petersen, E. F. (1997a). Phonetic intelligibility testing in dysarthria. Validity and reliability of listeners' perceptions. *Logopedics Phoniatrics & Vocology, 22*, 105–117.

Petersen, E. F. (1997b). *Test af Fonetisk Forståelighed.* Valby, Denmark: INHAKO.

Picheny, M. A., Durlach, N. I., & Braida, L. D. (1985). Speaking clearly for the hard of hearing I: Intelligibility differences between clear and conversational speech. *Journal of Speech and Hearing Research, 28*, 96–103.

Picheny, M. A., Durlach, N. I., & Braida, L. D. (1986). Speaking clearly for the hard of hearing II: Acoustic characteristics of clear and conversational speech. *Journal of Speech and Hearing Research, 29*, 434–446.

Picheny, M. A., Durlach, N. I., & Braida, L. D. (1989). Speaking clearly for the hard of hearing III: An attempt to determine the contribution of speaking rate to difference in intelligibility between clear and conversational speech. *Journal of Speech and Hearing Research, 32,* 600–603.

Platt, L. J., Andrews, G., Young, M., & Quinn, P. T. (1980). Dysarthria of adult cerebral palsy: I. Intelligibility and articulatory impairment. *Journal of Speech and Hearing Research, 23,* 28–40.

Rogers, C. L., Dalby, J., & Nishi, K. (2004). Effects of noise and intelligibility of Chinese accented English. *Language and Speech, 47,* 139–154.

Schiavetti, N. (1992). Scaling procedures for the measurement of speech intelligibility. In R. D. Kent (Ed.), *Intelligibility in speech disorders* (pp. 11–34). Philadelphia, PA: John Benjamins.

Schiltz, A. L. (1994). The effect of a multitalker babble noise on the speech intelligibility of females with amyotrophic lateral sclerosis. Unpublished Master's thesis, University of Wisconsin-Madison.

Sharp, D. J., Scott, S. K., & Wise, R. J. S. (2004). Monitoring and the controlled processing of meaning: Distinct prefrontal systems. *Cerebral Cortex, 14,* 1–10.

Shriberg, L. D., Austin, D., Lewis, B. A., McSweeny, J. L., & Wilson, D. L. (1997). The percentage of consonants correct (PCC) metric: Extensions and reliability data. *Journal of Speech, Language, and Hearing Research, 40,* 708–722.

Smith, L. E., & Nelson, C. L. (1985). International intelligibility of English. *World Englishes, 4,* 333–342.

Tikofsky, R. S. (1970). A revised list for the estimation of dysarthric single word intelligibility. *Journal of Speech and Hearing Research, 13,* 59–64.

Tikofsky, R. S., & Tikofsky, R. P. (1964). Intelligibility measures of dysarthric speech. *Journal of Speech and Hearing Research, 7,* 325–333.

Turner, G. S., Martin, H. , & de Jonge, R. (2008). Influence of amplification on word intelligibility and phonetic contrast errors in dysarthria. *Journal of Medical Speech-Language Pathology, 16,* 267–273.

Turner, G. S., Tjaden, K., & Weismer, G. (1995). The influence of speaking rate on vowel space and speech intelligibility for individuals with amyotrophic lateral sclerosis. *Journal of Speech, Language, and Hearing Research, 38,* 1001–1013.

Van Nuffelen, G., De Bodt, M., Wuyts, F., & Van de Heyning, P. (2009). The effect of rate control on speech rate and intelligibility of dysarthric speech. *Folia Phoniatrica et Logopaedica, 61,* 69–75.

Van Nuffelen, G., Middag, C., De Bodt, M., & Martens, J.-P. (2008). Speech technology-based assessment of phoneme intelligibility in dysarthria. *International Journal of Language & Communication Disorders, 30,* 1–15.

Walshe, M., Peach, R. K., & Miller, N. (2008). Dysarthria impact profile: Development of a scale to measure psychosocial effects. *International Journal of Language & Communication Disorders, 44,* 693–715.

Weismer, G. (1997). Motor speech disorders. In W. J. Hardcastle & J. Laver (Eds.), *The handbook of phonetic sciences* (pp. 191–219). Cambridge, MA: Blackwell.

Weismer, G. (2008). Speech intelligibility. In M. J. Ball, M. Perkins, N. Müller, & S. Howard (Eds.), *The handbook of clinical linguistics* (pp. 568–582). Oxford, UK: Blackwell.

Weismer, G., & Laures, J. S. (2002). Direct magnitude estimates of speech intelligibility in dysarthria: Effects of a chosen standard. *Journal of Speech, Language, and Hearing Research, 45,* 421–433.

Weismer, G., & Martin, R. E. (1992). Acoustic and perceptual approaches to the study of intelligibility. In R. D. Kent (Ed.), *Intelligibility in speech disorders: Theory, measurement and management* (pp. 68–118). Amsterdam, The Netherlands: John Benjamins.

Whitehill, T. L, & Ciocca, V. (2000). Perceptual-phonetic predictors of single-word intelligibility: A study of Cantonese dysarthria. *Journal of Speech, Language, and Hearing Research, 43,* 1451–1465.

World Health Organization. (2001) *International classification of functioning, disability, and health: ICF.* Geneva, Switzerland: World Health Organization.

Yorkston, K. M., & Beukelman, D. R. (1978). A comparison of techniques for measuring intelligibility of dysarthric speech. *Journal of Communication Disorders, 11,* 499–512.

Yorkston, K. M., Beukelman, D. R., & Hakel, M. (1996). *Speech intelligibility test for Windows.* Lincoln, NE: Communication Disorders Software.

Yorkston, K. M., Strand, E. A., & Kennedy, M. R. T. (1996). Comprehensibility of dysarthric speech: Implications for assessment and treatment planning. *American Journal of Speech-Language Pathology, 5,* 55–66.

Ziegler, W., Hartmann, E., & von Cramon, D. (1988). Word identification testing in the diagnostic evaluation of dysarthric speech. *Clinical Linguistics & Phonetics, 2,* 291–308.

Ziegler, W., Hartmann, E., & Wiesner, I. (1992). Dysarthriediagnostik mit dem "Münchner Verständlichkeits-Profil" (MVP) ó Konstruktion des Verfahrens und Anwendungen. *Nervenarzt, 63,* 602–608.

Ziegler, W., & Zierdt, A. (2008). Telediagnostic assessment of intelligibility in dysarthria: A pilot investigation of MVP-online. *Journal of Communication Disorders, 41,* 553–577.

Zraick, R. I., Davenport, D. J., Tabbal, S. D., Hutton, T. J., Hicks, G. M., & Patterson, J. H. (2004). Reliability of speech intelligibility ratings using the Unified Huntington Disease Rating Scale. *Journal of Medical Speech-Langage Pathology, 12,* 31–40.

Zraick, R. I., Dennie, T., Tabbal, S. D., Hutton, T. J., Hicks, G. M., & O'Sullivan, P. (2003). Reliability of speech intelligibility ratings using the Unified Parkinson Disease Rating Scale. *Journal of Medical Speech-Langage Pathology, 11,* 227–240.

3

Physiological Assessment

BRUCE E. MURDOCH, PH.D.

Introduction

Although perceptual evaluations remain the benchmark for the assessment of motor speech disorders, recent years have seen a quantum increase in the use of physiological instrumentation in the assessment and management of dysarthria and apraxia of speech. The so-called "physiological approach" to the assessment and treatment of motor speech impairment as espoused by Hardy (1967), Netsell (1986), and Murdoch (1996) evolved from the concept that assessment of the individual motor subsystems of the speech production mechanism (respiratory, laryngeal, velopharyngeal, and articulatory subsystems) was crucial in defining the underlying speech pathophysiology and, consequently, for enabling the development of optimal treatment programs (Abbs & De Paul, 1989; Murdoch, 1996).

More specifically, the inclusion of instrumental procedures as an adjunct to perceptual methods in the assessment and diagnosis of motor speech disorders enables clinicians to extend their senses and objectify their perceptual observations. In particular, physiological instrumentation has provided the clinician with the ability to determine the contributions of malfunctions in the various components of the speech production mechanism to the production of disordered speech. Indeed, modern instrumentation enables the clinician to assess and obtain information about the integrity and functional status of muscle groups at each stage of the speech production process from respiration through to articulation. Consequently, a growing level of appreciation exists among clinicians of the considerable advantages of instrumental analysis, which provides quantitative, objective data on a wide range of different speech parameters far beyond the scope of an auditory-based impressionistic judgment. Instrumental assessment can enhance the abilities of the clinician in all stages of clinical management including increasing the precision of diagnosis through more valid specification of abnormal functions that require modification; the provision of positive identification and documentation of therapeutic efficacy; and the expansion of options of therapy modalities, including the use of instrumentation in a biofeedback modality.

To be of maximum value in determining treatment priorities, physiological assessment should in most cases be comprehensive, covering as many components of the speech production mechanism as possible. In certain circumstances, however, such as conditions in which, based on perceptual findings, dysfunctioning of a specific component of the speech production mechanism is thought to underlie the observed speech disorder (e.g., dysfunctioning of the velopharyngeal valve leading to hypernasality), the physiological assessment may be restricted to those instruments capable of assessing the functioning of that component alone. A wide variety of different types of physiological instrumentation have been described in the literature for use in the assessment of different components of the speech production apparatus. Each of these instruments has been designed to provide information on a specific aspect of speech production including muscular activity, structural movements, airflows, and air pressures generated in various parts of the speech mechanism. It is the intent of the present chapter to provide the reader with an outline of the technological features of the more frequently used instrumental approaches to the assessment of the functioning of the respiratory system, larynx, velopharynx, and articulators and to highlight their

potential clinical value. A summary of the major physiological instruments used in the assessment of motor speech disorders is presented in Table 3–1.

Although at the time of this writing many of these techniques have not been incorporated into mainstream clinical use, each offers the potential to increase our understanding of the effects of neurological diseases on the functioning of specific components of the speech production apparatus. In future years, through the application of these techniques in research aimed at further elucidating the nature of the pathophysiological changes that underlie motor speech impairments, it is anticipated that a number of the instruments described in the following sections will become essential parts of our routine clinical examinations.

Physiological Assessment of Speech Breathing

The basic energy source for all speech and voice production is provided by the respiratory system, which regulates such important parameters as speech and voice intensity, pitch, linguistic stress, and the division of speech into units (e.g., phrases). Two major types of instruments are used in the assessment of speech breathing: (1) those that directly measure various lung volumes, capacities, and airflows (e.g., spirometers); and (2) those that indirectly measure respiratory function by monitoring the movements of the chest wall, the so-called kinematic assessments (e.g., mercury strain-gauges, magnetometers, respiratory inductance plethysmographs, strain-gauge belt pneumographs).

Table 3–1. Summary of the Major Physiological Instruments Available for Assessment of Components of Speech Production Mechanisms

Speech System	Instrument	Information Provided	Normative Data	Clinical Use
Respiratory Function	Direct Measures — Spirometer	Lung volumes and capacities (e.g., tidal volume, inspiratory capacity, FEV_1 etc.)	Available	Common in hospital respiratory units
	Kinematic Measures — Magnetometers; strain-gauge belt pneumographs; *respiratory inductance plethysmography (respitrace)	Speech breathing patterns, lung volumes, chest wall coordination, percent contribution of ribcage	RR	Respitrace system common in hospital respiratory units and speech science laboratories
Laryngeal Function	Direct Measures — Endoscopy (rigid, flexible, *videostroboscopy)	Movement of vocal folds during phonation: rigid endoscope—sustained vowels flexible endoscope—connected speech Videostroboscopy enables slow motion viewing of glottal cycle.	RR	Videostroboscopy in common use in hospital ENT departments
	High-speech photography	Finer details of glottal movement. Useful in cases of glottal fry, aperiodic voice, dichotic phonation	RR	Limited by significant cost and cumbersome equipment

continues

Table 3-1. *continued*

Speech System	Instrument		Information Provided	Normative Data	Clinical Use
Laryngeal Function	Direct Measures	Videokymography	Evaluation of vibrating abnormalities not analyzed by videostroboscopy (e.g., effects of scar tissue, subharmonic vibrations, multiple openings in glottal cycle)	RR	Limited by poor two-dimensional spatial resolution
		High-speech video	Onset and offset of vocal fold oscillation, diplophonia, vocal fold tension, stiffness	RR	Limited by poor image resolution at high speeds
		Electromyography	Activity of laryngeal musculature Surface electrodes—general muscle activity as in hyperfunctional dysphonia Needle electrodes—specific muscle function	RR	Limited—needle electrodes invasive, poor client comfort
	Indirect Measures	Electroglottography	Biomechanics of vibratory cycle: fundamental frequency, duty cycle, closing time	RR	Used in some clinics in association with videostroboscopy. Primarily a research tool
		Photoglottography	Analysis of glottal opening and closing	Not available	Rare

42

Speech System	Instrument	Information Provided	Normative Data	Clinical Use
Laryngeal Function	Aero-dynamics			
	Aerophone II	Airflow measures, mean flow rate, duration of phonation, subglottal pressure, glottal resistance, glottal efficiency, acoustic output power, etc	RR	Used in some hospital speech/language pathology clinics
	Pneumotachographs, hot-wire anemometers, oropharyngeal pressure catheters	Collectively, these techniques estimate vocal tract aerodynamics (e.g., laryngeal airways resistance, laryngeal/phonatory flow)	RR	Primarily used as research tools
Velopharyngeal Function	Electromyography	Activity of velopharyngeal muscles	Not available	Limited by highly invasive nature of needle electrodes
	Endoscopy	Direct observation of velopharyngeal valve (nasendoscopy preferable)	RR	Commonly used in hospital ENT departments
	Phototransduction	Estimates of velar elevation and pharyngeal wall movements	Not available	Limited by invasive nature of technique
	Radiographic procedures (cineradiography, high speed x-rays)	Observation of velar movements	RR	Used in hospital ENT departments. Limited by exposure to ionizing radiation
	Airflow/air pressure methods (e.g., pneumotachograph)	Nasal airflow measures	RR	Primarily used as research tools
	Accelerometers	Oral-nasal coupling index	RR	Primarily used as research tools

continues

43

Table 3–1. *continued*

Speech System	Instrument	Information Provided	Normative Data Available	Clinical Use
Velopharyngeal Function	*Nasometer	Nasality (nasalence)	Available	Relatively common use in hospital speech/language pathology departments
Articulatory Function	Strain-gauge systems	Movement and force generating capabilities of tongue, lips, jaw	RR	Primarily used as research tools
	Pressure and force transducers (e.g., Iowa Performance Instrument [IOPI])	Interlabial contact pressures, tongue force, and endurance	RR	IOPI system commonly used in hospital speech/language pathology departments
	Electromyography	Activity of articulatory musculature (e.g., presence of hypertonicity)	RR	Rare
	Cineradiography	Articulatory movements during speech	RR	Limited due to reliance on ionizing radiation
	Electropalatography	Tongue to palate contact patterns	RR	Used in some hospital speech/language pathology clinics; somewhat limited by high cost of artificial palates
	Electromagnetic articulography	Velocity, acceleration, deceleration, movement duration, and distance of movement of articulators	RR	Primarily used as a research tool

ENT = ear, nose and throat; * = most commonly used instrument; RR = no normative data but data collected from non-neurologically impaired controls reported in research articles.

Spirometric Assessments

Specifically designed for the evaluation of respiratory volumes and capacities, spirometers enable the clinician to obtain a number of valuable respiratory/airflow measures, including vital capacity, forced expiratory volume, functional residual capacity, inspiratory capacity, expiratory and inspiratory reserve volumes, as well as volume/flow relationships and tidal volume and respiration rate. Furthermore, the values of each of these respiratory parameters obtained by spirometric assessment can be compared to predicted values based on the client's age, height, and gender to determine whether their respiratory function is within normal limits. Although a variety of different types of spirometers are available, including wet spirometers, dry (hand-held) spirometers, mechanical spirometers, and electrical spirome-

ters, the basic principle of each is to measure and record the volumes of air blown into either a tube or fitted face mask, which is attached to the machine (Figure 3–1).

By far the most common spirometers used in contemporary clinical settings are the dry (hand-held) type as shown in Figure 3–1. Although measures of various respiratory volumes and capacities derived by these instruments provide valuable information as to the status of a client's respiratory system, their dependence on the use of physical encumbrances such as a mouthpiece, nose clip, or tightly fitted masks limits their application for determination of respiratory function during speech. Consequently, in the assessment of respiratory function in clients with dysarthria, clinicians and researchers predominantly have used respiratory kinematic measurement devices for the assessment of speech breathing.

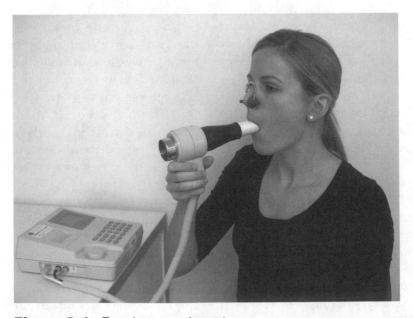

Figure 3–1. Respiratory spirometer.

Kinematic Assessments

Because they do not require the need for restrictive mouth pieces and nose clips that can interfere with natural speech production and respiratory patterns, kinematic procedures allow for more accurate measurements of breath support during speech production. Kinematic devices allow the clinician to infer the airflow/volume changes during respiration from rib cage and abdominal displacements. According to the kinematic theory, the chest wall is a two-part system consisting of the rib cage and diaphragm-abdomen arranged in mechanical parallel (Hixon, Goldman, & Mead, 1973). The rib cage and diaphragm-abdomen displace volume as they move, and, resultingly, their combined volume displacements equal that of the lungs. In essence, therefore, the kinematic analysis involves the simultaneous but independent recording of changes in the dimensions (e.g., circumference) of the rib cage and abdomen.

Three main types of kinematic instrumentation have been utilized in the assessment of speech breathing in speakers with dysarthria. These include the use of magnetometers (Hixon, Putnam, & Sharp, 1983; Hodge & Putnam-Rochet, 1989; Hoit, Banzett, Brown, & Loring, 1990; Hoit & Hixon, 1986; Hoit & Hixon, 1987; Hoit, Hixon, Altman, & Morgan, 1989; Hoit, Hixon, Watson, & Morgan, 1990; McFarland & Smith, 1992; Putnam & Hixon, 1984; Reich & McHenry, 1990; Solomon & Hixon, 1993; Stathopoulos, Hoit, Hixon, Watson, & Solomon, 1991; Stathopoulos & Sapienza, 1993), strain-gauge pneumograph systems (Manifold & Murdoch, 1993; Murdoch, Chenery, Bowler, &

Ingram, 1989a; Murdoch, Chenery, Stokes, & Hardcastle, 1991; Murdoch, Noble, Chenery, & Ingram, 1989b; Murdoch, Theodoros, Stokes, & Chenery, 1993), and respiratory-inductance plethysmography (available commercially as the Respitrace from Ambulatory Monitoring Inc., Ardsley, NY) (Bolick, Hixon, Watson, & Jones, 2004; Cahill, Theodoros, Murdoch, & MacMillan, 2003; Lane, Perkell, Svirsky, & Webster, 1991; Murdoch, Pitt, Theodoros, & Ward, 1999; Sperry & Klich, 1992; Warren, Morr, Putnam-Rochet, & Dalston, 1989; Winkworth, Davis, Adams, & Ellis, 1995). Using these various assessment techniques, specific details regarding lung volumes, breath patterns, and the relative contribution and degree of coordination of the chest wall muscles during speech breathing have been investigated.

Of the three major kinematic techniques used in the assessment of speech breathing, the Respitrace system is the most commonly available in contemporary clinical settings. This latter system senses movements of the chest wall via the changes in electrical inductance of a zigzag of wire embedded with elasticized straps positioned around the rib cage and abdominal regions (Figure 3–2). Oscillators positioned in the center of the chest wall anteriorly produce a frequency-modulated signal that passes through the wires of the chest bands, the frequency of which is related to the circumference of the chest wall. Changes in the size of the chest wall circumference alter the shape and, therefore, conductance of the zigzag wires of the straps, and consequently change the signal.

The linearized magnetometer system also has been used quite extensively for clinical and research purposes. The

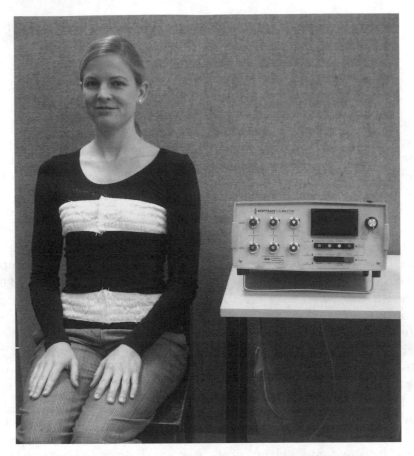

Figure 3–2. Respitrace system for kinematic assessment of speech breathing.

procedure involves the recording of the antero-posterior diameter changes of the rib cage and abdomen using linearized magnetometers incorporating two pairs of generator-sensor coils, one for the rib cage and one for the abdomen (Hoit et al., 1989). The generator coils of each pair are placed at the front of the torso at the levels of the sternal midlength and the abdomen, just over the umbilicus, while the sensor coils are placed at the corresponding levels on the back of the torso. The generator coil then is driven by an oscillator and produces an alternating electromagnetic field through the body including an alternating voltage in the sensor coil. The voltage that reaches the sensor coil is decreased by body diameter; therefore, the small changes in distance between the coils that occur during breathing are detected. As these voltage changes closely approximate linearity, the distance measurements obtained using this method are considered quite accurate. Although the level of electromagnetic radiation involved with using magnetometers does not pose a significant risk to most patients, subjects with cardiac pacemakers or other electronic implants are, however, advised to avoid this procedure.

The strain-gauge pneumograph method of kinematic assessment, while also being an easy kinematic device to use in comparison, has the added advantage of being safe to use with subjects who have cardiac pacemakers or other electronic implants. In this procedure, two strain-gauge belt pneumographs, which detect the circumferential changes, are wrapped around the subject's torso and fastened, one at the level of the sternal angle and the other at the level of (i.e., immediately over) the umbilicus. A strain-gauge transducer, which is a transducer that exhibits a change of some electrical property (most commonly resistance) when they are deformed or strained by an external force, is attached at the center of both straps anteriorly. Details of the temperature compensated strain-gauge transducer system can be found in Murdoch et al. (1989a). During respiration, the signals from the rib cage and the abdominal transducers record the increasing and decreasing circumferential changes of the rib cage and abdominal region, which occur during respiration.

Physiological Assessment of Laryngeal Function

Both direct and indirect techniques are employed in the physiological evaluation of laryngeal function. Direct techniques include endoscopic high-speed photography, high-speed video, videokymography, electromyography, and stroboscopic procedures. Indirect methods, on the other hand, include electroglottography (electrolaryngography) and aerodynamic examination.

Direct Examination of Vocal Function

Endoscopy, using a rigid endoscope, or nasoendoscopy, using a flexible fiberscope, both allow for direct observation of vocal fold movement. Both systems are telescopic type devices that function to illuminate the laryngeal area and allow visual inspection of the laryngeal region. The rigid endoscope is inserted through the mouth to the region of the orophyarynx, allowing direct observation of the vocal folds during phonation of sustained vowels. In comparison, the flexible fiberscope is inserted through the nasal cavity and then passed down through the pharyngeal area until the tip of the scope is positioned at approximately the level of the epiglottis to allow an unobstructed view of the vocal folds. As the oral cavity is not obstructed using the nasoendoscopic technique, visual record of laryngeal function can be obtained during normal speech production. Both the endoscope and nasoendoscope are connected to a video monitoring and recording system that allows the visual image of the vocal folds to be recorded for later viewing and analysis.

Videostroboscopy combines the use of a strobe light source in conjunction with the videoendoscopic procedures outlined previously. Using the stroboscopic technique, the movements of the focal folds during speech production can be slowed or stopped through the optical illusion of stroboscopy, making identification of vocal fold dysfunction much more easy. In essence, videostroboscopy involves the presentation of rapid flashes of light, which illuminate portions of the vibratory cycle of the vocal folds. Depending upon the frequency of the light pulses, this rapid sampling can give the clinician a clear view of the vocal folds at a particular phase of the glottal cycle or a slow motion view of the movement of the vocal folds through the whole vocal cycle. Although videostroboscopy currently is the most common technique used in clinical settings to assess vocal fold vibration, it does have a number of limitations. In particular, it is most useful with clients in whom the vocal folds vibrate in a periodic or pseudoperiodic fashion. The procedure is less optimal, however, for assessment of aperiodic vibration in that the frequency detection system of the stroboscope cannot track rapid, irregular changes effectively. The technique also may produce misleading data when the vocal folds produce more than one periodic source such as in diplophonia. A detailed description of the videostroboscopic technique, including its advantages and limitations, is presented in Reinhardt, Hawkshaw, and Sataloff (2005).

Other direct methods for assessment of vocal function include high-speed photography, videokymography (VKG), high-speed video, and electromyography. High-speed photography, which involves filming glottal movements at fast or ultrahigh speeds, allows for the finer details of glottal movement to be studied in a similar manner to stroboscopy. In particular, high-speed photography has been shown to provide useful and detailed information about vocal fold function, even in difficult circumstances in which videostroboscopy is limited, such as in aperiodic voices, dichotic phonation, and vocal fry. Despite its many advantages, however,

the use of this technique is limited due to the significant cost of the procedure. In addition, the cumbersome nature of the equipment and delay in processing make it impractical for clinical use. More recently introduced techniques such as VKG and high-speed video represent promising additions to the list of procedures available for visualizing movement of the vocal folds during speech. VKG visualizes the vocal folds using a line-scanning camera. Although introduced by Gall in 1984, it was not until 1996 that the system was developed sufficiently for practical clinical purposes (Svec & Schutte, 1996). The technique permits detailed evaluation of vibratory abnormalities that cannot be analyzed via videostroboscopy, such as the effect of scar tissue and outcomes of surgical treatment for scar, the presence of subharmonic vibrations, double or triple openings in a single glottal cycle, and irregular vocal-fold vibrations among others.

To circumvent a number of the limitations of high-speed photography, such as delayed processing, high-speed digital imaging was introduced in 1987. Several authors subsequently have reported on the usefulness of high-speed video (Eysholdt, Tigges, Wittenberg, & Proschel, 1996; Hess & Gross, 1993) with the technique being used to study parameters such as the normal onset and offset of vocal-fold oscillation, diplophonia, and vocal-fold tension, stiffness, and mass.

Electromyography (EMG), the study of electrical potential generated in skeletal muscles also has been used to examine the activity of the laryngeal musculature. Both surface (Boemke, Gerull, & Hippel, 1992; Milutinovic,

Lastovka, Vohradnik, & Janosevic, 1988) and needle electrodes (Hirano & Ohala, 1969; Shipp, Izdebski, Reed, & Morrissey, 1985; Watson, Schaefer, Freeman, Dembowski, Kondraske, & Roark, 1991) have been used in laryngeal muscle investigations. The information obtained from surface electrodes represents the global activity of the muscles of the laryngeal area and not specific muscle function. Consequently, surface electrodes are used when the muscle activity of the general laryngeal area is of interest, such as in cases of hyperfunction dysphonia. In contrast, needle electrodes are selected when specific information regarding individual laryngeal muscle function is required.

Indirect Examination of Vocal Function

Despite the obvious diagnostic and therapeutic advantages of direct observation of laryngeal function using the previously mentioned techniques, clinicians tend to forgo performing direct laryngeal observations due to the invasiveness of the procedures. Consequently, objective assessment of laryngeal function primarily is achieved through indirect approaches such as electroglottography, photoglottography, laryngeal aerodynamics, and spectrographic or acoustic analysis.

Electroglottography (EGG) is one of the most popular indirect methods of analyzing the glottal waveform as it is noninvasive, inexpensive, and easy to perform. Electroglottography makes use of the varying electrical impedance of the laryngeal structures as the vocal folds open and close, therefore making

it possible to investigate the vibratory patterns of the vocal folds (Motta, Cesari, Iengo, & Motta, 1990). It is, therefore, useful as an adjunctive technique in defining the deficit in laryngeal biomechanics at the level of the vibratory waveform. A number of different types of EGG instrumentation are available commercially, with one of the more commonly used versions being the Fourcin laryngograph interfaced with a Waveform Display System (Kay Elemetrics Model 6091) (Figure 3–3). In a similar manner to other EGG instruments, the Fourcin laryngograph provides a useful estimate of vocal-fold contact during the glottal cycle. Briefly, using the conductance of a 4-MHz signal transmitted and detected via two electrodes placed on the skin adjacent to the thyroid cartilage, a high frequency electric current then is passed between the electrodes with any tissue in the neck serving as a conductor. The conductance, which is reflected in the voltage, increases as the vocal folds make contact and decreases as they abduct, thereby reflecting the degree of vocal-fold contact and the vocal-fold vibratory patterns during phonation. These changes in conductance generate the laryngographic (Lx) waveform, which can be used to calculate a number of different parameters of vocal function including the fundamental frequency, the duty cycle, and closing time. It has been suggested by proponents of the EGG technique that different laryngeal pathologies yield specific Lx waveform shapes; however, this remains a topic for debate in the literature with many other authors advising caution when interpreting the results of EGG assessments. Despite this, many studies have

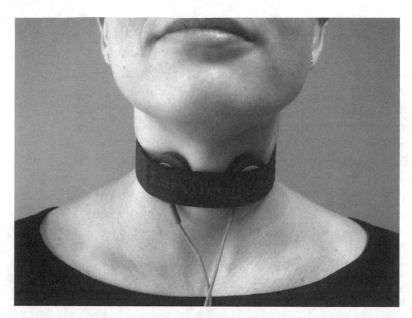

Figure 3–3. Client fitted with Fourcin laryngograph.

utilized EGG as part of the physiological assessment battery for investigating laryngeal function in dysarthric speakers of various etiologies (e.g., Cahill, Murdoch, & Theodoros, 2003; Murdoch, Manning, Theodoros, & Thompson, 1997; Murdoch, Thompson, & Stokes, 1994; Theodoros & Murdoch, 1994). Further, in some clinics, the technique is used in combination with videostroboscopy.

The photoglottographic technique is an indirect technique based on the theory that the glottis is a shutter through which light passes in proportion to the degree of the opening. In this technique, a bright light source is placed against the neck just below the cricoid cartilage, thereby illuminating the glottis, which suffuses the subglottal space with light. A pickup probe, which is situated in the pharynx, transmits the light that passes into the pharynx to a photosensor. The amount of light that is received at the photosensor should, therefore, be proportional to the area of the glottal opening. Photoglottography is not considered as clinically useful as EGG and, consequently, is not used routinely in many clinics.

Assessment of Vocal Tract Aerodynamics

A variety of different physiological instruments also are available for the examination of vocal-tract aerodynamics, such as subglottal air pressure, laryngeal airway resistance, and laryngeal/phonatory flow. Laryngeal/phonatory flow can be recorded using a number of different techniques including pneumotachographs, hot-wire anemometers, plethysmographs, electroaerometers, or using differential oropharyngeal pressure catheters. Each of these techniques and their various advantages can be found detailed in Miller and Daniloff (1993). Of these techniques, however, the pneumotachograph system possibly is the most frequently used technique to record airflow reported in the literature (Hoit & Hixon, 1992; Horii & Cooke, 1978; Netsell, Lotz, DuChane, & Barlow, 1991; Smitheran & Hixon, 1981) due to its excellent frequency response, linearity, and its relative insensitivity to turbulence in the breath stream (Miller & Daniloff, 1993). This technique, most frequently involves the use of a face-mask system, covering the mouth and nose of the subject, which is used to channel the airflow through to the pneumotachometer. In principle, a pneumotachograph is a differential pressure transducer that generates a pressure proportional to flow.

Measures of intra-oral pressure generally are recorded using a polyethylene tube inserted into the mouth of the client, just behind the lips, and connected to a differential pressure transducer. The recording of intra-oral pressure in this manner can also be used as an indirect measure of subglottal pressure as well as help determine a measure of laryngeal airway resistance. Direct recording of subglottal pressure during phonation requires the insertion of a hypodermic needle into the tracheal airway beneath the vocal folds. Due to the invasiveness of this latter procedure, Netsell and Hixon (1978) developed a less invasive procedure that involved the use of the intra-oral pressure catheter in conjunction with specific speech tasks (/pi/), to indirectly determine subglottal pressure. Essentially, during repetitions of the utterance /pi/, the oral pressure recorded during the occlusion phase of the voiceless stop consonant is considered a valid estimate of laryngeal subglottal pressure.

Unlike oral pressures or phonatory flow rates, laryngeal airway resistance cannot be measured directly. Rather, it is derived from calculating the ratio of translaryngeal pressure to translaryngeal flow (Smitheran & Hixon, 1981). In order to determine this aerodynamic variable, simultaneous recording of laryngeal airflow and oral air pressures is required, involving the use of face masks with oral catheters inserted through the mask. Details of the instrumentation involved in the assessment of laryngeal resistance can be found in Smitheran and Hixon (1981) and Hoit and Hixon (1992).

In addition to instrumentation specifically designed to record aspects of laryngeal aerodynamics, phonatory function analyzers also are available, which record and measure a number of aerodynamic parameters simultaneously. The Aerophone II, used in a number of studies (e.g., Frokjaer-Jensen, 1992; Murdoch et al., 1994; Theodoros & Murdoch, 1994) is one such device that utilizes both a hardware transducer system as well as transducers for recording airflows, pressures, and acoustic signals. The Aerophone II consists of a hand-held transducer module together with a powerful data acquisition and processing software program (Figure 3–4). Along with a number of other functions, the Aerophone II can provide a wealth of information about glottal functioning by providing detailed information on airflow, air pressures, and acoustic output and their interrelationships in running speech. This information enables the clinician to calculate maximum, minimum, and average sound pressure level, dynamic range,

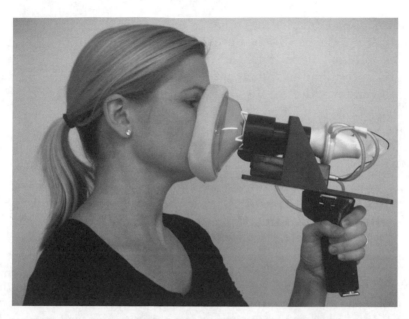

Figure 3–4. Aerophone II airflow measurement system.

volume of air used, duration of phonation, mean flow rate, a quotient of phonation, measures of subglottal pressure, glottal resistance, glottal aerodynamic input power, acoustic output power, and glottal efficiency during sustained phonation tasks and speech.

Acoustic Analysis of Vocal Function

Acoustic analysis of vocal function also can be performed using a number of software packages and dedicated systems. Various researchers have used acoustic analysis to examine fundamental frequency, frequency range, laryngeal perturbation measures (e.g., jitter, shimmer), voice amplitude, voice onset time, intonation contours, formant structure, and other aspects of phonation (Hartmann & von Cramon, 1984; Hillenbrand, Cleveland, & Erickson, 1994; Kent, Kent, Rosenbek, Weismer, Martin, Sufit, & Brooks, 1992; Kent & Kim, 2003; Kent & Read, 2002; Scherer, Gould, Titze, Meyers, & Sataloff, 1988). As with the analysis of aerodynamic parameters, however, the range of programs and dedicated devices for acoustic analysis of speech is wide, with a number of systems commercially available (Read, Buder, & Kent, 1992). As indicated earlier, discussion of the function and parameters measured by each of these systems is beyond this chapter. For further information concerning acoustic analysis of vocal function, the reader is referred to the following articles: Forrest & Weismer, 2009; Herman, 1989; Mann, 1987; Read, Buder, & Kent, 1990, 1992; Ryalls & Baum, 1990; Thomas-Stonell, 1989. Not only do these latter articles review the performance characteristics of a number of the systems marketed for acoustic speech analysis, they also provide capability and performance summaries for some of the acoustic systems, discuss the advantages and limitations of the various programs, outline and compare costs, detail vendor addresses (Read et al., 1992), as well as provide some considerations for the future generation of acoustic programs and devices.

Physiological Assessment of Velopharyngeal Function

Problems of nasality (hyper/hyponasality) and nasal emission have been identified as characteristic features of a number of different speech disorders. Hypernasality, however, commonly is an associated feature of dysarthric speech. In dysarthric speech, hypernasality is the result of improper function of the velopharyngeal valve, caused by a disturbance in the basic motor processes that regulate the contraction of the muscles of the soft palate and pharynx leading to a reduction in the force of their contractions and limitations of their range of movements (Darley, Aronson, & Brown, 1975). To objectively measure nasality in dysarthric speech and identify exactly how and to what degree the velopharyngeal valve is impaired, researchers have employed various different types of instrumentation designed to directly and indirectly measure the function of the velopharyngeal valve.

A wide range of instrumental techniques have been used to assess velopharyngeal function during speech—the main types being electromyographic, radiographic, fiberoptic, and ultrasonic methods, airflow and pressure techniques, and mechano-acoustic meth-

ods. Not all of the techniques, however, are suitable for routine clinical use.

Electromyography and Imaging Techniques

Electromyography

Investigations using electromyography (EMG) can provide significant information regarding specific activity and function of the velopharyngeal musculature during speech. However, despite the valuable information that can be obtained, the procedure is highly invasive, generally painful, disruptive of normal speech movements, and generally not feasible as a clinical tool. Surface electrodes also have been used to monitor the movements of the velum; however, although surface electrodes are slightly less invasive than hook-wire or intramuscular electrodes, their use is limited by the fact that they cannot be used to obtain specific information regarding the activity of individual muscles.

Endoscopic Procedures

Endoscopic or nasoendoscopic procedures have been used to observe directly the functioning of the velopharyngeal valve. This type of direct investigation can provide important information regarding deficits in timing and incoordination of velopharyngeal closure as well as identify sluggish, reduced, or incomplete palatal movement. Endoscopic procedures involve inserting the endoscope, which is a type of telescopic device, into the subject's mouth until the distal end lies in the oropharynx. From here, the function of the velopharyngeal port can be viewed directly. Nasoendoscopic procedures, in contrast, involve passing a thin, flexible, fiber-optic tube into the nasopharynx via the nasal passages allowing the velopharyngeal region to be viewed from above (Karnell, Linville, & Edwards, 1988; Niimi, Bell-Berti, & Harris, 1982). Although both techniques are comparable in the information they provide, the nasoendoscopic technique does not impair normal articulatory movements and, therefore, allows for the direct observation of velar movement during speech. Both the endoscope and the nasoendoscope can be used in conjunction with a video recording system (videoendoscopy / videonasoendoscopy) to allow for the image to be saved for later analysis.

Phototransduction

Phototransduction is another technique designed to evaluate velar movement. The photodetector system consists of a light source, a transmitting and a receiving optical fiber, and a light detector. The photodetection process involves the measurement of the intensity of light transmitted through the velopharyngeal port or reflected from the velar surface. The photodetector output is, therefore, a correlate of total velopharyngeal area, which reflects the function of both velar elevation and pharyngeal wall movement. Although phototransduction has been reported to accurately reflect velopharyngeal function when compared to cineradiographic and videoendoscopy procedures (Karnell, Seaver, & Dalston, 1988; Zimmermann, Dalston, Brown, Folkins, Linville, & Seaver, 1987), as in the case of most other direct assessments of velopharyngeal function, the invasive nature of the procedure limits the clinical use of this technique.

Radiographic Procedures

Radiographic assessments of velar function, such as cineradiography, a high-speed x-ray technique, also have been used by a number of researchers to observe palatial activity (Lock & Seaver, 1984; Williams & Eisenbach, 1981; Zimmermann et al., 1987). The x-ray film can be recorded at 150 frames per second (Lock & Seaver, 1984), which permits the recording of palatal movement relative to other articulatory movements typically in a single plane (e.g., midsagittal), during normal speech tasks. The use of this technique, however, is limited somewhat by the laborious analysis procedure and the degree of exposure of the patient to radiation.

Noninvasive Techniques

Due to the difficulties and invasive nature of many of the direct assessments of velar function, routine clinical assessments of nasality are conducted more frequently using indirect procedures that record the correlates of velopharyngeal function. From these indirect assessments, it is intended that inferences about the functioning of velopharynx can be drawn without the invasiveness and radiation risks of the more direct methods. The noninvasive instrumental assessments commonly are divided into two main groups: airflow / air-pressure methods and mechano-acoustic methods.

Airflow/Air-Pressure Methods

In that nasal airflow measures reflect many aspects of vocal tract function, including changing intraoral pressures, oral port constrictions, and nasal resistance, measures of nasal airflow cannot be used as an accurate index of the degree of nasalization. Despite this limitation, however, based on the principle that lowering the velum diverts part of the airstream through the nose, nasal airflow measures can be useful in the gross differentiation of good, fair, or poor velopharyngeal function.

Measures of nasal airflow can be achieved using a heated pneumotachograph. A number of authors (Andreassen, Smith, & Guyette, 1992; Dalston & Warren, 1986; Dalston, Warren, & Smith, 1990) have described an assessment technique that records both oral and nasal pressures as well as nasal airflow. Measuring nasal airflow and oral pressure at the same time can give a good indication of the functioning of the velopharyngeal muscles, as an incompetent velopharyngeal valve often can cause a severe reduction in oral pressures and an increase in nasal flow (Warren & Devereux, 1966). To use this pressure-flow technique, a catheter is placed in one nostril and secured by a cork to create a stagnant column of air. A second catheter is placed in the mouth, and both catheters are used to measure static air pressures, which are recorded by separate pressure transducers. The nasal airflow then is measured via a piece of plastic tubing placed in the other nostril and connected to the heated pneumotachograph.

Nasal airflow also can be estimated by simply using a pneumotachograph or a warm-wire anemometer fitted to a nasal mask (Hutters & Brondsted, 1992). A range of different mask systems have been described (Hoit, Watson, Hixon, McMahon, & Johnson, 1994), however, their basic design is to isolate and record nasal airflows. Although both techniques are comparable, the use of a nasal mask, as opposed to placing catheters in the nose, is conceivably less invasive and a more attractive option to the client.

Mechano-Acoustic Methods

Another noninvasive and indirect assessment of velopharyngeal function is the accelerometric method (Horii, 1980; Horii, 1983; Stevens, Kalikow, & Willemain, 1975; Theodoros, Murdoch, Stokes, & Chenery, 1993; Thompson & Murdoch, 1995). First discussed by Stevens et al. (1975), the accelerometric method is based on the principle that, as nasal sounds cause vibrations of the soft tissue of the nose, then an accelerometer (a transducer sensitive to vibration) placed on the nose could be used to detect nasalization. Later modified by Horii (1980, 1983), the accelerometric procedure currently involves the use of two miniature accelerometers to detect nasal and throat vibrations during speech. One miniature accelerometer is attached to the upper side of the nose over the lateral nasal cartilage just in front of the nasal bone, while the other is attached to the side of the neck over the lamina of the thyroid cartilage. The output signals from each accelerometer are amplified by a DC amplifier, and the amplified signals then are relayed to a computerized physiological data acquisition system. Horii (1980) proposed the use of a ratio of nasal accelerometric amplitude to voice amplitude as an index of nasal coupling. The HONC (Horii Oral-Nasal Coupling) index is the ratio of the amplitudes derived from the two separate accelerometers and is calculated during production of a range of nasal and non-nasal sounds. The accelerometric technique, involving the use of two accelerometers as outlined previously has been used by a number of researchers to examine nasality in dysarthric speakers (Theodoros, Murdoch, & Thompson, 1995; Thompson & Murdoch, 1995).

Other noninvasive mechano-acoustic assessments of nasality are based, not on vibration ratios, but rather the ratio of acoustic output from the oral and nasal cavities. The principle behind these techniques is based on the theory that as nasality is contingent upon the intermixing of phonic energy from the oral and nasal cavities, then a logical method to estimate nasality objectively is to separate and compare the sound energy from the mouth and the nose.

Although several instruments based on this principle have been devised, the system marketed as the Nasometer (Kay Elemetrics) is the one utilized in most contemporary clinics. The Nasometer is a computer-assisted instrument that provides objective measures of nasality during speech. Acoustic energy is detected by two directional microphones (one placed in front of the nares and the other in front of the mouth separated by a sound separator plate (Figure 3–5). The instrument yields a nasalance score made up of a ratio of nasal to oral plus nasal acoustic energy calculated as a percentage. The procedure allows for instantaneous calculation of the mean, standard deviation, and minimum and maximum nasalance scores and has been used by a number of researchers to investigate nasality in dysarthric speakers (Cahill, Murdoch, & Theodoros, 2001; Dalston & Seaver, 1992; Nellis, Neihman, & Lehman, 1992; Watterson, McFarlane, & Wright, 1993).

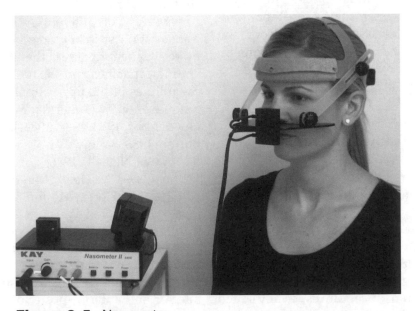

Figure 3–5. Nasometer.

Physiological Assessment of Articulation

The muscle groups of the lips, tongue, and jaw collectively represent what are termed the *articulators*. Although often grouped together due to their common influence over speech production at the articulatory stage, each of these structures functions independently and contributes differently to speech production. A variety of physiological instruments, therefore, have been developed in order to examine the degree of compression force exerted by each articulator during speech and nonspeech tasks, as well as to investigate force control properties, rate of individual articulatory movements, endurance capabilities of the individual articulators, and the movement patterns during speech production of each separate aspect of the articulatory system. Overall, the various physiological instruments developed to assess articulatory function fall into several categories, including strain-gauge transduction systems, pressure and force transduction systems, electromyography, imaging techniques, electropalatography and related methods, and electromagnetic articulation systems.

Strain-Gauge Transduction Systems

Strain-gauge transducers (variable resistors) have been the most frequently used type of instrumentation to record the movement and force generating capabilities of the articulators. Due to their high levels of sensitivity, strain-gauge transducers are especially suited to detecting the subtle changes in move-

ment that occur in speech production. In addition, they are relatively inexpensive, noninvasive, provide an immediate voltage analogue of movement, and can be adapted to assess lip, tongue, and jaw function during both speech and nonspeech tasks.

The basic configuration of many of the strain-gauge transduction systems described in the literature for use in assessing articulatory function involves the mounting of strain-gauges on either side of a flexible metal strip that is anchored at one end to a stable support to form a cantilever. The free end of the cantilever then can be moved by a force produced by either the lips, tongue, or jaw. This force resultingly bends the metal strip on which the gauges are attached, causing tension in the one strain-gauge mounted on the convex surface and compression of the one on the concave face. This displacement of the metal strip then is detected and recorded. An example of a strain-gauge system for estimating lip strength is shown in Figure 3–6.

A variety of different strain-gauge transduction systems have been used by researchers to assess the force generating capacities and the force control capabilities of the upper lip, lower lip, tongue, and jaw (Amerman, 1993; Barlow & Abbs, 1983, 1984, 1986; Barlow & Burton, 1988; Barlow, Cole, & Abbs, 1983; Barlow & Netsell, 1986; Langmore & Lehman, 1994; McHenry, Minton, & Wilson, 1994; McHenry, Minton, Wilson, & Post, 1994; McNeil, Weismer, Adams, & Mulligan, 1990; Wood, Hughes, Hayes, & Wolfe, 1992) as well as simultaneous movements of the upper lip, lower lip, and jaw in two dimensions (superior-inferior and anterior-posterior) during speech production (Abbs, 1973; Abbs,

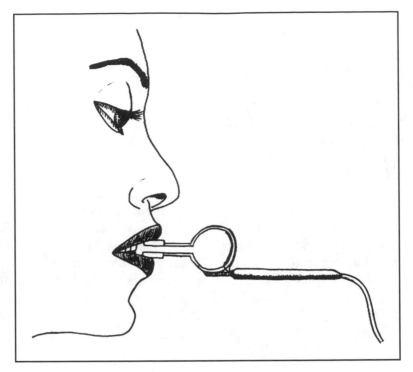

Figure 3–6. Example of strain-gauge system for measuring lip strength.

Folkins, & Sivarajan, 1976; Abbs & Netsell, 1973; Folkins & Abbs, 1976; Forrest & Weismer, 1995).

Pressure and Force Transduction Systems

In addition to strain-gauge transducers, pressure or force transducers also can provide valuable information regarding the functioning of the articulatory system. For example, a miniaturized pressure transducer has been used by a number of research groups to assess interlabial contact pressures during speech (Hinton & Luschei, 1992; Murdoch, Spenser, Theodoros, & Thompson, 1998; Thompson-Ward, Theodoros, Murdoch, & Cahill, 1999). Because of its small size, the transducer is capable of being placed between the lips to generate interlabial pressure measurements during speech production without interfering with normal articulatory movements. The transducer is interfaced with a dedicated software package designed to allow for investigations of combined upper and lower lip pressures, pressure control for maximum and submaximum pressure levels, and endurance and speech pressures during production of bilabial sounds.

Force transducers also have been used to examine tongue force and endurance capabilities. A commercially available instrument for estimating tongue strength and endurance is the Iowa Performance Instrument (IOPI), which consists of an air-filled rubber bulb attached to a pressure transducer (Figure 3–7). For testing, the bulb is placed in the mouth, and the subject is instructed to squeeze the bulb against the roof of the mouth with the tongue. When the bulb is squeezed by the tongue, the amount of pressure is displayed on a digital readout.

Either the IOPI or a similar system based on the IOPI has been used to assess tongue function in speakers with dysarthria associated with a range of neurological conditions (Murdoch et al., 1998; Robin, Goel, Somodi, & Luschei, 1992; Robin, Somodi, & Luschei, 1991; Theodoros, Murdoch, & Stokes, 1995; Ward, Theodoros, Murdoch, & Silburn, 2000).

Electromyography

Electromyography (EMG) is another technique that has commonly been used (primarily by researchers rather than clinicians) to examine articulator function. Using this technique, the momentary changes in electrical activity that occur when a muscle is contracting are recorded using various types of electrodes (e.g., surface, needle, hook-wire) placed either overlying (surface electrodes) or within (e.g., hook-wire and needle electrodes) the muscle. The data obtained from EMG assessment has proven useful for investigating the neurophysiological bases of various disorders, such as identifying the presence

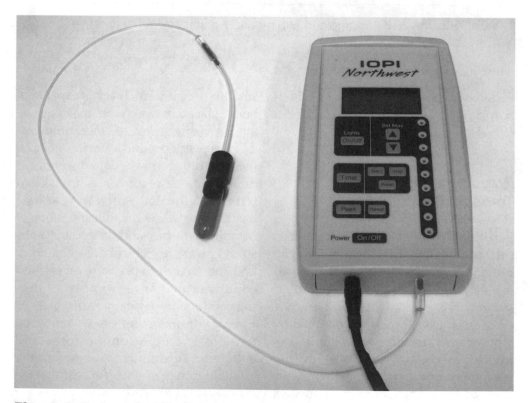

Figure 3–7. Iowa Oral Performance Instrument.

of increased muscle tone (hypertonicity) or abnormal variations in the activation or inhibition of muscle activity. In addition EMG has been used to record muscle activity simultaneously with the speech movement patterns of these same muscles in order to examine the motor control of the articulators. Examples of studies that have used EMG to examine articulatory function include those by Barlow and Burton (1988), McClean (1991), Moore, Smith, and Ringel (1988), and Shaiman (1989). For a review of EMG techniques used in the assessment of motor speech disorders, see Luschei & Finnegan (2009).

Imaging Techniques

Evaluating the movements of the tongue is much more difficult than assessing lip or jaw movement, due to the fact that the tongue functions within the confines of the mouth with only the anterior section directly observable. In addition, the complex muscular arrangement of the tongue allows an almost infinite combination of movements, which can occur at a very rapid rate. For these reasons, techniques such as ultrasound and cineradiography have proven useful for examining the complex patterns of lingual movement during speech. These types of imaging techniques, unlike other measurement devices actually provide information on the shape of the tongue. Considering that tongue position is crucial to the production of accurate vowel and consonant sounds, imaging techniques can provide very useful data on lingual positioning and function during speech in speech disordered subjects.

Cineradiography is a high-speed x-ray motion picture technique that records the lateral view of the mouth, nose, and pharynx. Using this technique, it is possible to view the articulatory structures during speech in order to identify gross deviations of articulatory movement such as reduced mobility of the tongue or soft palate (Folkins & Kuehn, 1982; Kent, Netsell, & Bauer, 1975). Unfortunately, due to its reliance on potentially harmful x-rays, cineradiography has fallen out of favor and has little potential for use as a routine clinical tool, especially for child cases. In contrast, ultrasonography involves the transmission of high-frequency sound waves through the body's tissues. Consequently, ultrasound is considered harmless and noninvasive, allowing tongue movement to be investigated for longer periods without harm or discomfort to the client. Unlike other imaging techniques, ultrasound reveals not only the surface displacement but also changes in soft tissue organization within the tongue in both the sagittal and coronal planes (Shawker & Sonies, 1984) and can be used to record lingual movements during production of vowels and most consonants (Stone, 1991).

Limitations with ultrasound include an inability to assess tongue tip movements and to view the movements of other structures (e.g., jaw, lips, etc.) besides the tongue using this technique. In addition, specialist training and some experience in viewing ultrasound scans is required in order to interpret the information provided by these scans accurately. Further, the need to place the ultrasound source below the lower jaw directly under the floor of the mouth may restrict natural jaw movement during speech. Despite these limitations, however, ultrasound has the potential to be a useful clinical tool for client evaluation.

Electropalatography and Related Methods

Electropalatography (EPG) is another technique for examining tongue function, which provides the clinician with information on the location and timing of tongue contacts with the palate during speech. In this technique, the client wears an acrylic palate with an array of contact sensors (varying from 32, 62, or 124) implanted on the surface (Hardcastle, Morgan-Barry, & Clark, 1985) (Figures 3–8a and 3–8b). When contact occurs between the tongue and any of the electrodes, a signal is conducted via lead-out wires to an external processing unit, which then displays the patterns of contact on a computer screen (Figure 3–9).

Traditional two-dimensional EPG is a well-established technique being used in many speech science laboratories and clinics (Hardcastle, 1996) for both the assessment and treatment of speech disordered populations, including individuals with motor speech disorders (Goozée, Murdoch, & Theodoros, 1999; Goozée, Murdoch, Theodoros, & Stokes, 2000; Hartelius, Theodoros, & Murdoch, 2005; McAuliffe, Ward, & Murdoch, 2007; Murdoch, Gardiner, & Theodoros, 2000), structural abnormalities such as cleft palate, hearing impairment, and children with developmental speech disorders (Hardcastle, 1996). Despite this, traditional two-dimensional EPG is limited by the nature of its display. The classic two-dimensional tongue to palate diagrams (see Figure 3–9) that represent the output of the system fail to demonstrate either the unique anatomical characteristics of the individual palates or the relative spacing between the touch sensitive electrodes. Given that it is well accepted that palatal shape varies widely from individual to individual (some individuals have narrow, high-arched palates while others have broad, flat palates) and that shape influences tongue to palate contacts during speech (Hiki & Itoh, 1986), this failure may cause the data derived from traditional two-dimensional EPG to be misinterpreted, especially when comparisons of the amount, location, and pattern of contacts are to be made between different speakers (e.g., narrow, high-arched palates are associated with an increased number of tongue to palate contacts due to closer proximity of the touch-sensitive electrodes).

In an attempt to provide a solution to the limitations of traditional two-dimensional EPG, researchers at the Centre for Neurogenic Communication Disorders Research, The University of Queensland, recently have developed a three-dimensional EPG system aimed at improving graphic representation of tongue to palate contacts by way of computer generated, interactive three-dimensional palatal models (Goozée, McAleer, Scott, & Murdoch, 2003). Although this latter system utilizes the same hardware and artificial acrylic palates as the traditional Reading EPG-3, it provides researchers and clinicians with the ability to visualize three-dimensional images of their client's tongue to palate contacts during speech (Figure 3–10).

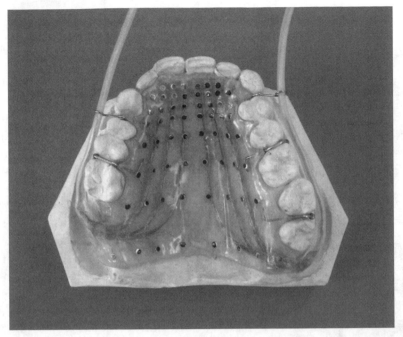

A

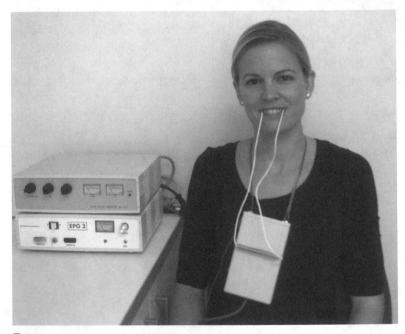

B

Figure 3–8. **A.** Acrylic electropalatography plate with imbedded touch sensors. **B.** Client fitted with an electropalatography plate.

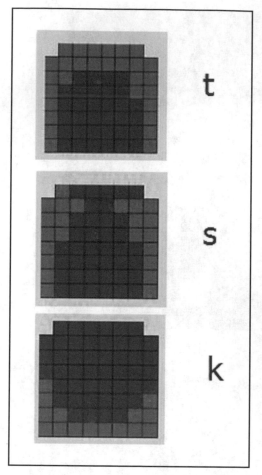

Figure 3–9. Electropalatographic contact pattern representing tongue contact with the palate.

Recently, steps have been taken to extend the capabilities of EPG to dynamic pressure sensing (Murdoch, Goozée, Veidt, Scott, & Meyers, 2004). A device that records the spatial, timing, and pressure features of tongue contacts against the hard palate during speech has the potential to extend the capabilities of researchers and clinicians in determining the physiological bases of tongue dysfunction in a variety of speech disorders. The prototype pressure-sensing palatograph (PPG) developed by Murdoch et al. (2004) has been reported to be capable of recording dynamic tongue to palate pressures during a variety of speech tasks. This tool has the potential to be a useful addition to the battery of instruments available to assess tongue function during speech in both normal and dysarthric speakers.

Electromagnetic Articulography

In recent years, the development and introduction of a technique called electromagnetic articulography (EMA) has provided a safe, noninvasive assessment

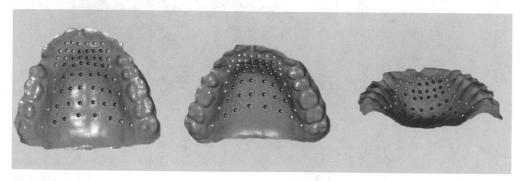

Figure 3–10. Three-dimensional electropalatography plate.

tool with which the dynamic aspects of articulatory dysfunction in various neurological speech disorders may be investigated. Importantly, the EMA technique does not require the use of ionizing radiation. Rather the EMA system tracks articulatory movements during speech using weak alternating electromagnetic fields. Transmitter coils, housed in a plastic helmet or cube and positioned around the head, generate alternating magnetic fields at different frequencies, which in turn induce alternating signals in small receiver coils temporarily glued to the tongue, upper and lower lip, and jaw. The position of the receiver coils in relation to the transmitter coils is sampled over time and plotted on a computer, providing a visual representation of articulator movements in real time. From this data, quantitive kinematic parameters can be derived including the velocity, acceleration, distance, and duration of movements of the lips, tongue, and jaw during speech production.

The first commercially available EMA system, the AG100 was developed by Carstens Medizinelektronik in Germany in 1988. Since that time, an upgraded EMA, the AG200 also has been released. In both the AG100 and AG200 EMA systems, the transmitter coils are housed in a helmet that fits around the client's head with the coils positioned in the midsaggital plane (Figure 3–11). Both of these systems plot movement of the articulators in two dimensions in the

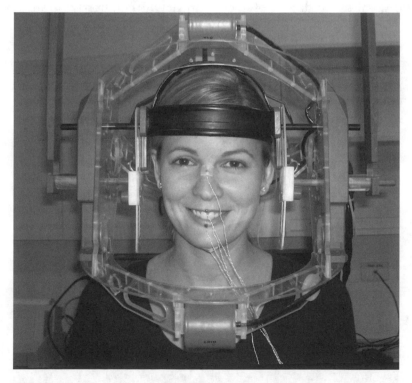

Figure 3–11. Client fitted with AG200 system.

midsaggital plane only. To date the two-dimensional EMA systems have been used to study articulatory kinematics in a range of normal and disorders speakers including children (Murdoch & Goozée, 2003), adults (Kuruvilla, Murdoch, & Goozée, 2007) with dysarthria subsequent to traumatic brain injury, adults with dysarthria poststroke (Chen, Murdoch, & Goozée, 2008), adults with apraxia of speech (Bartle-Meyer, Goozée, & Murdoch, 2009), and speech disordered children exhibiting differentiated and undifferentiated lingual gestures (Goozée, Murdoch, Ozanne, Cheng, Hill, & Gibbon, 2007).

Despite the ability of the AG100 and AG200 EMA systems to identify aberrant articulatory kinematics in speakers with motor speech disorders associated with a variety of neurological conditions, the greatest limitation of these systems is their restriction to tracing movements in the midsagittal plane. A major consequence of this limitation is that these EMA systems are not able to monitor substantial lateral deviations of the tongue and jaw from the midline (e.g., as occurs in flaccid dysarthria associated with unilateral lesioning of the XIIth cranial nerve) with error. To overcome this limitation, Carstens Medizinelektronik more recently has developed the AG500 EMA, which is capable of tracking articulatory movements in three dimensions. The AG500 EMA involves six transmitter coils housed within a plastic box-like helmet (Figure 3–12). Importantly, unlike the earlier EMA systems, the AG500 helmet does not restrict movement of the individual undergoing assessment, which facilitates the use of the instrument with children (who are more prone

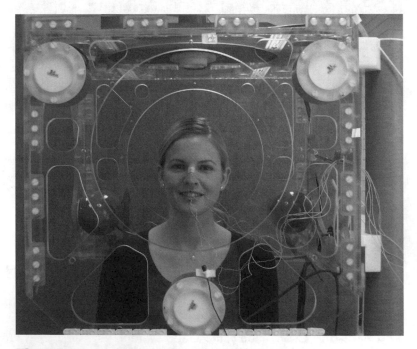

Figure 3–12. Client fitted with AG500 system.

to movement than adults) and persons with movement disorders (e.g., Parkinson's disease, Huntington's disease, etc.). Importantly, the AG500 EMA system allows not only full spatial recording of sensor movement, but also measurement of the sensor orientation. Consequently, unlike earlier EMA systems, lateral tongue and jaw movements provide a source of information rather than error. Given that the AG500 can track articulatory movements in three dimensions raises the possibility that movement signals (e.g., tongue movement) acquired by the AG500 may be able to be translated into visual representations (e.g., of tongue movement) that could be utilized in biofeedback therapy for the treatment of a range of articulatory disorders.

Summary

Although instrumentation has opened a whole new range of assessment techniques, physiological data should be integrated with data from other appraisal procedures (i.e., combine information from perceptual, physiological, and acoustic information) to ensure that an accurate diagnosis is made and that the subsequent remediation techniques are appropriate. In particular, the limitations of each of the instrumental procedures need to be kept in mind when making clinical decisions based on their findings. Despite the wide variety of objective instrumental measures available for documenting the physiology of speech production, to date, the clinical application of these techniques has been limited. Increasing the use of instrumentation in the clinical setting, for the purposes of both assessment and treatment, will require the implementation of training programs for the clinicians as well as an increase in clinical research projects designed to demonstrate the clinical utility of instrumental techniques and to validate the role of instrumentation in the management of neurological speech disorders.

Considering that it is accepted that the long-term advancement of intervention in dysarthria depends on the reliability and validity of assessments revealing the underlying motor pathophysiology of the disorder, investigation and the refinement of instrumental assessment techniques must, therefore, be a continuous process. The ultimate goal is to determine which tasks, and which types of instrumentation, provide the most salient data for each of the neurological groups. One important aspect of this process will be the generation of appropriate normative data for men, women, and children that can serve as a referent for the identification and interpretation of abnormal values. Currently, although normative data is available for some instruments (e.g., nasometer), it is not yet available for by far the majority of instruments described previously. When this information is available, the refinement of differential diagnosis and development of more effective treatment programs based on instrumental procedures will be possible.

References

Abbs, J. H. (1973). The influence of the gamma motor system on jaw movement during speech: A theoretical framework and some preliminary observations. *Journal of Speech and Hearing Research, 16,* 175–200.

Abbs, J. H., & De Paul, R. (1989). Assessment of dysarthria: The critical prerequisite to treatment. In M.M. Leahy (Ed.), *Disorders of communication: The science of intervention* (pp. 206–227). London, UK: Taylor and Francis.

Abbs, J. H., Folkins, J. W., & Sivarajan, M. (1976). Motor impairment following blockade of the infraorbital nerve. *Journal of Speech and Hearing Research, 19,* 19–35.

Abbs, J. H., & Netsell, R. W. (1973). An interpretation of jaw acceleration during speech. *Journal of Speech and Hearing Research, 16,* 421–425.

Amerman, J. D. (1993). A maximum-force-dependant protocol for assessing labial force control. *Journal of Speech and Hearing Research, 36,* 460–465.

Andreassen, M. L., Smith, B. E., & Guyette, T. W. (1992). Pressure-flow measurements for selected oral and nasal sound segments produced by normal adults. *Cleft Palate-Craniofacial Journal, 29*(1), 1–9.

Barlow, S. M., & Abbs, J. H. (1983). Force Transducers for the evaluation of labial, lingual, and mandibular motor impairments. *Journal of Speech and Hearing Research, 26,* 616–621.

Barlow, S. M., & Abbs, J. H. (1984). Orofacial fine motor control impairments in congenital spasticity: Evidence against hypertonus-related performance deficits. *Neurology, 34,* 145–150.

Barlow, S. M., & Abbs, J. H. (1986). Fine force and position control of select orofacial structures in the upper motor neurone syndrome. *Experimental Neurology, 94,* 699–713.

Barlow, S. M., & Burton, M. (1988). Orofacial force control impairments in brain-injured adults. *Association for Research in Otolaryngology Abstracts, 11,* 218.

Barlow, S. M., Cole, K. J., & Abbs, J. H. (1983). A new head-mounted lip-jaw movement transduction system for the study of motor speech disorders. *Journal of Speech and Hearing Disorders, 26,* 283–288.

Barlow, S. M., & Netsell, R. (1986). Differential fine force control of the upper and lower lips. *Journal of Speech and Hearing Research, 29,* 163–169.

Bartle-Meyer, C. J., Goozée, J. V., & Murdoch, B. E. (2009). Kinematic investigation of lingual movements in words of increasing length in acquired apraxia of speech. *Clinical Linguistics and Phonetics, 23,* 93–124.

Boemke, W., Gerull, G., & Hippel, K. (1992). Zur Elektromyographie des larynx mit hautoberflachenelektroden. *Folia Phoniatrica, 44,* 220–230.

Bolick, C. A., Hixon, T., Watson, P., & Jones, P. (2004). *Refinement of speech breathing in normal young children.* Paper presented at the bi-annual Conference on Motor Speech: Speech Motor Control. Albuquerque, NM.

Cahill, L., Murdoch, B. E., & Theodoros, D. G. (2001). Velopharyngeal function following severe traumatic brain injury in childhood: A physiological and perceptual analysis. *Asia Pacific Journal of Speech, Language and Hearing, 6,* 33–38.

Cahill, L., Murdoch, B. E., & Theodoros, D. G. (2003). Perceptual and instrumental analysis of laryngeal function following traumatic brain injury in childhood. *Journal of Head Trauma Rehabilitation, 18,* 268–283.

Cahill, L., Theodoros, D. G., Murdoch, B. E., & MacMillan, J. (2003). Physiological features of dysarthria in Friedreich's ataxia. *Asia Pacific Journal of Speech, Language and Hearing, 8,* 221–228.

Chen, Y. T., Murdoch, B. E., & Goozée, J. V. (2008). Electromagnetic articulographic assessment of tongue function in dysarthric and non-dysarthric speakers following stroke. *Journal of Medical Speech-Language Pathology, 16,* 22–32.

Dalston, R. M., & Seaver, E. J. (1992). Relative values of various standardized passages in the nasometric assessment of patients with velopharyngeal impairment. *Cleft Palate-Craniofacial Journal, 29*(1), 17–21.

Dalston, R. M., & Warren, D. W. (1986). Comparisons of Tonar II, pressure flow, and listener judgements of hypernasality in the assessment of velopharyngeal function. *Cleft Palate Journal, 32*(2), 108–115.

Dalston, R. M., Warren, D. W., & Smith, L. R. (1990). The aerodynamic characteristics of speech produced by normal speakers and cleft palate speakers with adequate velopharyngeal function. *Cleft Palate Journal, 27*(4), 393–401.

Darley, F. L., Aronson, A. E., & Brown, J. R. (1975). *Motor speech disorders.* Philadelphia, PA: W. B. Saunders.

Eysholdt, U., Tigges, M., Wittenberg, T., & Proschel, U. (1996). Direct evaluation of high-speed recordings of vocal fold vibrations. *Folia Phoniatrica et Logopaedica, 48,* 163–170.

Folkins, J. W., & Abbs, J. H. (1976). Additional observations on responses to resistive loading of the jaw. *Journal of Speech and Hearing Research, 19,* 820–821.

Folkins, J. W., & Kuehn, D. P. (1982). Speech Production. In N. J. Lass, L. V. McReynolds, J. L. Northern, & D. E. Yoder (Eds.), *Speech, language and hearing* (Vol. 1, 246–285). Philadelphia, PA: W. B. Saunders.

Forrest, K., & Weismer, G. (1995). Dynamic aspects of lower lip movement in Parkinsonian and neurologically normal geriatric speakers' production of stress. *Journal of Speech and Hearing Research, 38,* 260–272.

Forrest, K., & Weismer, G. (2009). Acoustic analysis of motor speech disorders. In M.R. McNeil (Ed.), *Clinical Management of sensorimotor speech disorders* (pp. 46–63). New York, NY: Thieme.

Frokjaer-Jensen, B. (1992). Data on air pressure, mean flow rate, glottal input and output energy, aerodynamic resistance, and glottal efficiency for normal and healthy voices. A preliminary study. *XXIInd World Congress of International Association of Logapedics and Phoniatrics.* Hanover, Germany.

Gall, V. (1984). Strip kymography of the glottis. *Archives of Otorhinolaryngology, 240,* 287–293.

Goozée, J. V., McAleer, T., Scott, D. H., & Murdoch, B. E. (2003). 3-D laser scanning of EPG palates: Benefits of using a 3-D EPG model in the analysis of tongue-to-palate contacts. *Proceedings of the 15th International Congress of Phonetic Sciences,* Barcelona, Spain.

Goozée, J. V., Murdoch, B. E., Ozanne, A. E., Cheng, Y., Hill, A., & Gibbon, F. (2007). Lingual kinematics and coordination in speech-disordered children exhibiting differentiated versus undifferentiated lingual gestures. *International Journal of Language & Communication Disorders, 42,* 703–724.

Goozée, J. V., Murdoch, B. E., & Theodoros, D. G. (1999). Electropalatographic assessment of articulatory timing characteristics in dysarthria following traumatic brain injury. *Journal of Medical Speech-Language Pathology, 7,* 209–222.

Goozée, J. V., Murdoch, B. E., Theodoros, D. G., & Stokes, P. D. (2000). Kinematic analysis of tongue movements in dysarthria following traumatic brain injury using electromagnetic articulography. *Brain Injury, 14,* 153–174.

Hardcastle, W. J. (1996). Current developments in instrumentation for studying supraglottal structures. In M. J. Ball & M. Duckworth (Eds.), *Advances in clinical phonetics* (pp. 27–49). Amsterdam: John Benjamins.

Hardcastle, W. J., Morgan-Barry, R. A., & Clark, C. J. (1985). Articulatory and voicing characteristics of adult dysarthric and verbal dyspraxic speakers: An instrumental study. *British Journal of Disorders of Communication, 20,* 249–270.

Hardy, J. C. (1967). Suggestions for physiological research in dysarthria. *Cortex, 3,* 128–156.

Hartelius, L., Theodoros, D. G., & Murdoch, B. E. (2005). Use of electropalatography in the treatment of disordered articulation following traumatic brain injury: A case study. *Journal of Medical Speech-Language Pathology, 13*, 189–204.

Hartmann, E., & von Cramon, D. (1984). Acoustic measurement of voice quality in central dysphonia. *Journal of Communication Disorders, 17*, 425–440.

Herman, G. (1989). MacADIOS and Mac-Speech Lab as instructional tools. *CUSH: Journal for Computer Users in Speech and Hearing, 5*(2), 62–72.

Hess, M. M. & Gross, M. (1993). High-speed, light-intensified digital imaging of vocal fold vibrations in high optical resolution via indirect microlaryngoscopy. *Annals of Otorhinolarygology, 102*, 502–507.

Hiki, S., & Itoh, H. (1986). Influence of palate shape on lingual articulation. *Speech Communication, 5*, 141–158.

Hillenbrand, J., Cleveland, R. A., & Erickson, R. L. (1994). Acoustic correlates of breathy vocal quality. *Journal of Speech and Hearing Research, 37*, 769–778.

Hinton, V. A., & Luschei, E. S. (1992). Validation of a modern miniature transducer for measurement of interlabial contact pressures during speech. *Journal of Speech and Hearing Research, 35*, 245–251.

Hirano, M., & Ohala, J. (1969). Use of hooked-wire electrodes for electromyography of the intrinsic laryngeal muscles. *Journal of Speech and Hearing Research, 12*, 362–373.

Hixon, T. J., Goldman, M., & Mead, J. (1973). Kinematics of the chest wall during speech production: Volume displacements of the rib cage, abdomen, and lung. *Journal of Speech and Hearing Research, 16*, 78–115.

Hixon, T. J., Putnam, A. H., & Sharp, J. T. (1983). Speech production with flaccid paralysis of the rib cage, diaphragm and abdomen. *Journal of Speech and Hearing Disorders, 48*, 315–327.

Hodge, M. M., & Putnam-Rochet, A. (1989). Characteristics of speech breathing in young women. *Journal of Speech and Hearing Research, 32*, 466–480.

Hoit, J. D., Banzett, R. B., Brown, R., & Loring, S. H. (1990). Speech breathing in individuals with cervical spinal cord injury. *Journal of Speech and Hearing Research, 33*, 798–807.

Hoit, J. D., & Hixon, T. J. (1986). Body type and speech breathing. *Journal of Speech and Hearing Research, 29*, 313–324.

Hoit, J. D., & Hixon, T. J. (1987). Age and speech breathing. *Journal of Speech and Hearing Research, 30*, 351–366.

Hoit, J. D. & Hixon, T. J. (1992). Age and laryngeal airway resistance during vowel production in women. *Journal of Speech and Hearing Research, 35*, 309–313.

Hoit, J. D., Hixon, T. J., Altman, M. E., & Morgan, W. J. (1989). Speech breathing in women. *Journal of Speech and Hearing Research, 32*, 353–365.

Hoit, J. D., Hixon, T. J., Watson, P. J., & Morgan, W. J. (1990). Speech breathing in children and adolescents. *Journal of Speech and Hearing Research, 33*, 51–69.

Hoit, J. D., Watson, P. J., Hixon, K. E., McMahon, P., & Johnson, C. L. (1994). Age and velopharyngeal function during speech production. *Journal of Speech and Hearing Research, 37*, 295–302.

Horii, Y. (1980). An accelerometric approach to nasality measurement: A preliminary report. *Cleft Palate Journal, 17*, 254–261.

Horii, Y. (1983). An accelerometric measure as a physical correlate of perceived hypernasality in speech. *Journal of Speech and Hearing Research, 26*, 476–480.

Horii, Y., & Cooke, P. A. (1978). Some airflow, volume, and duration characteristics of oral reading. *Journal of Speech and Hearing Research, 21*, 470–481.

Hutters, B., & Brondsted, K. (1992). A simple nasal anemometer for clinical purposes. *European Journal of Disorders of Communication, 27*(2), 101–119.

Karnell, M. P., Linville, R. N., & Edwards, B. A. (1988). Variations in velar position over time: A nasal videoendoscopic study. *Journal of Speech and Hearing Research, 31*, 417–424.

Karnell, M. P., Seaver, E. J., & Dalston, R. M. (1988). A comparison of the photodetector and endoscopic evaluations of velopharyngeal function. *Journal of Speech and Hearing Research, 31,* 503–510.

Kent, J. F., Kent, R. D., Rosenbek, J. C., Weismer, G., Martin, R., Sufit, R., & Brooks, B. R. (1992). Quantitative description of the dysarthria in women with amyotrophic lateral sclerosis. *Journal of Speech and Hearing Research, 35,* 723–733.

Kent, R., & Kim, Y-J. (2003). Toward an acoustic typology of motor speech disorders. *Clinical Linguistics & Phonetics, 17,* 227–245.

Kent, R., & Read, C. (2002). *The acoustic analysis of speech.* San Diego, CA: Singular.

Kent, R., Netsell, R., & Bauer, L. L. (1975). Cineradiographic assessment of articulatory mobility in the dysarthrias. *Journal of Speech and Hearing Disorders, 40,* 467–480.

Kuruvilla, M., Murdoch, B. E., & Goozée, J. V. (2007). Electromagnetic articulography assessment of articulatory function in adults with dysarthria following traumatic brain injury. *Brain Injury, 21,* 601–613.

Lane, H., Perkell, J., Svirsky, M., & Webster, J. (1991). Changes in speech breathing following cochlear implant in postlingually deafened adults. *Journal of Speech and Hearing Research, 34,* 526–533.

Langmore, S. E. & Lehman, M. E. (1994). Physiologic deficits in the orofacial system underlying dysarthria in amyotrophic lateral sclerosis. *Journal of Speech and Hearing Research, 37,* 28–37.

Lock, R. B., & Seaver, E. J. (1984). Nasality and velopharyngeal function in five hearing impaired adults. *Journal of Communication Disorders, 17,* 47–64.

Luschei, E.S., & Finnegan, E.M. (2009). Electromyographic techniques for the assessment of motor speech disorders. In M. R. McNeil (Ed.), *Clinical management of sensorimotor speech disorders* (pp. 100–115). New York, NY: Thieme.

Manifold, J. A. Y., & Murdoch, B. E. (1993). Speech breathing in young adults: Effect of body type. *Journal of Speech and Hearing Research, 36,* 657–671.

Mann, V. (1987). Review of DSPS realtime signal lab by Robert Morris. *ASHA, 29,* 64–65.

McAuliffe, M. J., Ward, E. C., & Murdoch, B. E., (2007). Intra-participant variability in Parkinson's disease: An encephalographic examination of articulation. *Advances in Speech Language Pathology, 9,* 13–19.

McClean, M. (1991). Lip muscle EMG responses to oral pressure stimulation. *Journal of Speech and Hearing Research, 34,* 248–251.

McFarland, D. H., & Smith, A. (1992). Effects of vocal task and respiratory phase on prephonatory chest wall movements. *Journal of Speech and Hearing Research, 35,* 971–982.

McHenry, M. A., Minton, J. T., & Wilson, R. L. (1994). Increasing the efficiency of articulatory force testing of adults with traumatic brain injury. In J. A. Till, K. M. Yorkston, & D. R. Beukelman (Eds.), *Motor speech disorders: Advances in assessment and treatment* (pp. 135–146). Baltimore, MD: Paul H. Brooks.

McHenry, M. A., Minton, J. T., Wilson, R. L., & Post, Y. V. (1994). Intelligibility and non-speech orofacial strength and force control following traumatic brain injury. *Journal of Speech and Hearing Research, 37,* 1271–1283.

McNeil, M. R., Weismer, G., Adams, S., & Mulligan, M. (1990). Oral structure non-speech motor control in normal, dysarthric, aphasic and apraxic speakers: Isometric force and static position control. *Journal of Speech and Hearing Research, 33,* 255–268.

Miller, C. J., & Daniloff, R. (1993). Airflow measurements: Theory and utility of findings. *Journal of Voice, 7*(1), 38–46.

Milutinovic, Z., Lastovka, M., Vohradnik, M., & Janosevic, S. (1988). EMG study of hyperkinetic phonation using surface electrodes. *Folia Phoniatrica, 40,* 21–30.

Moore, C. A., Smith, A., & Ringel, R. L. (1988). Task specific organization of activity in human jaw muscles. *Journal of Speech and Hearing Research, 31,* 670–680.

Motta, G., Cesari, U., Iengo, M., & Motta, G. (1990). Clinical application of electroglottography. *Folia Phoniatrica, 42,* 111–117.

Murdoch, B. E. (1996). Physiological rehabilitation of disordered speech following closed head injury. In B. P. Uzzell & H. H. Stonnington (Eds.), *Recovery after traumatic brain injury* (pp. 163–184). Mahwah, NJ: Lawrence Erlbaum.

Murdoch, B. E., Chenery, H. J., Bowler, S., & Ingram J. C. (1989a). Respiratory function in Parkinson's subjects exhibiting a perceptible speech deficit: A kinematic and spirometric analysis. *Journal of Speech and Hearing Disorders, 54,* 610–626.

Murdoch, B. E., Chenery, H. J., Stokes, P. D., & Hardcastle, W. J. (1991). Respiratory kinematics in speakers with cerebellar disease. *Journal of Speech and Hearing Research, 34,* 768–780.

Murdoch, B. E., Gardiner, F., & Theodoros, D. G. (2000). Electropalatographic assessment of articulatory dysfunction in multiple sclerosis: A case study. *Journal of Medical Speech-Language Pathology, 8,* 359–364.

Murdoch, B. E., & Goozée, J. V. (2003). EMA analysis of tongue function in children with dysarthria following traumatic brain injury. *Brain Injury, 17,* 79–93.

Murdoch, B. E., Goozée, J. V., Veidt, M., Scott, D., & Meyers, I. A. (2004). Introducing the pressure-sensing palatograph: The next frontier in electropalatography. *Clinical Linguistics & Phonetics, 18,* 433–445.

Murdoch, B. E., Manning, C. Y., Theodoros, D. G., & Thompson, E. C. (1997). Laryngeal and phonatory dysfunction in Parkinson's disease. *Clinical Linguistics & Phonetics, 11,* 245–266.

Murdoch, B. E., Noble, J., Chenery, H., & Ingram, J. (1989b). A spirometric and kinematic analysis of respiratory function in pseudobulbar palsy. *Australian Journal of Human Communication Disorders, 17,* 21–35.

Murdoch, B. E., Pitt, G., Theodoros, D. G., & Ward, E. C. (1999). Real-time visual biofeedback in the treatment of speech breathing disorders following childhood traumatic brain injury: Report of one case. *Pediatric Rehabilitation, 3,* 5–20.

Murdoch, B. E., Spenser, T., Theodoros, D. G., & Thompson, E. C. (1998). Lip and tongue function in multiple sclerosis: a physiological analysis. *Motor Control, 2,* 148–160.

Murdoch, B. E., Theodoros, D. G., Stokes, P. D., and Chenery, H. J. (1993). Abnormal patterns of speech breathing in dysarthric speakers following severe closed head injury. *Brain Injury, 7*(4), 295–308.

Murdoch, B. E., & Thompson, E. C., & Stokes, P. D. (1994). Phonatory and laryngeal dysfunction following upper motor neurone vascular lesions. *Journal of Medical Speech-Language Pathology, 2*(3), 177–189.

Nellis, J. L., Neihman, G. S., & Lehman, J. A. (1992). Comparison of nasometer and listener judgements of nasality in the assessment of velopharyngeal function after pharyngeal flap surgery. *Cleft Palate-Craniofacial Journal, 29*(2), 157–163.

Netsell, R. (1986). *A neurologic view of the dysarthrias.* San Diego, CA: College-Hill Press.

Netsell, R., & Hixon, T. J. (1978). A noninvasive method for clinically estimating subglottal air pressure. *Journal of Speech and Hearing Disorders, 63,* 326–330.

Netsell, R., Lotz, W. K., DuChane, A. S., & Barlow, S. M. (1991). Vocal tract aerodynamics during syllable productions: Normative data and theoretical implications. *Journal of Voice, 5,* 1–9.

Niimi, S., Bell-Berti, F., & Harris, K. S. (1982). Dynamic aspects of velopharyngeal closure. *Folia Phoniatrica, 34,* 246–257.

Putnam, A. H. B., & Hixon, T. J. (1984). Respiratory kinematics in speakers with motor neurone disease. In M. R. McNeil, J. C. Rosenbek, & A. E. Aronson (Eds.), *The dysarthrias: Physiology, acoustics, perception, management* (pp. 37–67). San Diego, CA: College-Hill Press.

Read, C., Buder, E., & Kent, R. D. (1990). Speech analysis systems: A survey. *Journal of Speech and Hearing Research, 33,* 363–374.

Read, C., Buder, E., & Kent, R. D. (1992). Speech analysis systems: An evaluation. *Journal of Speech and Hearing Research, 35,* 314–332.

Reich, A. R., & McHenry, M. A. (1990). Estimating respiratory volumes from rib cage and abdominal displacements during ventilatory and speech activities. *Journal of Speech and Hearing Research, 33,* 467–475.

Reinhardt, J. H., Hawkshaw, M. J., & Sataloff, R. T. (2005). The clinical voice laboratory. In R. T. Sataloff (Ed.), *Clinical assessment of voice* (pp. 33–71). San Diego, CA: Plural.

Robin, D. A., Goel, A., Somodi, L. B., & Luschei, E. S. (1992). Tongue strength and endurance: Relation to highly skilled movements. *Journal of Speech and Hearing Research, 35,* 1239–1245.

Robin, D. A., Somodi, L. B., & Luschei, E. S. (1991). Measurement of strength and endurance in normal and articulation disordered subjects. In C. A. Moore, K. M. Yorkston, & D. R. Beukelman (Eds.), *Dysarthria and apraxia of speech: Perspectives on management* (pp. 173–184). Baltimore, MD: Paul H. Brooks.

Ryalls, J., & Baum, S. (1990). Review of three software systems for speech analysis: CSpeech, Bliss, and CSRE. *Journal of Speech-Language Pathology & Audiology, 13,* 59–60.

Scherer, R. C., Gould, W. J., Titze, I. R., Meyers, A. D., & Sataloff, R. T. (1988). Preliminary evaluation of selected acoustic and glottographic measures for clinical phonatory function analysis. *Journal of Voice, 2*(3), 230–244.

Shaiman, S. (1989). Kinematic and electromyographic responses to perturbation of the jaw. *Journal of the Acoustical Society of America, 86*(1), 78–88.

Shawker, T. H., & Sonies, B. C. (1984). Tongue movement during speech: A real-time ultrasound evaluation. *Journal of Clinical Ultrasound, 12,* 125–133.

Shipp, T., Izdebski, K., Reed, C., & Morrissey, P. (1985). Intrinsic laryngeal muscle activity in a spastic dysphonia patient. *Journal of Speech and Hearing Disorders, 50,* 54–59.

Smitheran, J. R., & Hixon, T. J. (1981). A clinical method for estimating laryngeal airway resistance during vowel production. *Journal of Speech and Hearing Disorders, 46,* 138–146.

Solomon, N., & Hixon, T. (1993). Speech breathing in Parkinson's disease. *Journal of Speech and Hearing Research, 36,* 294–310.

Sperry, E. E., & Klich, R. J. (1992). Speech breathing in senescent and younger women during oral reading. *Journal of Speech and Hearing Research, 36,* 1246–1255.

Stathopoulos, E. T., Hoit, J. D., Hixon, T. J., Watson, P. J., & Solomon, N. P. (1991). Respiratory and laryngeal function during whispering. *Journal of Speech and Hearing Research, 34,* 761–767.

Stathopoulos, E. T., & Sapienza, C. (1993). Respiratory and laryngeal function of women and men during vocal intensity variation. *Journal of Speech and Hearing Research, 36,* 64–75.

Stevens, K. N., Kalikow, D. N., & Willemain T. R. (1975). A miniature accelerometer for detecting glottal waveforms and nasalization. *Journal of Speech and Hearing Research, 18,* 594–599.

Stone, M. (1991). Imaging the tongue and vocal tract. *British Journal of Disorders of Communication, 26,* 11–23.

Svec, J. G., & Schutte, H. K. (1996). Videokymography: High speed line canning of vocal fold vibration. *Journal of Voice, 10,* 201–205.

Theodoros, D. G., & Murdoch, B. E. (1994). Laryngeal dysfunction in dysarthric speakers following severe closed-head injury. *Brain Injury, 8*(8), 667–684.

Theodoros, D. G., Murdoch, B. E., & Stokes, P. (1995). A physiological analysis of articulatory dysfunction in dysarthric speakers following severe closed head injury. *Brain Injury, 9*(3), 237–254.

Theodoros, D., Murdoch, B. E., Stokes, P. D., & Chenery, H. J. (1993). Hypernasality in dysarthric speakers following severe closed head injury: A perceptual and instrumental analysis. *Brain Injury, 7*, 59–69.

Theodoros, D. G., Murdoch, B. E., & Thompson, E. C. (1995). Hypernasality in Parkinson's disease: A perceptual and physiological analysis. *Journal of Medical Speech-Language Pathology, 3*, 73–84.

Thomas-Stonell, N. (1989). Speechviewer review. *Journal of Speech-Language Pathology & Audiology, 14*, 49–52.

Thompson, E. C., & Murdoch, B. E. (1995). Disorders of nasality in subjects with upper motor neurone type dysarthria following cerebrovascular accident. *Journal of Communication Disorders, 28*, 261–276.

Thompson-Ward, E. C., Theodoros, D. G., Murdoch, B. E., & Cahill, L. (1999). Use of a miniature lip transducer system in the assessment of patients with Parkinson's disease. *Journal of Medical Speech-Language Pathology, 7*, 175–179.

Ward, E. C., Theodoros, D. G., Murdoch, B. E., & Silburn, P. (2000). Changes in maximum capacity tongue pressure in surgical and non-surgical patients with Parkinson's disease following the Lee Silverman Voice Treatment Program. *Journal of Medical Speech-Language Pathology, 8*, 331–335.

Warren, D. W., & Devereux, J. L. (1966). An analog study of cleft palate speech. *Cleft Palate Journal, 3*, 103–114.

Warren, D. W., Morr, K. E., Putnam-Rochet, A., & Dalston, R. M. (1989). Respiratory response to a decrease in velopharyngeal resistance. *Journal of the Acoustical Society of America, 86*(3), 917–924.

Watson, B. C., Schaefer, S. D., Freeman, F. J., Dembowski, J., Kondraske, G., & Roark, R. (1991). Laryngeal electromyographic activity in adductor and abductor spasmodic dysphonia. *Journal of Speech and Hearing Research, 34*, 473–482.

Watterson, T., McFarlane, S. C., & Wright, D. S. (1993). The relationship between nasalance and nasality in children with cleft palate. *Journal of Communication Disorders, 26*, 13–28.

Williams, W. N., & Eisenbach, C. R. (1981). Assessing VP function: The lateral still technique vs. cinefluorography. *Cleft Palate Journal, 18*(1), 45–50.

Winkworth, A. L., Davis, P. J., Adams, R. D., & Ellis, E. (1995). Breathing patterns during spontaneous speech. *Journal of Speech and Hearing Research, 38*, 124–144.

Wood, L. M., Hughes, J., Hayes, K. C., & Wolfe, D. L. (1992). Reliability of labial closure force measurements in normal subjects and patients with CNS disorders. *Journal of Speech and Hearing Research, 35*, 252–258.

Zimmermann, G., Dalston, R. M., Brown, C., Folkins, J. W., Linville, R. N., & Seaver, E. J. (1987). Comparison of cineradiographic and photodetection techniques for assessing velopharyngeal function during speech. *Journal of Speech and Hearing Research, 30*, 564–569.

4

Assessment of Prosody

RUPAL PATEL, PH.D.

Introduction

Prosody is a complex phenomenon that pertains to the stress, intonation, and rhythm of speech. Variations in pitch, loudness, length, and pause can be quantified in term of fundamental frequency (F0), intensity, duration, and silence, respectively, in the acoustic stream (cf. Bolinger, 1989; Lehiste, 1970, 1976; Netsell, 1973). These acoustic cues can be employed individually or in some combination to convey a variety of linguistic and communicative functions such as to signal given versus new information, to distinguish different kinds of speech acts (e.g., questions versus statements), to contrast the meaning of an utterance, and to convey affective state (cf. Bolinger, 1961; Brewster, 1989; Crystal, 1978, 1979; Cutler, Dahan, & van Donselaar, 1997; Shattuck-Hufnagel & Turk, 1996; Williams & Stevens, 1972). While prosody previously had been thought of as merely an overlaid signal on top of the "meaningful" segmental units, the interconnections between prosodic cues and speech segments now are acknowledged widely and prosody is beginning to be viewed as the scaf-folding that binds different levels of phonetic description together.

Prosodic modulation is evident in early communicative gestures, such as infant cries and babbles (Gilbert & Robb, 1996; Kent & Bauer, 1985; Kent & Murray, 1982; Lind & Wermke, 2002, Protopapas & Eimas, 1997; Wermke, Mende, Manfredi, Bruscaglioni, 2002). In fact, over the past few decades, some researchers have suggested that typical development of prosodic control precedes and may facilitate segmental control (Bloom, 1973; Crystal, 1978; Katz, Beach, Jenouri, & Verma, 1996; Mac-Neilage & Davis, 1993; Menyuk & Bernholtz, 1969; Snow 1994). Conversely, breakdowns in prosody can have a significant impact on speech intelligibility and naturalness in both developing and adult populations (cf. Barnes, 1983; Boutsen & Christman 2002; Darley, Aronson, & Brown, 1969; Kent & Rosenbek, 1982; Odell & Shriberg, 2001; Shriberg, Aram, & Kwiatkowski, 1997a, 1997b, 1997c; Yorkston, Beukelman, Minifie, & Sapir, 1984, Yorkston, Beukelman, Strand & Bell, 1999).

It is acknowledged widely that dysprosody is a perceptual hallmark of dysarthria (cf. Darley, Aronson, &

Brown, 1969, 1975; Duffy, 2005; Kent & Rosenbek, 1982; Lowit-Leuschel & Docherty, 2000; Robin, Klouda & Hug, 1991), and apraxia of speech (cf. Boutsen & Christman, 2002; Davis, Jakielski & Marquardt, 1998; Square-Storer, Darley, & Sommers, 1988; McNeil, Robin, & Schmidt, 1997; Odell & Shriberg, 2001; Shriberg et al., 1997a, 1997b, 1997c; Velleman & Shriberg, 1999). Rather than focusing on differences between healthy and impaired speakers, recent work has taken an alternative approach focused on characterizing residual prosodic *control* that can be leveraged to improve intelligibility and overall communicative effectiveness (cf. Patel, 2002, 2003, 2004; Patel & Campellone, 2009; Ramig, Sapir, Fox, & Countryman, 2001; Whitehill, Patel, & Lai, 2008; Yorkston et al., 1984; Yorkston et al., 1999). Thus, a comprehensive understanding of an individual's prosodic abilities *and* impairment is essential to any assessment of motor speech function.

Unlike standardized tests for the assessment of segmental intelligibility in dysarthria (e.g., *Assessment of Intelligibility of Dysarthric Speech*, Yorkston & Beukelman, 1981; Word Intelligibility Test, Kent, Weismer, Kent, & Rosenbek, 1989) and syllable and word error patterns in apraxia of speech (e.g., Kaufman Speech Praxis Test for Children, Kaufman, 1995; *Screening Test for Developmental Apraxia of Speech–Second Edition*, Blakeley, 2000; *ABA-2: Apraxia Battery for Adults–Second Edition*, Dabul, 2000), less agreement exists regarding the stimuli, methods, and dimensions of prosodic assessment. This is due in part to the multidimensional nature of prosody and the variability of its manifestation. For example, the same cues

that are important for linguistic prosody also are used to convey affective and attitudinal states (Bolinger, 1989; Lehiste, 1976; Wymer, Lindman, & Booksh, 2002; Williams & Stevens, 1972). Additionally, individual speakers differ in the set of acoustic cues used to signal prosodic contrasts (see Howell, 1993 and Peppe, Maxim, & Wells, 2000, for examples in healthy speakers and Patel, 2003; Patel & Campellone, 2009; Patel & Salata, 2006; Patel & Watkins, 2007; and Yorkston et al., 1984, for examples of speakers with motor speech impairment). This chapter is aimed at appraising conventional practices of assessing prosody in motor speech disorders in order to pose possible avenues to advance such practices.

Assessment of prosody in motor speech disorders is influenced by the (1) goals/purpose of assessment; (2) prosodic dimensions studied; (3) analysis methods—perceptual, physiological, acoustic, linguistic, and so on; and (4) stimuli and task variables—word versus phrase production, read versus conversational speech, imitation versus spontaneous speech, and so on. Each of these factors is explored in further detail in the subsequent sections.

Hallmarks of Dysprosody in Motor Speech Disorders

Prosodic control in dysarthria typically has been characterized in terms of reduced precision and flexibility compared to nonimpaired speech. Slowed or abnormally accelerated rate, monopitch, monoloudness, reduced ability to vary stress within words and sentences, and poor phrasing are among the prosodic traits of various dysarthrias (cf. Barnes, 1983; Canter, 1963; Darley, et al., 1969, 1975; Duffy, 2005; Kent & Rosenbek, 1982; Rosenbek & LaPointe, 1985; Yorkston et al., 1984). Prosodic errors also are prevalent in apraxia of speech with slow rate, equal and excess stress, silent pauses at initiation of words or between syllables, reduced variation in F0 and loudness, and difficulty signaling lexical and emphatic stress (Shriberg et al., 1997a, 1997b, 1997c; Wertz, LaPointe, & Rosenbek, 1991). Note that these prosodic disturbances may reflect the motor deficit itself as well as, or in addition to, the impact of compensation (Wertz et al., 1991).

Purposes of Assessing Prosody

Examination of prosodic deficits can serve several purposes including assisting in differential diagnosis, specifying severity, and determining the need and focus of treatment. The clinician's motivations play a critical role in choosing tasks and the methods of analysis. If the primary goal is differential diagnosis, the clinician may select stimuli and tasks that highlight the difference between speakers with dysarthria and those with apraxia of speech. For example, emphatic stress may help differentiate childhood apraxia of speech from dysarthria (Shriberg, Kwiatkowski & Rasmussen, 1990).

Alternatively, if the goal of examination is to characterize the type and degree of impairment, a variety of tasks may be chosen. In order to assess severity of dysfunction, it would be helpful

to have comparative norms. Unlike well-established norms for acquisition of segmental control and the vast literature on the acoustic patterns of speech sounds (see Kent, 1997; Kent & Read, 2002; Creaghead, Newman, & Secord, 1989), developmental norms of prosodic control are lacking, and the acoustic fingerprints of prosodic contrasts are heavily debated. For example, although F0 is thought to be the primary cue for signaling questions versus statements and contrastive stress, some have argued that duration and/or intensity cues are at least as salient (Cooper, Eady, & Mueller, 1985; Eady & Cooper, 1986; Fry, 1955, 1958; Huss, 1978; Sluijter & van Heuven, 1996a, 1996b).

A thorough assessment of prosodic function also can be used to determine the need and focus of intervention. Although prosody traditionally has been thought of as the "icing on the cake," something to address when all the segmental elements are in order, mounting evidence demonstrates that establishing appropriate prosody may facilitate accurate segmental control and improve speech naturalness (Bellaire, Yorkston, & Beukelman, 1986; Hartelius, Wising & Nord, 1997; LeDorze, Dionne, Ryalls, Julien, & Quellet, 1992; Patel & Campellone, 2009; Yorkston, Beukelman, & Bell, 1988; Yorkston et al., 1999). Melodic Intonation Therapy is a treatment approach that incorporates prosody and leverages it to improve intelligibility in individuals with apraxia of speech (Helm-Estabrooks, Nicholas, & Morgan, 1989; Schlaug, Marchina, & Norton, 2008).

Lacking from most clinical protocols is the goal of assessing residual function in order to document *ability*. Understanding how speakers with motor speech impairment signal prosodic contrasts can inform treatments targeted at the speaker as well as at the listener. Even when acoustic patterns differ from healthy speakers, it may be possible to shape the speaker's behavior to be optimally contrastive (Patel & Campellone, 2009; Patel & Salata, 2006, Whitehill, Patel, & Lai, 2008; Yorkston et al., 1984).

What to Assess

Although prosodic impairments in motor speech disorders have been documented as far back as the 1600s (see Duffy, 2007, for a historical overview of motor speech disorders), systematic description of prosodic deficits were initially posited by Darley et al. (1969, 1975) in their seminal work on dysarthria. Among the 38 dimensions of speech and voice analysis undertaken by Darley et al. (1969, 1975) four pertained to pitch, five to loudness, and ten to prosody. Each dimension was rated on a 7-point scale with 1 representing normal and 7 representing severe deviation from normal. Perceptual judgments were based on short speech samples (approximately 30 seconds) of either read ("Grandfather" passage) or conversational speech. In the initial set of 212 patients, Darley et al. (1969, 1975) noted two main clusters of prosodic impairment: (1) prosodic excess, which included prolonged intervals, excess and equal stress, prolonged phonemes and slow rate; and (2) prosodic insufficiency that included monopitch, monoloudness, and reduced stress. Additionally, they noted that some deviant prosodic dimensions co-occurred across dysarthria subtypes and etiologies.

In what has come to be known as the "Mayo protocol," Darley et al.'s, (1969, 1975) prosodic dimensions have been classified into five broad categories: pitch, loudness, rate, phrasing, and stress (Duffy, 2005). This taxonomy also is used to assess prosodic function in apraxia of speech (Prosody-Voice Screening Profile (PVSP), Shriberg, et al., 1990). Given that prosody largely is the result of respiratory and phonatory behaviors, considerable overlap exists in the tasks and functions assessed across subsystems of speech production. Thus, aspects of breath support and phrasing that traditionally are classified as respiratory functions (Weismer, 2007) also have direct impact on prosody. Similarly, considerable overlap exists between voicing characteristics and prosody. For example, level and variation of pitch and loudness are cited by Buder (2007) in his recent review of assessment of voice production in motor speech disorders.

How to Assess Prosody

Perceptual Analysis

As with any aspect of motor speech assessment, auditory-perceptual judgments of prosody are held as the gold standard. In fact, Duffy (2005, 2007) argues that acoustic and/or physiological abnormalities in the absence of deviant perceptual features are insufficient to warrant diagnosis and treatment.

Commonly used assessment protocols such as the Mayo Protocol and standardized tests of motor speech impairment assess only a subset of the prosodic dimensions described previously. In the Mayo approach, deviant speech characteristics are rated on a five-point scale (0 = normal, 1 = mild, 2 = moderate, 3 = marked, and 4 = severely deviant) and pitch and loudness level also are marked to indicate excessively high or low values (Duffy, 2005). Although the rating scale is straightforward, the relative nature of the judgments requires considerable experience with patients with motor speech impairment in order to differentiate between disorders and dysarthria subtypes.

Given the considerable overlap between dysarthria subtypes along segmental and prosodic dimensions (cf. Chenery, Murdoch & Ingram, 1988; Chenery, Ingram, Murdoch, 1990), several research groups have attempted to alter the rating scale to capture the severity of dysfunction and/or the frequency and type of errors noted along each dimension (Chenery, 1998; Chenery et al., 1988, 1990; FitzGerald, Murdoch, & Chenery, 1987; Ludlow & Bassich, 1983). For example, Ludlow and Bassich (1983) used a 13-point scale to judge pitch level, loudness level, and overall rate in which 7 represented normal or expected level, 1 represented extreme low measures (too low, too soft), and 13 represented extreme high values (too high or too loud). Results indicated that the altered scale was helpful in differentiating among patients with Parkinson's disease and Shy Drager Syndrome. Similarly, Chenery and Murdoch and colleagues (Chenery, 1998; Chenery et al., 1988, 1990; FitzGerald et al., 1987) found it useful to scale dimensions such as shortness of breath on a scale of 1–4 to indicate severity of dysfunction, presence of glottal fry on a scale of 1–5 to indicate frequency of occurrence, and

pitch on a 7-point scale to categorize it in terms of high, low, or normal.

Standardized assessment batteries of dysarthria (Frenchay Dysarthria Assessment (FDA), Enderby, 1983, and (FDA-2), Enderby & Palmer, 2008; *Dysarthria Examination Battery* (DEB), Drummond, 1993; Dysarthria Profile, Robertson, 1982) include some prosodic tasks but fail to probe across all prosodic dimensions. For example, in the FDA, the main prosodic feature assessed is rate (words/minute), using a spontaneous speech sample. In the Dysarthria Profile, rate and rhythm are assessed while producing months of the year and in short conversation. Additionally, the ability to vary sentence level stress is assessed via imitation of short sentences. In the DEB, read and spontaneous speech samples are used to assess rate, average F0 range, and sentence duration.

In contrast, the Prosody-Voice Screening Protocol (PVSP) Shriberg et al., 1990) consists of a list of 32 prosody-voice codes used to classify utterances with inappropriate prosody or voice. Although some of the dimensions assessed are posited to be diagnostic indicators of apraxia of speech, the protocol also can be used to assess prosody in speakers with dysarthria. The prosodic codes are divided into three broad categories including phrasing, rate, and stress, while voice codes pertain to loudness, pitch, and quality. Phrasing, rate, pitch, and loudness are coded based on a conversational speech sample. Phrasing includes seven codes that consider disruptions of the flow of words or phrase groups. Rate includes four codes that classify speaking rate and pause time as too slow or too fast relative to an appropriate rate of 4–6 syllables/second for adult conversational speech. Pitch and loudness are coded as too high, too low, or appropriate. The ability to imitate lexical and emphatic stress is assessed using perceptual and acoustic measures obtained from a standardized set of words and sentences. The specificity of the coding scheme, the standardization of stimuli used, and the quantitative measures (e.g., Lexical Stress Ratio) used to describe dysfunction make the PVSP a highly sensitive tool for assessing prosodic control in motor speech disorders. Although the protocol requires extensive training and experience, several reports of its use with children and adults have been made (McSweeny & Shriberg, 2001; Odell & Shriberg, 2001).

Assessment of prosody in children with motor speech disorders is particularly difficult given limited age-appropriate standardized tests and stimulus materials. Prosodic assessment in developmental dysarthria relies primarily on nonstandardized protocols such as the Mayo motor speech exam, maximum phonation tasks, and measures of speaking rate in imitated sentences or spontaneous speech (Hodge & Wellman, 1999; Strand & McCauley, 1999; Wit, Maassen, Gabreels & Thoonen, 1993). Structure and function of the respiratory and phonatory systems supporting prosodic control can be assessed using the Pre-Speech Assessment Scale (Morris, 1982) in toddlers, the Robbins & Klee (1987) protocol in young children (2.5–6.5 years old), and by the DCOME-T (Dworkin & Culatta, 1995) for older children. There are, however, few resources for assessing word, sentence, and discourse level prosody in children with dysarthria.

Despite a lack of agreement on the core characteristics of childhood apraxia of speech (Caruso & Strand, 1999; Davis,

et al., 1998; Forrest, 2003; Shriberg, et al., 1997a), there are several standardized batteries for diagnosing developmental apraxia (e.g., Kaufman Speech Praxis Test for Children, Kaufman, 1995; *Screening Test for Developmental Apraxia of Speech—Second Edition*, Blakely, 2000; *Verbal Dyspraxia Profile*, Jelm, 2001; Verbal Motor Production Assessment for Children (VMPAC), Hayden & Square, 1999). However, few of these diagnostic batteries assess prosodic function in a comprehensive manner. Moreover, a recent review indicated that only the VMPAC met psychometric criteria of reliability and validity (McCauley & Strand, 2008).

The ever-changing nature of motor speech impairment in children poses a challenge for designing valid tests (Shriberg et al., 2003; Strand, 2002; Yorkston et al., 1999). This is especially true for assessing prosodic ability given that impairments are most notable at conversational and discourse levels, which may be beyond the child's expressive abilities. Thus prosodic impairments may be disproportionately higher in children with some expressive ability compared to those with more severe or limited speech production abilities (Caruso & Strand, 1999).

Although the prosodic dimensions outlined by Darley et al. (1969, 1975) and those incorporated in standardized protocols are readily available and help guide the clinician in terms of the behaviors to assess, as with any perceptual measure, an element of subjectivity exists that impacts reliability and validity. Moreover, it is not uncommon that prosodic disturbances can be confounded by other impairments such as resonatory and articulatory disorders

(Brancewicz & Reich, 1989; Hoodin & Gilbert, 1989; Lethlean, Chenery, & Murdoch, 1990). Poor rates of agreement have been noted between clinicians (both experienced and inexperienced) on differential diagnosis using perceptual measures (Kearns & Simmons, 1988; Kent, 1996; Sheard, Adams, & Davis, 1991; Zeplin & Kent, 1996; Zyski & Weisiger, 1987). Thus, the importance of structured listening experiences to train clinicians in performing perceptual analyses of prosodic control cannot be emphasized enough (Duffy & Kent, 2001; Kent, Kent, Duffy, & Weismer, 1998; Rosenbek & LaPointe, 1985). Additionally, given that prosodic impairment is most notable at the conversational level, it is difficult to obtain controlled samples and common metrics of assessment. Further efforts aimed at developing standardized stimuli and rating scales are required. Along these lines, a pressing need exists for developmentally appropriate assessments of prosodic function (Duffy, 2007; Hodge & Wellman, 1999; McCauley & Strand, 2008). On a theoretical note, there is an inherent bias in perceptual scales to identify prosodic abnormality rather than to document residual ability. Perhaps the use of instrumental analyses may help quantify not only the type and degree of dysprosody, but also the speaker's arsenal of compensatory behaviors.

Instrumental Analysis

Acoustic and physiological measures of prosodic function provide objective data that can supplement perceptual findings and, thereby, aid in diagnosis and monitoring of treatment efficacy

(Netsell, 1986; Netsell & Rosenbek, 1985; Peterson & Marquardt, 1981; Wertz & Rosenbek, 1992). Although instrumentation for assessing physiological function is not as readily available in the clinical setting, it is possible to assess respiratory and phonatory function through clinical observation using well-defined tasks. Weismer (2007) outlines methods for assessing speech breathing including estimating lung volume usage, vocal level, and chest wall contributions through noninstrumental clinical observation. Given that phrasing and stress patterning are tied intricately to respiratory functions (Hammen & Yorkston, 1996; Murdoch, Theodoros, Stokes, & Chenery, 1993), a careful examination of speech breathing behaviors is essential for assessing prosody.

Acoustic analysis is a powerful tool for improving the precision of diagnosis and for providing objective measures to document treatment progress. Advances in digital technologies now allow for acoustic analyses on any computer. Although many clinics may still have stand-alone systems such as the Visi-Pitch (KayPentax) or the Computerized Speech Laboratory (CSL, KayPentax), numerous freeware and shareware acoustic analysis programs are available (e.g., Wavesurfer, Praat, Audacity). Within the last decade of research in motor speech disorders, the Praat speech analysis toolkit (Boersma & Weenink) has become used widely. After the software is downloaded, all that is required is a high-quality microphone and a computer with a sound card. Prosodic features can be viewed readily and measured using the acoustic waveform and/or spectrographic displays. Macrofunctions that calculate mean, range, standard deviation, and other descriptive statistics for F0 and intensity contours of selected portions of an acoustic waveform that make it easy to obtain objective measures of prosodic control.

Now that software is readily available and affordable for use in clinical settings, the main barriers include lack of experience and poor consensus on which acoustic cues should be examined. Commonly measured features include mean F0, peak F0, range of F0, variance in F0, slope of F0, mean intensity, peak intensity, range of intensity, vowel/syllable/word duration, silence duration, mean length of breath group

(cf. Bunton, Kent, Kent, & Rosenbek, 2000; Forrest & Weismer, 1997; Leuschel & Docherty, 1996; Lowit-Leuschel & Docherty, 2000; Kent & Kim, 2003; Kent, Weismer, Kent, Vorperian, & Duffy, 1999; Patel, 2003, 2004; Patel & Campellone, 2009; Schlenck, Bettrich, & Willmes, 1993; Skodda, Rinsche, & Schiegel, 2009; Yorkston et al., 1984). The acoustic feature(s) chosen depend on the spoken task and the purpose of the measurement (see Figure 4–1 for an illustration of possible acoustic features). For example, if the goal is to quantify prosodic range in a speaker with dysarthria, one

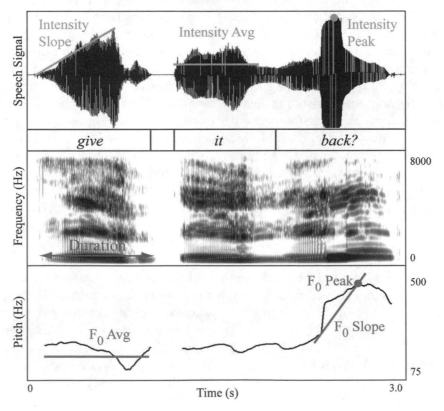

Figure 4–1. Composite Praat screenshot displaying the acoustic waveform (*top panel*), spectrogram (*middle panel*), and F0 contour (*bottom panel*). A subset of possible quantitative measures are illustrated in the overlay (See Color Plate 1).

can compare the change in F0 within an utterance (particularly on the last syllable) of questions versus statements. To examine stress patterning, one can compare the peak F0 and intensity of stressed words to unstressed words within an utterance.

Although there certainly are benefits to using acoustic methods, the speech of individuals with motor speech impairments sometimes can pose particular challenges (see Baken, 1987; Kent & Kim, 2003; and Read, Buder, & Kent, 1992 for reviews of acoustic analysis systems and considerations). Specifically, tracking F0 in children, women, and individuals with speech impairment can be difficult. Pitch breaks and errors in tracking are not uncommon, and, thus, qualitative analysis via auditory and visual inspection is essential (Liss & Weismer, 1992). Additionally, hypernasality among motor speech impairments can reduce acoustic contrasts on a spectrogram leading to poor measurement accuracy. Microphone placement also is an important consideration for intensity measurements (Baken, 1987). When possible, a head-worn microphone should be used to maintain a constant mouth-to-microphone distance.

Despite advances in instrumentation and measurement techniques, physiological and acoustic measurements are not yet widely used in clinical settings. There is a need for providing clinicians with more hands-on practice with readily available acoustic software (see Ingram, Bunta, & Ingram, 2004, for a clinician-friendly tutorial on using digital sound files for transcription, analysis, and treatment). Demystifying instrumentation and acoustic analysis for the clinician would have significant impact on accountability and outcome measurement. As Duffy (2007) notes, these efforts will take root only, however, if they are time efficient and can offer additional benefit compared to perceptual measures alone. In this respect, methods for automating prosodic analysis are particularly attractive (DiCicco, 2009; DiCicco & Patel, 2008; van Santen, Tucker Prud'hommeaux, & Black, 2009).

Stimuli and Task Variables That Impact Prosodic Assessment

Prosodic control is highly task dependent. Many researchers have noted the importance of using a variety of structured and nonstructured tasks to obtain a comprehensive profile of the client's prosodic abilities (Kent & Kim, 2003; Leuschel & Docherty, 1996; Peppe & McCann, 2003; Schlenck et al., 1993; Shriberg et al., 1990; Ziegler, 2003). Table 4–1 provides examples of stimuli and measurement features for each prosodic dimension compiled across various sources.

The ability to modulate stress within a word can be useful for signaling noun/verb contrasts (PROtest versus protest) and compound noun/noun phrase (blackboard versus blackboard) contrasts. Darkins, Fromkin, and Benson (1988) noted that healthy speakers decreased F0 on the second word of compound nouns but not for noun phrases, a distinction that speakers with dysarthria due to Parkinson's disease could not make. Although speakers with motor speech impairments have difficulty marking such contrasts, few assessment protocols include such tasks.

Table 4–1. Sample Behaviors/Tasks to Assess Each Prosodic Dimension and Corresponding Physiologic/Acoustic Measures

Prosodic Dimension	Behaviors/Tasks to Assess	Example(s) of Physiological or Acoustic Measures
Stress	Overall stress pattern in connected speech	Examine stress modulation in connected speech as a function of F0, intensity, and duration variation
	Appropriate stress variation in connected speech	Measure change in F0, intensity, and duration for stressed versus unstressed words
	Lexical stress in trochaic words	Calculate the lexical stress ratio; divide stress (i.e., peak or average F0, intensity, and duration) on the first syllable by stress on the second syllable
	Emphatic stress within a sentence	Compare mean/peak F0, intensity, and duration of a given word in stressed and unstressed positions
Rate	Overall rate	Average duration of sentence or number of words per second
	Rate maintenance	Compare rate at beginning and end of connected speech sample or reading passage
	Short rushes of speech	Number of syllables per breath
	Fluctuations of rate	Compare rate within utterance or connected speech sample
Phrasing and breath patterning	Disturbed breath support— excessive shoulder elevation	Examine changes in lung volume at sentence and conversational levels using visual inspection or via instrumentation (i.e., respiratory inductance plethysmography [Respitrace])
	Audible inspiration	Presence of inhalatory stridor or audible inspiration in acoustic waveform
	Length of breath group	Number of syllables per breath group
	Naturalness/appropriateness of pauses at phrase boundaries	Frequency of pauses at appropriate phrase junctures; length of pause

Table 4–1. *continued*

Prosodic Dimension	Behaviors/Tasks to Assess	Example(s) of Physiological or Acoustic Measures
Loudness	Appropriateness of loudness level	Mean intensity level in connected speech sample; too high, normal or too low for age, sex, and speaking context
	Loudness maintenance	Change in intensity level within a connected speech sample
	Loudness variation	Change in intensity level between stressed and unstressed words in pragmatically loaded sentences
	Abnormal loudness variation	Presence of sudden bursts of loudness
Pitch	Pitch steadiness	Mean F0 variation in connected speech
	Appropriateness of pitch level	Mean F0 in connect speech: scale as too high, normal, or too low for age, sex, and speaking context
	Pitch variation within an utterance	Change in F0 between stressed and unstressed words within pragmatically loaded sentences (e.g., question-statement, contrastive stress)
	Pitch breaks	Frequency of pitch breaks; frequency of glottal fry

Stress patterning of trochaic words (e.g., ladder, bathtub) also may provide a window into motor speech impairment. Shriberg and colleagues have noted that children with apraxia of speech either overstress or understress syllables in trochaic words (Shriberg, et al., 2003; Shriberg, Ballard, Tomblin, Duffy, Odell, & Williams, 2006; Odell & Shriberg, 2001). They noted that the lexical stress ratio, obtained by dividing stress on the first syllable by stress on the second syllable, was useful in differentiating between children with apraxia of speech and those without (Shriberg et al., 2003, 2006). At present, the PVSP is the only test protocol in motor speech disorders to assess lexical stress. The PEPS-C (Profiling Elements of Prosodic Systems—Child Version, Peppe & McCann, 2003), a test used primarily for assessing prosody in children with language impairment, also assesses lexical stress.

At the phrasal level, modulation of prosodic cues can be used to signal question-statement distinctions (He plays the piano. versus He plays the piano?) and to contrast alternative meanings of an utterance ("JOHN lives near me", i.e., not *Bill*, from "John lives NEAR me", i.e., not *far*). In English, declarative statements are marked by falling intonation, whereas declarative questions generally are marked by rising phrase-final intonation (Cruttenden 1981; Lieberman, 1967). Although speakers with dysarthria have restricted F0 range for signaling questions (Le Dorze, Ouellet, & Ryalls, 1994; Le Dorze, Ryalls, Brassard, Boulanger, & Ratte, 1998), some speakers appear to retain the ability to mark the contrast by modifying duration (Patel, 2002, 2003). In other words, rather than signaling questions with an increasing terminal F0 contour, speakers marked the final syllable with increased duration. Moreover, unfamiliar listeners were able to perceive and utilize this cue trade to accurately classify statements and questions produced by speakers with dysarthria (Patel, 2002). Speakers with dysarthria due to cerebral palsy show similar cue compensations for signaling contrastive stress within an utterance (Patel & Campellone, 2009; Weismer & Ingrisano, 1979; Yorkston et al., 1984). Although healthy speakers mark stressed words by increasing fundamental frequency, intensity, and duration relative to unstressed words (Bolinger, 1961; Eady & Cooper, 1986; Lehiste, 1970; Morton & Jassem, 1965), speakers with dysarthria rely more heavily on duration cues (Patel & Campellone, 2009; Weismer & Ingrisano, 1979; Yorkston et al., 1984). These findings highlight the importance of not only documenting differences between healthy and impaired speakers but also understanding the manner in which speakers with dysarthria manifest prosodic contrasts. If speakers can convey prosodic contrasts in a consistent albeit nonstandard manner, perhaps this residual ability can be leveraged for communication. With the exception of the Emphatic Stress Task in the PVSP, most motor speech assessments do not assess phrase level prosody in a systematic manner.

Read and conversational samples are the most common tasks for assessing prosody in connected speech. The "Grandfather" passage is the most widely used and consists of 115 words that contain most of the phonemes of standard American English (Fairbanks, 1960). Decreased range and variation of F0 and intensity commonly are cited deficits noted in reading samples of speakers with dysarthria (Canter, 1963; Darley et al., 1975; Flint, Black, Campbell-Taylor, Gailey, & Levinton, 1992; Kent & Rosenbek, 1982; Metter & Hanson, 1986). Often overlooked are the errors and dysfluencies present in read samples due to the use of dated vocabulary and language in the passage (e.g., Banana oil!). Although these errors may be due to motor deficits, they also may be due to cognitive-linguistic demands imposed by the reading passage itself. Although several research groups have devised novel passages to elicit utterances with prosodic variation (Brown & Docherty, 1995; Lowit, Brendel, Dobinson, & Howell, 2006), further efforts are required to design a contemporary passage that contains stimuli aimed specifically at assessing and differentiating among motor speech impairments.

While reading passages provide structured and controlled contexts (e.g., controlled phonetic content, syntactic structure, and utterance length) for assessing and reassessing connected speech, Leuschel & Docherty (1996) warn that prosodic modulation during reading is not representative of more naturalistic tasks such as conversation. Additional confounds to assessing prosody using read speech include the variability across speakers in reading ability and the fact that written text may pace the speaker or otherwise serve to mask prosodic abnormalities. Duffy (2007) argues that conversational and narrative samples are the most important for assessing the integrated behavior of all of the speech subsystems (respiration, phonation, articulation, resonance, and prosody). Creative methods to elicit naturalistic conversational samples are required.

What We Can Learn About Prosodic Assessment from Neighboring Fields

Assessment of prosodic control in motor speech impairment can be informed by adjacent disciplines and disorders that impact prosody. The ToBI framework used by linguistics to transcribe intonational patterns of spoken language (Beckman, Hirschberg, & Shattuck-Hufnagel, 2005) is based on the autosegmental-metrical (AM) theory (Pierrehumbert, 1980) and has potential for examining prosodic control in motor speech impairment (see Kent & Kim, 2003; Mennen, Schaeffler, Watt, & Miller, 2008; Penner, Miller, Hertrich, Ackermann, & Schumm, 2001; Penner, Miller, Hertrich, Ackermann, & Schumm, 2006; Shattuck-Huffnagel, Patel, & Veilleux, 2007, for recent work on dysarthric speech). Rather than quantifying into-

nation in terms of F0 values, the transcription scheme attempts to describe intonation patterns using tone (L for low, H for high) and break indices (% for boundary, * for accents, etc.). This qualitative analysis may be particularly helpful for motor speech disorders given the difficulty in obtaining error-free F0 contours. Drawbacks to using this approach include the level of training required to learn the ToBI coding system (Brugos, Shattuck-Huffnagel, & Veilleux, 2006) and the time involved in the analysis itself (see Chapter 12, "Assessment of Intonation," by Kuschmann, Miller, Lowit, & Mennen, this volume, for more information on this analysis approach).

There have been several recent advances in the assessment of prosody in language impairment that also could be leveraged for motor speech disorders. In particular, the PEPS-C (Profiling Elements of Prosodic Systems—Child Version; Peppe & McCann, 2003) is a comprehensive battery of tasks aimed at assessing comprehension and production of prosody at various task levels. Computerized and paper formats of the test are available to assess four main prosodic functions: turn-taking, affect, chunking, and focus. The stimuli have been standardized and normed on several groups of children and adults with language impairment (Peppe, McCann, Gibbon, O'Hare, & Rutherford, 2006, 2007). The use of picture stimuli to offer choices between contrastive prosodic pairs also enables the use of this test with nonreaders.

Along similar lines, van Santen, Tucker Prud'hommeaux, & Black (2009) have developed an automated assessment of prosodic production. The tasks and stimuli included are variants of tasks in the PEPS-C and those used by

Paul, Augustyn, Klin, & Volkmar (2005). For example, lexical stress, emphatic stress, focus, and phrasing are among the tasks used. Pattern recognition-based automatic algorithms have been implemented to analyze spoken responses to each task. Although tuning the algorithms to annotate recordings from individuals with motor speech disorders is not trivial, this work is a significant step forward in bringing automated analyses of prosody into the clinical setting.

Summary

Upon surveying current practices on assessing prosody in motor speech disorders and reviewing related research evidence, several overarching themes emerge. First, assessment of prosody requires multiple levels of analyses (e.g., perceptual, acoustic, physiologic, etc.) and a variety of spoken tasks (e.g., word, sentence, discourse). Second, there is a need for standardized and developmentally appropriate stimuli and test batteries that guide clinicians through the assessment process. Moreover, tailoring graduate curricula to include structured practice with perceptual and instrumental analysis of prosody is essential for attaining respectable levels of intra- and inter-clinician reliability. Third, full or semi-automatic processes that facilitate assessment would enhance the likelihood of comprehensive assessment practices in the clinical setting. Finally, assessment should include examinations of both control *and* impairment in order to leverage residual prosody to improve communicative effectiveness.

References

Baken, R. J. (1987). *Clinical measurement of speech and voice.* Boston, MA: College-Hill Press.

Barnes, G. J. (1983) Suprasegmental and prosodic considerations in motor speech disorders. In W. Berry (Ed.), *Clinical dysarthria* (pp. 57–68). San Diego, CA: College-Hill Press.

Beckman, M., Hirschberg, J., & Shattuck-Hufnagel, S. (2005). The original ToBI system and the evolution of the ToBI framework. In Jun, S. (Ed.), *Prosodic typology: The phonology of intonation and phrasing* (pp. 9–54). Oxford: Oxford University Press.

Bellaire, K., Yorkston, K. M., & Beukelman, D. R. (1986). Modification of breath patterning to increase naturalness of a mildly dysarthric speaker. *Journal of Communication Disorders, 19,* 271–280.

Blakely, R. W. (2000). *Screening Test for Developmental Apraxia of Speech—Second Edition,* Austin, TX: Pro-Ed.

Bloom, L. (1973). *One Word at a Time.* The Hague, The Netherlands: Mouton.

Boersma, P., & Weenink, D. (2008). *PRAAT: A system for doing phonetics by computer* (Version 5.1.11). [Computer software]. Amsterdam, The Netherlands: Institute of Phonetic Sciences.

Bolinger, D. (1961). Contrastive accent and contrastive stress. *Language, 37,* 83–96.

Bolinger, D. (1989). *Intonation and its uses: Melody in grammar and discourse.* Stanford, CA: Stanford University Press.

Boutsen, F. R., & Christman, S.S., (2002). Prosody in apraxia of speech. *Seminars in Speech and Language, 23,* 245–256.

Brancewicz, T. M., & Reich, A. R. (1989). Speech rate reduction and "nasality" in normal speakers. *Journal of Speech and Hearing Research, 32,* 837–848.

Brewster, K. (1989). The assessment of prosody. In K. Grundy (Ed.), *Linguistics in Clinical Practice* (pp. 168–185). London, UK: Taylor & Francis.

Brown, A., & Docherty, G. J. (1995). Phonetic variation in dysarthric speech as a function of sampling task. *European Journal of Disorders of Communication*, 30(1), 17-35.

Brugos, A., Shattuck-Hufnagel, S., Veilleux, N. (2006), A ToBi Tutorial. Open Courseware, Massachusetts Institute of Technology. Retrieved January 17, 2008, from http://ocw.mit.edu/OcwWeb/Electrical-Engineering-and-Computer-Science/6911January—IAP-2006/CourseHome/.

Buder, E. (2007). Voice production and dysfunction in motor speech disorders. In G. Weismer (Ed.), *Motor Speech Disorders* (pp. 121–150). San Diego, CA: Plural Publishing.

Bunton, K., Kent, R. D., Kent, J. F., & Rosenbek, J. C. (2000). Perceptuo-acoustic assessment of prosodic impairment in dysarthria. *Clinical Linguistics & Phonetics*, 14(1), 13–24.

Canter, G. (1963). Speech characteristics of patients with Parkinson's disease: I. Intensity, pitch, and duration. *Journal of Speech and Hearing Disorders, 28,* 221–229.

Caruso, A. J., & Strand, E. A. (1999). Motor speech disorders in children: Definitions, background, and a theoretical framework. In A. J. Caruso & E. A. Strand (Eds.), *Clinical management of motor speech disorders in children* (pp. 1–27). New York, NY: Thieme.

Chenery, H. (1998). Perceptual analysis of dysarthric speech. In B. E. Murdoch (Ed.), *Dysarthria: A physiological approach to assessment and treatment* (pp. 36–67). Cheltenham, U.K.: Stanley Thornes.

Chenery, H. J., Ingram, J. L., & Murdoch, B. E. (1990). Perceptual analysis of the speech in ataxic dysarthria. *Australian Journal of Human Communication Disorders, 18,* 19–28.

Chenery, H. J., Murdoch, B. E., & Ingram, J. C. L. (1988). Studies in Parkinson's disease: Perceptual speech analyses. *Australian Journal of Human Communication Disorders, 16,* 17–29.

Cooper, W. E., Eady, S. J., & Mueller, P. R. (1985). Acoustical aspects of contrastive stress in question-answer contexts. *Journal of the Acoustical Society of America, 77*(6), 2142–2156.

Creaghead, N. A., Newman, P. W., & Secord, W. A. (1989). *Assessment and remediation of articulation and phonological disorders* (2nd ed.). Toronto, ON: Collier Macmillan Canada.

Cruttenden, A. (1997). *Intonation* (2nd ed.). Cambridge, UK: Cambridge University Press.

Crystal, D. (1978). The analysis of intonation in young children. In F. D. Minifie and L. L. Lloyd (Eds.), *Communication and cognitive abilities—early behavioral assessment* (pp. 257–271). Baltimore, MD: University Park Press.

Crystal, D. (1979). Prosodic development. In P. Fletcher & M. Garman (Eds.), *Language acquisition* (pp. 174–197). Cambridge, UK: Cambridge University Press.

Cutler, A., Dahan, D., & van Donselaar, W. (1997). Prosody in the comprehension of spoken language: A literature review. *Language and Speech, 40,* 141–201.

Dabul, B. L. (2000). *ABA-2: Apraxia battery for adults* (2nd ed.). Austin, TX: ProEd.

Darley, F. L., Aronson, A. E., & Brown, J. R. (1969). Differential diagnostic patterns of dysarthria. *Journal of Speech and Hearing Research, 12,* 246–269.

Darley, F. L., Aronson, A. E., & Brown, J. R. (1975). *Motor speech disorders*. Philadelphia, PA: W.B. Saunders.

Darkins, A., Fromkin, V., & Benson, D. (1988). A characterization of the prosodic loss in Parkinson's disease. *Brain & Language, 34,* 315–327.

Davis, B., Jakielski, K., & Marquardt, T. (1998). Developmental apraxia of speech: Determiners of differential diagnosis. *Clinical Linguistics & Phonetics, 12,* 25–45.

DiCicco, T. (2009). *Optimization of acoustic feature extraction from dysarthric speech.* Unpublished doctoral dissertation, MIT.

DiCicco, T., & Patel, R. (2008). Automatic landmark analysis of dysarthric speech.

Journal of Medical Speech Language Pathology, 16(4), 213–221.

Drummond, S. S. (1993). *Dysarthria examination battery.* San Antonio, TX: Communication Skill Builders.

Duffy, J. R. (2005). *Motor speech disorders: Substrates, differential diagnosis and management* (2nd ed.). St. Louis, MO: Mosby.

Duffy, J. R. (2007). History, current practice and future trends and goals. In G. Weismer (Ed.), *Motor speech disorders* (pp. 7–56). San Diego, CA: Plural Publishing.

Duffy, J. R., & Kent, R. D. (2001). Darley's contribution to the understanding, differential diagnosis, and scientific study of the dysarthrias. *Aphasiology, 15,* 275–289.

Dworkin, J. P., & Culatta, R. (1995). *Dworkin-Culatta Oral Mechanism Exam-Treatment (DCOME-T).* Nicholasville, KY: Edgewood Press.

Eady, S. J., & Cooper, W. E. (1986). Speech intonation and focus location in matched statements and questions. *Journal of the Acoustical Society of America, 80*(2), 402–415.

Enderby, P. (1983). *Frenchay dysarthria assessment.* San Diego, CA: College-Hill Press.

Enderby, P. & Palmer, R. (2008). *Frenchay dysarthria assessment* (2nd ed.). Austin, TX: Pro-Ed.

Fairbanks, G. (1960). *Voice and articulation drillbook.* New York, NY: Harper.

FitzGerald, F., Murdoch, B., & Chenery, H. (1987). Multiple sclerosis: Associated speech and language disorders. Australian *Journal of Human Communication Disorders, 15*(2), 15–33.

Flint, A., Black, S., Campbell-Taylor, I., Gailey, G., & Levinton, C. (1992). Acoustic analysis in the differentiation between Parkinson's Disease and major depression, *Journal of Psycholinguistic Research, 21,* 383–399.

Forrest, K. (2003). Diagnostic criteria of developmental apraxia of speech used by clinical speech language pathologists. *American Journal of Speech Language Pathology, 12,* 376–380.

Forrest, K., & Weismer, G. (1997). Acoustic analysis of dysarthric speech. In M. R. McNeil (Ed.), *Clinical management of sensorimotor speech disorders* (pp. 63–80). New York, NY: Thieme.

Fry, D. (1955). Duration and intensity as physical correlates of linguistic stress. *Journal of the Acoustical Society of America, 27,* 765–768.

Fry, D. (1958). Experiments in the perception of stress. *Language and Speech, 1*(2), 126–152.

Gilbert, H., & Robb, M. (1996). Vocal fundamental frequency characteristics of infant hunger cries: Birth to 12 months. *International Journal of Pediatric Otorhinolaryngology, 34,* 237–243.

Hammen, V. L., & Yorkston, K. M. (1996). Respiratory patterning and variability in dysarthric speech. In D. A. Robin, K. M. Yorkston, & D. R. Beukelman (Eds.), *Disorders of motor speech: Assessment, treatment and clinical characterization* (pp. 181–192). Baltimore, MD: Paul H. Brookes.

Hartelius, L., Wising, C., & Nord, L. (1997). Speech modification in dysarthria associated with multiple sclerosis: An intervention based on vocal efficiency, contrastive stress and verbal repair strategies. *Journal of Medical Speech-Language Pathology, 5,* 113–140.

Hayden, D., & Square, P. (1999). *Verbal motor production assessment for children.* San Antonio, TX: The Psychological Corporation.

Helm-Estabrooks, N., Nicholas, M., Morgan, A. (1989). *Melodic intonation therapy* [Manual and instructional videotape]. Chicago, IL: Riverside.

Hodge, M. M., & Wellman, L. (1999). Management of children with dysarthria. In A. J. Caruso & E. A. Strand (Eds.), *Clinical management of motor speech disorders in children* (pp. 209–280). New York, NY: Thieme.

Hoodin, R., & Gilbert, H. (1989). Nasal airflows in parkinsonian speakers. *Journal of Communication Disorders, 22,* 169–180.

Howell, P. (1993). Cue trading in the production and perception of vowel stress. *Journal of the Acoustical Society of America, 94*(4), 2063–2072.

Huss, V. (1978). English word stress in the post-nuclear position. *Phonetica, 35,* 86–105.

Jelm, J. M. (2001). *Verbal Dyspraxia Profile.* DeKalb, IL: Janelle.

Katz, W. F., Beach, C. M., Jenouri, K., & Verma, S., 1996. Duration and fundamental frequency correlates of phrase boundaries in productions by children and adults. *Journal of the Acoustical Society of America, 99,* 3179–3191.

Kaufman, N. R. (1995). *Kaufman Speech Praxis Test for Children.* Austin, TX: Pro-Ed.

Kearns, K P., & Simmons, N. N. (1988). Interobserver reliability and perceptual ratings: more than meets the ear. *Journal of Speech and Hearing Research, 31,* 131–136.

Kent, R. D. (1996). Hearing and believing: some limits to the auditory-perceptual assessment of speech and voice disorders. *American Journal of Speech Language Pathology, 5,* 7–23.

Kent, R. D. (1997). *The speech sciences.* San Diego, CA: Singular.

Kent, R. D., & Bauer, H. R. (1985). Vocalizations of one-year-olds. *Journal of Child Language, 12,* 491–526.

Kent, R. D., Kim, Y.-J. (2003). Toward an acoustic typology of motor speech disorders. *Clinical Linguistics & Phonetics, 17,* 427–445.

Kent, R. D., Kent, J. F., Duffy, J. R., & Weismer, G. (1998). The dysarthrias: Speech-voice profiles, related dysfunctions, and neuropathology. *Journal of Medical Speech Language Pathology, 6,* 165–211.

Kent, R. D., & Murray, A. D. (1982). Acoustic features of infant vocalic utterances at 3, 6, and 9 months. *Journal of the Acoustical Society of America, 72*(2), 353–365.

Kent, R. D., & Read, C. (2002). *Acoustic analysis of speech.* San Diego, CA: Singular.

Kent, R. D., & Rosenbek, J. C. (1982). Prosodic disturbance and neurological lesion. *Brain & Language, 15,* 259–291.

Kent, R. D., Weismer, G., Kent, J. F., & Rosenbek, J. C. (1989). Toward phonetic intelligibility testing in dysarthria. *Journal of Speech and Hearing Disorders, 54,* 482–499.

Kent, R. D., Weismer, G., Kent, J. F., Vorperian, H. K., & Duffy, J. R. (1999) Acoustic studies of dysarthric speech: Methods, progress, and potential. *Journal of Communication Disorders, 32,* 141–186.

LeDorze, G., Dionne, L., Ryalls, J., Julien, M., & Quellet, L. (1992). The effects of speech and language therapy for a case of dysarthria associated with Parkinson's disease. *European Journal of Disorders of Communication, 27,* 313–324.

Le Dorze, G., Ouellet, L., & Ryalls, J. (1994). Intonation and speech rate in dysarthric speech, *Journal of Communication Disorders, 27,* 1–17.

Le Dorze, G., Ryalls, J., Brassard, C., Boulanger, N., & Ratte, D. (1998). A comparison of the prosodic characteristics of the speech of people with Parkinson's disease and Friedrich's ataxia with neurologically normal speakers, *Folia Phoniatrica et Logopaedica, 50,* 1–9.

Lehiste, I. (1970). *Suprasegmentals.* Cambridge, MA: MIT Press.

Lehiste, I. (1976). Suprasegmental features of speech. In N. J. Lass (Ed.), *Contemporary issues in experimental phonetics* (pp. 225–239). New York, NY: Academic Press.

Lethlean, J., Chenery, H., & Murdoch, B. (1990). Disturbed respiratory and prosodic function in Parkinson's disease: A perceptual and instrumental analysis. *Australian Journal of Human Communication Disorders, 18,* 83–97.

Leuschel, A., & Docherty, G. J. (1996). Prosodic assessment of dysarthria. In D. A. Robin, K. M. Yorkston, and D. R. Beukelman (Eds), *Disorders of motor speech: Assessment, treatment and clinical characterization* (pp. 155–178). Baltimore, MD: Paul H. Brookes.

Lieberman, P. (1967). *Intonation, perception and language.* Cambridge: MIT Press.

Lind, K., & Wermke, K. (2002). Development of the vocal fundamental frequency of spontaneous cries during the first 3 months. *International Journal of Pediatric Otorhinolaryngology, 64*(2), 97–104.

Liss, J.M., & Weismer, G. (1992). Qualitative acoustic analysis in the study of motor speech disorders. *Journal of the Acoustical Society of America, 92,* 2984–2987.

Lowit, A., Brendel, B., Dobinson, C., & Howell, P. (2006). An investigation into the influences of age, pathology, and cognition on speech production. *Journal of Medical Speech Language Pathology, 14*(4), 253–262.

Lowit-Leuschel, A. & Docherty, G. (2000). Dysprosody. In R. D. Kent & M. J. Ball (Eds), *Voice quality measurement* (pp. 59–72). San Diego, CA: Singular.

Ludlow, C. L., & Bassich, C. J. (1983). Relationships between perceptual ratings and acoustic measures of hypokinetic speech. In M. R. McNeil, J. C. Rosenbek, & A. E. Aronson (Eds.), *The dysarthrias: physiology, acoustics, perception, management* (pp. 163–195). San Diego, CA: College-Hill Press.

MacNeilage, P. F., & Davis, B. L. (1993). Acquisition of speech production: Frames then content. In M. Jeannerod (Ed.), *Attention and performance XIII: Motor representation and control* (pp. 453–475). Hillsdale, NJ: Lawrence Erlbaum.

McCauley, R. J., & Strand, E. A. (2008). A review of standardized tests of nonverbal oral and speech motor performance in children. *American Journal of Speech-Language Pathology, 17,* 81–91.

McNeil, M. R., Robin, D. A., & Schmidt, R. A. (1997). Apraxia of speech: Definition, differentiation and treatment. In M. R. McNeil (Ed.), *Clinical management of sensorimotor speech disorders* (pp. 311–344). New York, NY: Theime.

McSweeny, J. L., & Shriberg, L. D. (2001). Clinical research with the prosody-voice screening profile. *Clinical Linguistics & Phonetics, 15*(7), 505–528.

Mennen, I., Schaeffler, F., Watt, N., & Miller, N. (2008). An auto-segmental-metrical investigation of intonation in people with Parkinson's Disease. *Asia Pacific Journal of Speech, Language, and Hearing, 11*(4), 205–219.

Menyuk, P., & Bernholtz, N. (1969). Prosodic features and children's language production. *MIT Quarterly Progress Report, 93,* 216–219.

Metter, J., & Hanson, W. (1986). Clinical and acoustic variability in hypokinetic dysarthria. *Journal of Communication Disorders, 19,* 347–366.

Morris, S. E. (1982). *Pre-Speech Assessment Scale (0–2 years).* Clifton, NJ: JA Preston Corp.

Morton, J., & Jassem, W. (1965). Acoustic correlates of stress. *Language and Speech, 8,* 159–181.

Murdoch, B. E., Theodoros, D. G., Stokes, P. D., & Chenery, H. J. (1993). Abnormal patterns of speech breathing in dysarthric speakers following severe closed head injury. *Brain Injury, 7,* 295–308.

Netsell, R. (1973). Speech Physiology. In F. Minifie, T. J. Hixon, & F. Williams (Eds.), *Normal aspects of speech, hearing, and language* (pp. 211–234). Englewood Cliffs, NJ: Prentice-Hall.

Netsell, R. (1986). *A neurobiologic view of speech production and the dysarthrias.* San Diego, CA: College-Hill Press.

Netsell, R., & Rosenbek, J. C. (1985). Treating the dysarthrias. In J. Darby (Ed.), *Speech and language evaluation in neurology: Adult disorders* (pp. 363–392). New York, NY: Grune and Stratton.

Odell, K. H., & Shriberg, L. D. (2001). Prosody-voice characteristics of children and adults with apraxia of speech. *Clinical Linguistics & Phonetics, 15,* 275–307.

Patel, R. (2002). Prosodic control in severe dysarthria: preserved ability to mark the question-statement contrast. *Journal of Speech, Language and Hearing Research, 45,* 858–870.

Patel, R. (2003). Acoustic characteristics of the question-statement contrast in severe dysarthria due to cerebral palsy. *Journal of Speech, Language and Hearing Research, 46*(6), 1401–1415.

Patel, R. (2004). The acoustics of contrastive prosody in adults with cerebral palsy. *Journal of Medical Speech-Language Pathology, 12,* 189–193.

Patel, R., & Campellone, P. (2009). Production and identification of contrastive stress in dysarthria. *Journal of Speech, Language and Hearing Research, 52,* 206–222.

Patel, R., & Salata, A. (2006). Using computer games to mediate caregiver-child communication for children with severe dysarthria. *Journal of Medical Speech Language Pathology, 14*(4), 279-284.

Patel, R., & Watkins, C. (2007). Stress identification in speakers with dysarthria due to cerebral palsy: An initial report. *Journal of Medical Speech Language Pathology, 15*(2), 149–160.

Paul, R., Augustyn, A., Klin, A., & Volkmar, F. (2005). Perception and production of prosody by speakers with autism spectrum disorders. *Journal of Autism and Developmental Disorders, 35,* 201–220.

Penner, H., Miller, N., Hertrich, I., Ackermann, H., & Schumm, F. (2001). Dysprosody in Parkinson's disease: An investigation of intonation patterns. *Clinical Linguistics & Phonetics, 15,* 551–566.

Penner, H., Miller, N., Hertrich, I., Ackermann, H., & Schumm, F. (2006). Is impaired intonation in speakers suffering from Parkinson's disease caused at a motor or at a planning level? *Journal of the Neurological Sciences, 248*(1–2), 279.

Peppe, S., Maxim, J., & Wells, B. (2000). Prosodic variation in southern British English. *Language and Speech, 43*(3), 309–334.

Peppe, S., & McCann, J. (2003), Assessing intonation and prosody in children with atypical language development: The PEPS-C test and the revised version. *Clinical Linguistics & Phonetics, 17,* 345–354.

Peppe, S., McCann, J., Gibbon, F., O'Hare, A., & Rutherford, M. (2006). Assessing prosodic and pragmatic ability in children with high functioning autism. *Journal of Pragmatics, 38,* 1776–1791.

Peppe, S., McCann, J., Gibbon, F., O'Hare, A., & Rutherford, M. (2007). Receptive and expressive prosodic ability in children with high functioning autism. *Journal of Speech, Language and Hearing Research, 50,* 1015–1028.

Peterson, H., & Marquardt, T. (1981). *Appraisal and diagnosis of speech and language disorders.* Englewood Cliffs, NJ: Prentice-Hall.

Pierrehumbert, J. (1980). *The phonetics and phonology of English intonation.* Unpublished doctoral dissertation, Massachusetts Institute of Technology.

Protopapas, A., & Eimas, P. D. (1997). Perceptual differences in infant cries revealed by modifications of acoustic features. *Journal of the Acoustical Society of America, 102*(6), 3723–3734.

Ramig, L. O., Sapir, S., Fox, C., & Countryman, S. (2001). Changes in vocal loudness following intensive voice treatment (LSVT) in individuals with Parkinson's Disease: A comparison with untreated patients and normal age-matched controls. *Movement Disorders, 16,* 79–83.

Read, C., Buder, E. H., & Kent, R. D. (1992). Speech analysis systems: An evaluation. *Journal of Speech and Hearing Research, 35,* 314–332.

Robbins, J., & Klee, T. (1987). Clinical assessment of oropharyngeal motor development in young children. *Journal of Speech and Hearing Research, 52,* 271–277.

Robertson, S. J. (1982). *Dysarthria profile.* Tuscon, AZ: Communication Skill Builders.

Robin, D. A., Klouda, G., & Hug, L. (1991). Neurogenic disorders of prosody. In M. P. Cannito & D. Vogel (Eds), *Treating disordered speech motor vontrol: For clinicians by clinicians* (pp. 241–271). Austin, TX: Pro-Ed.

Rosenbek, J. C., & LaPointe, L. L. (1985). The dysarthrias: Description, diagnosis, and treatment. In D. F. Johns (Ed.), *Clinical management of neurogenic communication disorders* (2nd ed., pp. 97–152). Boston, MA: Little Brown.

Schlaug. G., Marchina, S., & Norton A. (2008). From singing to speaking: Why patients with Broca's aphasia can sing and how that may lead to recovery of expressive language functions. *Music Perception, 25,* 315–323.

Schlenck, K. J., Bettrich, R., & Willmes, Z. K. (1993). Aspects of disturbed prosody in dysarthria. *Clinical Linguistics & Phonetics, 7,* 119–128.

Shattuck-Hufnagel, S., Patel, R., & Veilleux, N. (2007). Prosodic labeling of adult dysarthric speech. *Proceedings of the Conference on Speech Prosody in Atypical Populations,* Reading, UK, April 2007.

Shattuck-Hufnagel, S., & Turk, A. E. (1996). A prosody tutorial for investigators of auditory sentence processing. *Journal of Psycholinguistic Research, 25*(2), 193–247.

Sheard, C., Adams, R. D., & Davis, P. J. (1991). Reliability and agreement of ratings of ataxic dysarthric speech samples with varying intelligibility. *Journal of Speech and Hearing Research, 34,* 285–293.

Shriberg, L. D., Aram, D. M., & Kwiatkowski, J. (1997a). Developmental apraxia of speech: I. Descriptive and theoretical perspectives. *Journal of Speech, Language and Hearing Research, 40,* 273–285.

Shriberg, L. D., Aram, D. M., & Kwiatkowski, J. (1997b). Developmental apraxia of speech: II. Toward a diagnostic marker. *Journal of Speech, Language and Hearing Research, 40,* 286–312.

Shriberg, L. D., Aram, D. M., & Kwiatkowski, J. (1997c). Developmental apraxia of speech: III. A subtype marked by inappropriate stress. *Journal of Speech, Language and Hearing Research, 40,* 313–337.

Shriberg, L. D., Ballard, K. J., Tomblin, J. B., Duffy, J. R., Odell, K, H., & Williams, C. A. (2006). Speech, prosody, and voice characteristics of a mother and daughter with a 7;13 translocation affecting FOXP2. *Journal of Speech, Language and Hearing Research, 49,* 500–525.

Shriberg, L. D., Campbell, T. F., Karlsson, H. B., Brown, R. L., McSweeny, J. L., & Nadler, C. J. (2003). A diagnostic marker for childhood apraxia of speech: The lexical stress ratio. *Clinical Linguistics & Phonetics, 17,* 549–574.

Shriberg, L. D., Kwiatkowski, J., & Rasmussen, C. (1990). *The prosody-voice screening profile.* Tuscon, AZ: Communication Skill Builders.

Skodda, S., Rinsche, H., & Schlegel, U. (2009). Progression of dysprosody in Parkinson's disease over time—a longitudinal study. *Movement Disorders, 24*(5), 716–722.

Sluijter, A., & van Heuven, V. (1996a). Acoustic correlates of linguistic stress and accent in Dutch and American English. In *Proceedings of the international conference on spoken language processing 1996* (pp. 630–633). Philadelphia: Applied Science and Engineering Laboratories, Alfred I. duPont Institute.

Sluijter, A., & van Heuven, V. (1996b). Spectral balance as an acoustic correlate of linguistic stress. *Journal of the Acoustical Society of America, 100*(4), 2471–2485.

Snow, D., 1994. Phrase-final syllable lengthening and intonation in early child speech. *Journal of Speech and Hearing Research, 37,* 831–840.

Square-Storer, P., Darley, F., & Sommers, R. T. (1988). Nonspeech and speech processing skills in patients with aphasia and apraxia of speech. *Brain & Language, 33,* 65–85.

Strand, E. A. (2002). Childhood apraxia of speech: Suggested diagnostic markers for the younger child. In L. Shriberg & T. Campbell (Eds.), *Proceedings of the 2002 childhood apraxia of speech research symposium* (pp. 75–80). Carlsbad, CA: The Hendrix Foundation.

Strand, E. A., & McCauley, R. J. (1999). Assessment procedures for treatment planning in children with phonologic and motor speech disorders. In A. J.

Caruso & E. A. Strand (Eds.), *Clinical management of motor speech disorders in children* (pp. 73–107). New York, NY: Thieme.

Theodoros, D. G., Murdoch, B. E., Stokes, P. D., & Chenery, H. J. (1993). Hypernasality in dysarthric speakers following severe closed head injury: A perceptual and instrumental analysis. *Brain Injury, 7*, 59–69.

van Santen, J. P. H., Tucker Prud'hommeaux, E., & Black, L. M. (2009). Automated assessment of prosody production. *Speech Communication, 51*, 1082–1097.

Velleman, S. L., & Shriberg, L. D. (1999). Metrical analysis of children with suspected developmental apraxia of speech and inappropriate stress. *Journal of Speech, Language and Hearing Research, 42*, 1444–1460.

Weismer, G. (2007). Speech breathing in motor speech disorders. In G. Weismer (Ed.), *Motor speech disorders* (pp. 93–120). San Diego, CA: Plural Publishing.

Weismer, G., & Ingrisano, D. (1979). Phrase-level timing patterns in English: Effects of emphatic stress location and speaking rate. *Journal of Speech and Hearing Research, 22*(3), 516–533.

Wermke, K., Mende, W., Manfredi, C., & Bruscaglioni, P. (2002). Developmental aspects of infant's cry melody and formants. *Medical Engineering & Physics, 24*(7–8), 501–514.

Wertz, R. T., LaPointe, L. L., & Rosenbek, J. C. (1991). *Apraxia of speech in adults: The disorder and its management.* San Diego, CA: Singular.

Wertz, R. T., & Rosenbek, J. C. (1992). Where the ear fits: A perceptual evaluation of motor speech disorders. *Seminars in Speech and Language, 13*, 39–54.

Whitehill, T., Patel, R., Lai, J. (2008). The use of prosody by children with severe dysarthria: A Cantonese extension study. *Journal of Medical Speech Language Pathology, 16*(4), 293–301.

Williams, C., & Stevens, K. N. (1972). Emotions and speech: Some acoustical correlates. *Journal of the Acoustical Society of America, 52*, 1238–1250.

Wit, J., Maassen, B., Gabreels, F. J. M., & Thoonen, G. (1993). Maximum performance tests in children with developmental spastic dysarthria. *Journal of Speech and Hearing Research, 36*, 452–459.

Wymer, J. H., Lindman, L. S., & Booksh, R. L. (2002). A neuropsychological perspective of aprosody: Features, function, assessment and treatment. *Applied Neuropsychology, 9*(1), 37–47.

Yorkston, K. M, & Beukelman, D. R. (1981). *Assessment of intelligibility of dysarthric speech.* Tigard, OR: CC Publications.

Yorkston, K. M, Beukelman, D. R., & Bell, K. (1988). *Clinical management of dysarthric speakers.* San Diego, CA: College-Hill Press.

Yorkston, K. M., Beukelman, D. R., Minifie, F., & Sapir, S. (1984). Assessment of stress patterning. In M. McNeil, J. Rosenbek, & A. Aronson (Eds.), *The dysarthria: Physiology, acoustics, perception, management* (pp. 131–162). Austin, TX: Pro-Ed.

Yorkston, K. M., Beukelman, D. R., Strand, E. A., & Bell, K. (1999). *Management of motor speech disorders in children and adults* (2nd ed.). Austin, TX: Pro-Ed.

Zeplin, J., & Kent, R. D. (1996). Reliabilty of auditory-perceptual scaling of dysarthria. In D. A. Robin, K. M. Yorkston, & D. R. Beukelman (Eds.), *Disorders of motor speech: Recent advances in assessment, treatment and clinical characterization* (pp. 145–154). Baltimore, MD: Paul H. Brookes.

Ziegler, W. (2003). Speech motor control is task specific: Evidence from dysarthria and apraxia of speech. *Aphasiology, 17*, 3–36.

Zyski, B. J., & Weisiger, B. E. (1987). Identification of dysarthria types based on perceptual analysis. *Journal of Communication Disorders, 20*, 367–378.

5

The Psychosocial Impact of Acquired Motor Speech Disorders

MARGARET WALSHE, PH.D.

Introduction

Over the past decade, there have been numerous calls for research on the psychosocial impact of acquired motor speech disorders on the speaker. One of the many reasons for this is the fact that the ICF framework (World Health Organization, 2001) has drawn considerable attention to the dearth of literature in this area (see Chapter 1, "The ICF Framework and its Relevance to the Assessment of People with Motor Speech Disorders," Hartelius and Miller, this volume). A second reason is that the field of aphasiology, which is allied closely with acquired motor speech disorders, has forged ahead with significant advances in understanding the psychological and social impacts of aphasia, the development of aphasia-friendly outcome measures in this domain, and an exploration of different methodologies and frameworks to assist people to 'live with' their aphasia.

The growing sense that motor speech disorders is somewhat lagging behind in this area is confirmed by an electronic database search (PubMed, EMBASE, CINAHL, PsychInfo, Web of Science, 1995–2010) which retrieved a handful of articles on the area in dysarthria with no relevant results for apraxia of speech (AOS) contrasting with a larger body of research on aphasia. How can one explain this apparent inequity? Lack of research cannot be attributed to incidence and prevalence. Although it is acknowledged that AOS is less prevalent than dysarthria and aphasia, dysarthria is the most commonly acquired communication disorder (Enderby & Emerson, 1995) representing a significant proportion of communication disorders in medical speech-language pathology clinics (Duffy, 2005). It could be argued that people with aphasia encounter greater challenges with regard to communication and, therefore, require more urgent attention. However, without true evidence that this is the case, the argument is not supported.

In this chapter, the reader is urged to consider the evidence that motor speech disorders can have a negative impact on the speaker and to reflect on the application and relevance of current knowledge to clinical practice. The available evidence is small, and the nature and extent of motor speech disorders is diverse. The speech characteristics of AOS and dysarthria differ, although many common characteristics exist (Wambaugh et al., 2006). Within AOS and dysarthria, the disorders can range from minimal changes in speech intelligibility, apparent only to the speaker or trained listener, to the complete absence of speech. The speech disorders can be degenerative and unpredictable or stable and improving. They can exist in association with depression, cognitive impairment, right hemisphere language disorder, aphasia, physical disability, and hearing impairment. Although throughout the chapter the primary focus remains with the speaker, the psychosocial impact on those close to the individual also is given consideration. The argument for increasing the current body of knowledge on the topic is made throughout. Finally, the reader is provided with food for thought regarding directions for future research.

A Framework for Examining Psychosocial Impact

As Brumfitt (2006) and Parr (2001) acknowledge, the term "psychosocial impact" is a multidimensional construct. Some authors consider it as synonymous with quality of life (QOL), subjective and psychological well-being, and levels of societal participation. Consequently, one of the key difficulties associated with research on the topic is a lack of clarification of the term "psychosocial" (Byng, Pound & Parr, 2000; Brumfitt, 2006; Herrmann, 1997). In this chapter, the term is taken literally as the psychological and social consequences of a motor speech disorder with QOL, subjective well-being, and societal participation, viewed predominantly as consequences or factors that contribute to psychosocial impact (Figure 5–1).

Byng, Pound, & Parr's (2000) framework for examining psychosocial effects is used broadly to direct the discussion. They categorize the effects as follows:

(a) Effects on the person
(b) Effects on lifestyle
(c) Effects on others in the immediate social context

Effects on the person incorporate psychological effects, effects on identity, self-concept, self-esteem, relationships, and roles with resulting impact on communication behavior and societal participation, well-being, and QOL. Effects on lifestyle include changes in employment status, leisure activities, social networks, and social inclusion as well as perceptions of barriers to communication. These effects result also in changes to societal participation, subjective well-being, and QOL. Effects on others in the immediate social context consider the psychological and social effects of motor speech disorders on other people close to the person (i.e., family, close friends, etc.).

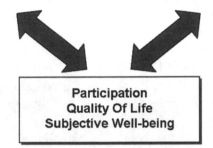

Figure 5–1. A framework for examining psychosocial impact.

The Effects on the Person: Psychological Effects

The emerging research and personal accounts from people with acquired motor speech disorders, specifically dysarthria, confirm that individuals can suffer anxiety and depression, experience a number of negative emotions in response to their speech disorders, and undergo changes to self-perception. Although these topics are discussed separately in the following sections, they are all strongly linked.

Anxiety and Depression

Sapir and Aronson (1990) as well as Brumfitt (2010) discuss the presence of anxiety and depression in people with acquired communication disorders. Symptoms of anxiety are psychological

as well as physical. Psychological characteristics of anxiety can include fearful anticipation, difficulty with concentration, constant worrying, heightened alertness, sleep disturbances, feelings of guilt, and negative thoughts. Physical characteristics typically involve fatigue, headaches, a feeling of tightness in the chest, breathlessness, irritability, loss of appetite, nausea, heart palpitations, muscular tension, and sweating. Anxiety can coexist with depression. Symptoms of depression include feelings of low mood for long periods of time; tiredness; difficulty concentrating; feelings of numbness, emptiness, and hopelessness; feeling guilty; and experiencing negative thoughts.

In neurological conditions in which anxiety and depression can arise, researchers distinguish between the emotional responses linked with the structural and/or neurobiochemical events caused by the neurological condition (primary depression) and reactions associated with consequences of the condition (secondary depression). Code and Herrmann (2003) include a third category, tertiary depression, which they suggest is provoked by psychosocial alterations and insufficient coping strategies. Depression (primary, secondary, and tertiary) is common in people with medical conditions associated with motor speech disorders. There are extensive accounts of depression following stroke (see Starkstein & Robinson, 1988; Turner-Stokes & Hassan, 2002) as well as traumatic brain injury (TBI) (Gouick & Gentleman, 2004). Dysarthria and AOS are both common consequences of stroke and TBI; therefore, depression and motor speech disorders must coexist. Depression also is prevalent in other conditions that give rise to dysarthria and AOS such as amyotrophic lateral sclerosis (ALS) (Hunter, Robinson, & Neilson, 1993; Montgomery & Erikson, 1987), multiple sclerosis (MS) (Wallin, Wilken, Turner, Williams, & Kane, 2006) and Parkinson's Disease (PD) (Murray, 1996; Remy, Doder, Lees, Turjanski, & Brooks, 2005). How much the presence of a motor speech disorder causes or contributes to secondary and tertiary depression is unknown. Further research is needed to clarify this relationship and explore specifically the distinctions between primary, secondary, and tertiary depression in people with motor speech disorders. Although people with acquired motor speech disorders might not have clinical depression, they may say that they are "depressed" and report feelings of sadness or loneliness among other negative emotions (Dickson, Barbour, Brady, Clark, & Paton, 2008; Miller, Noble, Jones, Allcock & Burn, 2008; Walshe & Miller, in press).

Negative Emotions

Qualitative studies involving people with dysarthria have referred to negative emotions in their accounts of living with a speech impairment. Three main categories of emotions can be identified: (1) emotions relating directly to the motor speech disorder itself (2) emotions relating to communication situations; and (3) emotions relating to consequences of the speech disorder and its associated medical condition on the person, his/her lifestyle, and quality of life (Table 5–1).

Not all feelings are negative. In Miller et al.'s (2008) study one person with communication impairment and PD was very upbeat regarding communication. This was linked with having received a definitive diagnosis of the disease and taking a positive approach to its management. Dickson et al., (2008), explored the psychosocial impact of dysarthria, interviewing 24 people with varying severities of dysarthria following stroke. One person, who prior to his stroke frequently worked away from home, reported having a new, more appreciative outlook on life. These positive feelings, that are not unusual in the chronic illness literature, may be in some way linked to acceptance and adaptation of the communication impairment and are considered again later in this chapter.

Changes to Perception of Self

"Self-identity," "self-esteem," "sense of self," "self-concept," and "self" are used interchangeably in the literature resulting in some confusion. In this chapter, "self" encompasses identity, self-concept,

Table 5–1. Negative Emotions Associated with Motor Speech Disorders

Emotions	Authors
Emotions Relating to Speech Disorder	
Worry about speech difficulties	Hartelius, Elmberg, Holm, Lövberg & Nikolaidis (2008)
Fear about getting "words out"	Dickson, Barbour, Brady, Clark, & Paton (2008); Miller, Noble, Jones, & Burn (2006)
Anger that speech is different	Dickson et al. (2008)
Self-hate due to inability to speak properly	Dickson et al. (2008)
Annoyance	Walshe & Miller (in press)
Helplessness regarding speech intelligibility	Dickson et al. (2008)
Emotions Relating to Communication Situations	
Embarrassment	Dickson et al. (2008), Miller et al. (2006), Walshe & Miller (in press)
Frustration	Dickson et al. (2008); Walshe & Miller (in press)
Lack of confidence	Dickson et al. (2008); Walshe & Miller (in press)
Worry and fear before speaking	Walshe & Miller (in press)
Nervous/uncomfortable in situations involving communication	Walshe & Miller (in press)
Inadequacy in response to listener reaction	Walshe & Miller (in press)
Angry/upset/hurt/frustrated by listener reaction	Walshe & Miller (in press); Dickson et al. (2008)
Feeling stupid in response to listener reaction	Dickson et al. (2008)
Emotions Relating to Consequences of the Speech Disorder and Its Associated Medical Condition on the Person and Quality of Life	
Worry about communication generally and in the future	Hartelius et al. (2008); Walshe & Miller (in press)
Upset thinking of the past	Yorkston et al. (2007)
Loss of independence generally	Walshe & Miller (in press)
Loneliness and feelings of isolation	Walshe & Miller (in press)
Depression	Dickson et al. (2008)

and self-esteem. Baumeister (1995) defines the identity component of self as:

> *A cluster of meaningful definitions that become attached to the body, including a name, social roles, membership of various groups, and various other attributes.* (p. 52)

Baumeister calls attention to the importance of unity and continuity in understanding identity. Rosenberg (1987) proposes that identity is based on feelings of personal sameness, suggesting that events, conditions, or circumstances that threaten one's sense of personal sameness could result in *depersonalization*, which he defines as, "the loss of a sense of personal identity, characteristically accompanied by a sense of unreality." (p. 193)

Stroke or TBI as well as progressive neurological conditions such as ALS, MS, and PD, all of which give rise to motor speech disorders, can threaten "one's sense of personal sameness" and result in depersonalization. This is evident in two notable accounts of the experience of a motor speech disorder after stroke provided by Robin Cant (1997) and Robert McCrum (1998). Cant, a social scientist and university lecturer, suffered a stroke resulting in a motor speech disorder (possibly dysarthria) and hemiplegia. Cant describes a feeling of depersonalization following his stroke:

> *It was almost as if I was one of the visitors visiting myself, and looking at my unfamiliar damaged body. It was as though the person confined to bed was someone else and I was going through the motions of explaining how they were feeling for them.* (p. 298)

McCrum, an editor and well-known author, also suffered a stroke resulting in a motor speech disorder. The enormity of the impact of stroke on McCrum's sense of identity is emphasized by the following extract:

> *. . . the cruel fact is that this former self is irretrievably shattered into a thousand pieces, and try as one may to glue those bits together again, the reconstituted version of the old self will never be better than a cracked, imperfect assembly, a constant mockery of one's former, successful individuality.* (p. 151)

Having an identity is a prerequisite for social interaction. Interacting with other people requires that one has some understanding of "you" and "I." With regard to impact of speech impairment and identity, McCrum (1998) states,

> *Limitations of mobility and articulacy strike at the heart of who one is as a person.* (p. 195)

The link between verbal communication and identity is emphasized throughout the literature (Brumfitt, 1993; Duchan, Maxwell, & Kovarsky, 1999; Fransella, 1972). Brumfitt and Clarke (1983) suggest:

> *Loss of speech may be experienced not simply as an external loss apparent to everyone but also a mutilation of the person's identity or even a contradiction of his/her self-definition.* (p. 91)

Exploring the relationship between motor speech disorder and identity is therefore important. More than half the people interviewed by Dickson et al., (2008) had negative changes in identity.

Walshe (2003a) explored the psychosocial impact of dysarthria in 31 people with dysarthria arising mainly from progressive neurological conditions and also found negative changes in identity. In both studies, speakers felt they were "not the same person" now. The altered perceptual quality of their speech and voice was commented on: "It doesn't sound like me," was a recurring theme across the studies and suggests that for individuals whose voice and speech are core tenets of identity, the impact can be significant.

Along with identity, people also have a great deal of beliefs or knowledge about themselves. This is their self-concept. Markus and Nurius (1987) define self-concept as a collection of self-knowledge and self-conceptions, formed through personal experiences and interpretation of the environment. One's self-concept can define and determine interaction with the environment. Symbolic interactionists such as Cooley (1902) and Mead (1925, 1934) believed that self-concept is purely a product of social interaction and that the appraisals of others shape self-concept.

Essentially, self-concept involves how we think of ourselves now, how we imagine ourselves in the future, and the way we thought about ourselves in the past. Although self-concept is relatively stable, it is also susceptible to change as the individual encounters new roles, situations, and life-transitions (Demo, 1992). The onset of of a motor speech disorder may be one such transition. Other factors that might influence changes in self-concept include interpersonal factors (Baumeister, 1995). Thus, a change in interpersonal relationships or in the nature of that relationship

(e.g., following motor speech disorder) might affect self-concept.

Studies to date suggest that people with dysarthria experience changes to self-concept. Hartelius, Elmberg, Holm, Lövberg and Nikolaidis (2008) evaluated speech difficulties as perceived by 55 people with dysarthria arising from a range of progressive and nonprogressive conditions found that 53% of participants agreed with the statement, "My speech difficulties negatively affect my self-image." Walshe (2003b) examined changes in self-concept of 31 people with acquired progressive neurological conditions and dysarthria, using a modified version of the Head Injury Semantic Differential Scale (Tyerman & Humphrey, 1984). Individuals had to rate themselves on 20 given constructs (self-confident, lack of confidence, self-conscious, unself-conscious, etc.). People were asked to rate themselves first with respect to how they viewed themselves six months prior to the onset of dysarthria and, second, over the two weeks prior to the interview. Results indicated that dysarthria could have a negative impact on the speaker with individuals demonstrating statistically significant changes in 18 of the 20 constructs examined. Only two constructs (friendly–unfriendly and intelligent–stupid) remained unchanged. Miller et al., (2008) also used a semantic differential scale to examine self-perception of communication changes in a group of 104 people with dysarthria and PD. They found that speakers perceived themselves more negatively as communicators since the onset of PD. However, people still perceived themselves as friendly, caring, and of value. This notion that people still perceived themselves as "friendly" in both studies suggests that the speakers were still interested in communicating despite their negative self-concept as communicators.

The impact of change in self-concept has implications for interaction and participation in communication situations and in society generally. Baumeister describes how people generally hold positive and often exaggerated opinions of themselves. He states that people will seek opportunities to make a good impression and will avoid events that present them in a less positive and favorable light. Shrauger and Schoeneman (1979) and Layder (1993) contend that it is the perception of how other people appraise individuals that is important in considering self-concept. This notion of others' appraisal is significant in interpreting what influences self-concept for people with motor speech disorders.

Concerns regarding listeners' reactions to speech are recurrent themes in speakers' accounts of dysarthria. Cant (1997) worried that people who did not know him might perceive him differently:

> For me my voice was vital for my work. It was the essential "tool" of my trade, and I feared students would view me differently. Would they see me as second best? Less worthy? Defective? Would they hear my disability rather than the content of what I was saying? (p. 300)

The fear that listeners will perceive the speaker as "drunk" or "stupid" or "on drugs" also is persistent (Cant, 1997; Dickson et al., 2008; Miller et al., 2006; Walshe & Miller, in press).

One of the core features of self-concept is self-esteem. Self-esteem is the generalized or global evaluation of the self. It can be subdivided into two main processes: self-evaluation and self-worth. Self-evaluation involves the comparison between Real Self and Ideal Self (i.e., differences between how the person perceives him or her self now and how he or she would like to be). This provides important information with regard to motivation and realistic expectations from therapy. Self-worth involves feeling that self is important and useful. Vickery, Sepehri and Evans (2008) found that low self-esteem is associated with the impact of stroke. Both McCrum and Cant refer to self-esteem in their autobiographical accounts and both do so with specific reference to speech therapy. McCrum (1998) refers to speech therapy as "one of the battlegrounds" between himself and his wife:

> I found it humiliating to have to accept that, though my thought processes seemed unimpaired, my utterances needed help from a speech therapist. The failure of articulation seemed such a fundamental failure, and one that went to the core of my self-esteem. (p. 73)

Cant (1997) states,

> . . . I found speech therapy to be the most stressful of all the therapies. Perhaps this is because one's self-esteem is more damaged by not being able to pronounce words properly. (p. 301)

This raises the question of whether we, as clinicians, do much in therapy to help rebuild the speakers' self-esteem, and this issue is taken up later again in considering psychosocial impact in clinical practice.

Knowing the impact of a motor speech disorder on identity, self-concept and self-esteem can uncover a greater understanding of the nature and extent of psychological impact on the speaker. Although the literature would suggest that there are many common themes in terms of impact of motor speech disorders, it is acknowledged that the reaction can be highly individual (Walshe, 2003a). Understanding changes in self-perception should help explain individual reactions and help analyze methods of coping and adapting to speech disorders. Charmaz (1983) and Nettleton (1995), among others, discuss the fact that identity and self-concept can change over time as people learn to live with their conditions, and Cant concludes his account by stating, "I think I can live with the new me" (p. 304). It is important to track the evolution of changes in identity, self-concept, and self-esteem in people with motor speech disorders and reflect on what gives rise to positive change.

Relationship Changes

A further psychological effect of motor speech disorders that can add to psychological impact is changes to relationships. It is established that acquired communication disorders such as aphasia impact negatively on relationship and friendships (Davidson, Howe, Worrall, Hickson, & Togher, 2008). People with motor speech disorders also can experience changes in relationships.

Some people with dysarthria in Dickson et al.'s study (2008) said that they could no longer keep up with conversations with friends and family, including spouses, and as a result felt "left out" and "different." People in other studies reported arguments with spouses and family members because

the speaker was said to mumble or because the listener was not attending (Miller, Noble, Jones, & Burn, 2006). In Walshe & Miller's study (in press) many of people interviewed reported negative changes in relationships with either spouses or friends since the onset of their dysarthria. Relationships with young children can be difficult as evident from accounts in Dickson et al.'s study. One individual felt she had not bonded with her youngest child because of her speech difficulties. In addition, she perceived that his speech was underdeveloped because of her reduced communicative interactions with him. Another person with dysarthria and young children decided that he did not want to see them until his speech was intelligible, as he did not want to embarrass them. Whether relationships with younger family members are more problematic for people with motor speech disorders than relationships with spouses or adult family members is unknown. This information would be important in planning support services and may help understand individual psychological reactions to motor speech disorders.

Relationship changes are not always negative. In some instances, the speech disorder and the condition associated with the disorder often can bring the families closer together and strengthen relationships (McCrum, 1998).

Role Changes

Relationship changes can arise as a result of role changes, particularly within the family. Changes in role can occur because of motor speech difficulty. These roles can involve taking up the role of homemaker while the spouse becomes the breadwinner or taking over other roles, which require verbal interaction (e.g., carrying out financial transactions, etc.) (Walshe & Miller, in press). However, these roles can resume for people whose speech is improving. In Dickson et al.'s (2008) study, some participants resumed some previously fulfilled social and recreational roles as their speech improved. This may not be an option for people with progressive degenerative dysarthria and requires further consideration.

In summary, motor speech disorders can be associated with anxiety and depression as well as changes in self-perception. Further psychological effects are changes to relationships and roles. How these psychological changes impact on levels of participation, subjective well-being, and quality of life is considered next.

Consequences of Psychological Effects

The psychological consequences of a motor speech disorder can directly impact on speech production. In Hartelius, et al's 2008 study, 49% of participants agreed with the statement, "my speech difficulties get worse when I am angry or sad." This is a familiar complaint. Griffin and Greene (1994) describe the negative impact of a spouse's reaction to her husband's dysarthric speech, claiming that a decrease in speech intelligibility occurred in this man's speech following a series of negative comments made by his wife.

Participation is influenced directly by psychological reactions. Participation,

as discussed by Yorkston and Baylor (Chapter 6, "Measurement of Communicative Participation," this book), is defined as the involvement in life situations (WHO, 2001). Communication for participation is defined as: "holding a conversation, starting and sustaining an interchange of thoughts and ideas, carried out by means of spoken, written, sign or other forms of language, with one or more people one knows or who are strangers in formal or casual settings" (WHO, 2001: p. 135)

The psychological impact of a speech disorder can affect participation. The literature suggests that anxiety and depression can result in withdrawal from social interactions. People with motor speech disorders who have experienced changes to self-perception may limit participation in an attempt to live with their speech disorder. Avoidance of speaking situations can result in social isolation as individuals reduce levels of societal participation and involvement in situations in which verbal communication is likely. Situations in which negative feedback is anticipated may be avoided as negative feedback, or perceived negative feedback, can have a detrimental effect on self-esteem. People with acquired dysarthria reveal that they have changed their communication behavior and limited societal participation in an attempt to cope with their speech disorder (Dickson et al., 2008; Miller et al., 2006; Walshe & Miller, in press). Changes in communication behavior include the following:

(1) Adopting the role of bystander or listener in communication situations rather than be involved in interaction. This change is reported regularly (Dickson et al., 2008; Miller et al., 2006;

Walshe, 2003a) and arises from a fear of negative evaluation and lack of confidence in participating in conversation. The following extract from Miller et al., (2006) illustrates this point:

> *I don't speak unless I have to as I'm frightened I don't get my words out, and if I go to the hospital my wife comes and does all the talking.* (p. 237)

(2) Avoidance of communication situations is common, particularly when they involve interaction with strangers, situations in which the speaker will have to speak against background noise, speak under pressure, or when there is speed demanded in delivery of a message. There is a belief that under these environmental conditions, communication will fail. This expectation is accompanied by a fear of negative evaluations. Speakers perceive that listeners are attending to speech production rather than message content.

> *Frequently, the qualities of speech affect the value placed on its content. There is even a sense in which poorly pronounced and slurred words are seen to be the consequence of not making an effort to talk properly.* (Cant, 1997; p. 300)

(3) Talking on the telephone is avoided regularly by people with dysarthria (Dickson et al., 2008; Walshe & Miller, in press). The lack of visual clues for the listener means that speakers are less likely to be understood. Listeners' perceptions that they are drunk or frequent listener requests for repetition result in many avoiding this speaking situation.

The psychological impact of motor speech disorders also results in changes to the style of communication. People avoid words they perceive as difficult, report a reluctance to engage in small talk, tell jokes, argue, or engage in camaraderie (Beukelman, Yorkston, & Reichle, 2000; Miller et al., 2006; Walshe & Miller, in press). One person with MS and dysarthria (UC) who participated in Yorkston et al.'s (2007) qualitative study on satisfaction with communicative participation, describes changes to her communication:

> *Needless to say (having to think about communication) has taken a lot of quality away from communication. And I tend not to engage in extra chat, that is talking just to talk, to socialize.* (p. 443)

People also tend to keep their communications short. Shortening the intended message is a common practice in people with motor speech disorders, mainly because of timing and time pressure. Higginbotham and Wilkins (1999) discuss this issue with reference to augmentative and alternative communication (AAC) users, but it could be applied to other individuals with less severe speech disorders. They state,

> *It happens all too often that augmented communicators overvalue the time of others in relation to the value of their own communication desires and needs. The result may be that they do not communicate at all or keep their contributions as minimal and "practical" as possible.* (p. 57).

Changing the style of communication and avoidance of people and communication situations is not specific to motor speech disorders and is pervasive in other acquired communication disorders such as aphasia and spasmodic dysphonia (Jordan & Kaiser, 1996; Papathanasiou, MacDonald, Whurr,

Brookes, & Jahanshahi, 1997). This avoidance behavior can be a direct result of difficulty speaking but often the behavior, not unlike that of people who stutter, is in response to anxiety regarding speech production and fear of negative evaluations.

In summary, reduced levels of participation can be associated with changes to communication style and behavior as well as withdrawal from communication. These can arise from negative changes in self-perception as well as depression and anxiety. Participation also can be affected by relationship tensions and role changes within the family. This can lead to further loneliness and isolation. Consequently, reduced participation and changes in relationships and roles within the family must impact on quality of life. There is no real consensus on how quality of life is defined, and for the purposes of this discussion, the following definition is used, "an individual's perception of their position in life in the context of the culture and value systems in which they live and in relation to their goals, expectations, standards, and concerns." (World Health Organization Quality of Life Group, 1995: p. 1405).

Quality of life and subjective well-being are strongly interlinked. Subjective well-being includes happiness, life satisfaction, morale, and positive affect (Diener, 2009). The psychological effects of motor speech disorders on quality of life and well-being are relatively unexplored, but it is known that psychological factors such as clinical depression are related to increased mortality, functional dependence, poor improvement and participation in rehabilitation, longer stays in hospital, poor cognitive function, reduced social activity, and

failure to return to work (Turner-Stokes & Hassan, 2002). How these factors must be considered in clinical practice is taken up later in the chapter.

Effects on Lifestyle: Social Factors

Little is known about the direct impact of motor speech disorders on the lifestyle of the individual. Effects on lifestyle include changes in employment status, leisure activities, social networks, and social inclusion and perceptions of barriers to communication.

Change in employment does occur for people with dysarthria as a result of their speech disorder (Walshe & Miller, in press). These changes will depend on the severity of the impairment and the nature of the person's premorbid employment. People whose career requires clear articulate and intelligible speech (e.g., teachers, sales personnel, telemarketers, receptionists, lecturers, etc.) can find it difficult to return to work or remain in their current employment. Garcia, Laroche, and Barrette (2002) examined the perceived barriers to work re-integration for a group of people with a range of communication disorders. Thirteen of the 78 participants had dysarthria. Garcia et al. (2002) identified a range of personal and environmental factors that influence work reintegration. Personal factors for people with dysarthria included not having inflection or assertiveness in their voices and anticipation of what people might think of them and their disorder. Organizational factors such as noise, telephone use, speaking to bosses, and communication with clients were all identified as problematic. Issues related to employers' expectations on efficiency also were identified as well as the speed at which tasks were requested. Finally, the perceptions of the attitudes of others also were considered a significant barrier to work re-integration. Problems with work re-integration might result in people taking lower paid positions. One participant in Walshe and Miller's study (in press) had ALS and was forced to give up his job as an architect because of his dysarthria and to take a lower paid position in which interaction with clients was not required.

A dearth of research exists on changes to social networks following the onset of a motor speech disorder. It is known that people with aphasia communicate with fewer friends and have smaller social networks when compared with people without aphasia (Cruice, Worrall, & Hickson, 2006; Davidson et al., 2008) and much emphasis often is placed on social network size. The growth of social network sites (e.g., Facebook, MySpace, etc.) has incited popular interest on the size and characteristics of one's social networks (Lewis, Kaufman, Gonzalez, Wimmer, & Christakis, 2008). Russell (1996) among others suggests that it is not the size of the network but rather the person's perceptions of the quality of the relationships within that network that is important. Changes to size and quality of the interactions within social networks for people with motor speech disorders would seem to be important for future research.

Little also is known about individuals' perceptions of social inclusion and exclusion. Using qualitative methods, Parr (2007) examined social exclusion in 20 people with severe aphasia many years after their stroke. She found evidence of social exclusion at three levels:

1. Infrastructural level (e.g., limited access to employment, inadequate income, access to housing, health, education services, information, and communication technology, etc.).
2. Interpersonal level (e.g., limited associations with groups and places in society such as family, neighbors, friends, work colleagues, etc.).
3. Personal level (e.g., alienation, lack of identity, low self-esteem, dependence, etc.)

Leisure activities that involve verbal communication and interaction may change as a result of motor speech disorders.

Consequences of Social Effects

Social consequences of a motor speech disorder can impact on participation, well-being, and quality of life (QOL). The nature and extent of this impact is difficult to quantify in the absence of any significant work in the area of motor speech disorders. It is hypothesized that there may be changes in social life depending on the age or life stage of the individual. Dalemans, De Witte, Wade, and Von den Heuvel (2008) carried out a systematic review of the literature on social participation of working age (20–65 years) people with aphasia but were unable to reach any firm conclusions due to methodological limitations of included studies and a failure for many to define "participation."

Younger people (i.e., <65 years) with motor speech disorders must face different challenges to older people (i.e.,

>65 years) in terms of the social effects of a disorder. Loss of employment or change in employment status can have financial implications for individuals and their families with significant implications for lifestyle. There also can be a stigma attached to being unemployed, particularly if the motor speech disorder is not obvious or severe. Breakwell (1986), in her studies on unemployment, states that isolation is common in the unemployed and particularly in the 25–55 year age group. Loss of employment also has implications for loss of social contacts and social networks, which can further reduce participation and impact on subjective well-being and quality of life.

Older people (i.e., >65 years) with acquired motor speech disorders can face a number of different social challenges compared to younger people. They already may be retired, have grown up children, and have different financial situations, but they can still face significant changes associated with aging that impact QOL. These changes can include moving to residential care, experiencing the loss of a spouse, and developing health conditions related to aging, all exacerbated by the presence of communication difficulty.

Psychosocial Impact on Others in the Immediate Social Context

Few studies have examined specifically the psychological impact of communication disorders on people close to the individual. Many have instead focused on the impact of the medical condition that can give rise to motor speech disorders. For example, Buschenfeld, Morris, and Lockwood (2009) looked at the

experience of partners of young stroke survivors (<60 years) two to seven years after stroke. Three of the nine people interviewed were partners of people who had communication difficulty following stroke. In addition, one was the partner of someone with severe aphasia. These partners reported major changes in their own lives since their spouses' or partners' strokes. These included restrictions in social life, changes to roles and relationships, and changes to employment. Buschenfeld et al. (2009) concluded that caring impacts on partners' sense of self and identity. In this instance, it was not possible to separate out the findings for partners of people with communication impairment, but other researchers (Bakes, Kroenke, Plue, Perkins, & Williams, 2006; Rombough, Howse, & Bartfay, 2006) have compared the burden of care experienced by caregivers of people with and without aphasia and concluded that caring for an individual with a communication impairment can be more detrimental to mental health and QOL.

The severity of the communication disorder must play a role. Michallet, Tetreault, and Le Dorze (2003) looked at the impact of severe aphasia on spouses. These spouses perceived themselves to be stressed due to changes in lifestyle, communication changes, interpersonal relationships, leisure activities, responsibilities, and finances.

Specific medical conditions, because of the nature of the illness, also could give rise to a reduction in caregivers' social networks. Roland, Jenkins, and Johnson (2010) looked at changes in the social networks of spouses of people with PD. They found that loss of social interactions involving work and loss of interactions with related friends and family were primarily due to the unpredictability of the spouse's PD symptoms, strict medical regimens, and the person with PD's general discomfort in social interactions. This suggests that a number of variables can influence reductions in caregivers' and spouses' social networks. The presence of a speech disorder is another variable. The extent to which the motor speech disorder exacerbates the problem is unknown.

A case for providing support for these caregivers can be made clearly from the current body of research in the area of aphasia and chronic illness. In the absence of any substantial evidence, the case is harder to make for caregivers of people with motor speech disorders, and further investigation is required.

Considering Psychosocial Impact in Clinical Practice

Undoubtedly, clinicians consider psychosocial impact in clinical practice, albeit often informally. Brumfitt (2006) surveyed 521 speech-language pathologists (SLPs) on their views on psychosocial aspects of aphasia management. Although the response rate was low (33%), the majority of respondents (97%) stated that psychosocial aspects were either important or very important to the overall management of their clients. Only 23% of respondents stated that they were not prepared for the challenge of managing psychosocial effects. Brumfitt reflects that although clinicians reported an interest in this area, not many assessed psychosocial impact routinely. It is suggested that the first challenge for SLPs is to know what and how to assess psychosocial impact.

Assessment Considerations

Three key considerations exist for assessment of psychosocial impact of acquired motor speech disorders. First, assessment should be holistic, incorporating psychological and social factors and the consequences of these factors for the individual and those within his immediate environment (see Figure 5–1). Second, one should consider the impact of the motor speech disorder in the context of other medical, environmental, and personal factors. Finally, assessments should be valid and reliable providing credible outcome data.

Assessment of Psychological Effects

Screening for depression and anxiety should be undertaken if the clinician perceives these to be present. The rationale for screening is that clinical depression and anxiety disorders frequently are undiagnosed and can be amenable to treatment. The U.S. Preventive Services Task Force (USPSTF) (2009) has issued a Recommendation Statement on screening for depression in adults. It recommends a brief two–question screening test:

Q1: "Over the past two weeks, have you felt down, depressed, or hopeless?"

Q2: "Over the past two weeks, have you felt little interest or pleasure in doing things?"

Thomas (2010) provides a good overview of assessments for anxiety and depression for people with acquired communication impairments that may assist clinicians in examining this area. Aphasia-friendly assessments for people with aphasia are included as motor speech disorders and aphasia can co-exist.

The USPSTF also recommends that screening should take place "when staff-assisted care supports are in place to assure accurate diagnosis, effective treatment, and follow-up" (p. 784). In reviewing the evidence for intervention for depression, the task force found good evidence that treating depression in adults and older adults, identified through screening in primary care settings, with antidepressants, psychotherapy, or both decreases clinical morbidity.

Assessment should consider an evaluation of changes in self-perception. Assessment of self-concept often is carried out to gain further insight into identity and self-esteem. McAdams (1993) and Hill (1997) discuss the fact that a sense of personal identity is created and maintained through telling one's life story. This life story is created from the perceptions of one's past, present, and future life. Assessing self-concept through looking at Past Self and Present Self can be seen as a way of accessing particular aspects of identity at a specific point in time (Ellis-Hill & Horn, 2000). Assessing self-concept also provides some information on self-esteem as it is one component of self-concept.

Semantic differential scales have been used to explore self-concept (see Walshe, 2003b; Miller et al., 2008). Assessments of self-esteem include the Visual Analogue Self-esteem Scale (Brumfitt & Sheeran, 1999) and the Rosenberg Self-Esteem Scale (Rosenberg, 1965). Scales under development that examine the effect of dysarthria on the speaker include the Dysarthria Impact Profile

(Walshe, Peach, & Miller, 2009). This scale explores five domains: (1) the effect of dysarthria on me as a speaker, (2) accepting my dysarthria, (3) how I feel others react to my speech, (4) how dysarthria affects my communication with others, and (5) dysarthria relative to other worries and concerns. Other self-report instruments, such as the "Living with Dysarthria" questionnaire (Hartelius et al., 2008) examine some important domains discussed previously, for example, how emotions, situations, and persons affect communication and roles in which the speaker feels restricted.

Assessment of Social Effects

Surprisingly few tools are available that specifically examine the physical, environmental, and attitudinal barriers that can exist for the person with motor speech disorders. The Situational Intelligibility Survey (Berry & Saunders, 1983), although devised as a checklist for people with hearing impairment, frequently is used to explore environmental barriers to communication. Other checklists such as the Communication Effectiveness Survey (modified CETI) (Yorkston, Beukelman, Strand, & Bell, 1999; Ball, Beukelman, & Pattee, 2004) can be used to examine the speaker's perception of communication effectiveness in different settings, highlighting for SLPs the barriers to effective communication. Donovan, Velozo, and Rosenbek (2007) have further developed the Communicative Effectiveness Survey (CES) and are establishing its psychometric properties.

Regarding assessment of barriers to resuming employment, including questions on changes and evaluating barriers to re-integration back into employment is important particularly for younger individuals who are not yet retired and who wish to return to work. Environmental factors, based on Garcia, et al's. (2002) work can be explored with individuals. Questions should examine both the organizational barriers (task demands, communication environment, etc.) as well as societal barriers (attitudes of work colleagues and clients, awareness of the disorder, socio-economic supports, etc.).

In investigating the social networks of people with aphasia, Cruice, et al. (2006), used the Social Activities Checklist (SOCACT; Cruice, 2001 in Worrall & Hickson, 2003) and social network analysis (Antonucci & Akiyama, 1987) to examine social network change. They are suitable for people with motor speech disorders. *The Social Networks: A Communication Inventory for Individuals with Complex Communication Needs and their Communication Partners* (Blackstone & Berg, 2003) also can be used with people with motor speech disorders, particularly those with severe impairment who use AAC systems.

Assessment of Psychosocial Impact on Others in the Immediate Social Context

Conscious consideration of the impact of a motor speech disorder on those close to the individual may be sufficient to direct attention here and consider the support systems available. However, the Carer Communication Outcome After Stroke (Carer COAST) scale (Long, Hesketh, & Bowen, 2009) is useful in directing discussion on caregiver burden. It has been piloted by the authors on caregivers of people

with dysarthria and aphasia, and although further work is required on establishing its psychometric properties, it does show promise in clinical practice.

Assessment of Impact of Psychological and Social Effects

The psychosocial impact of motor speech disorders on participation, QOL, and well-being are considered in this section. Assessments of societal participation are limited, and the development of the Communication Participation Item Bank described by Yorkston and Baylor in Chapter 6 of this volume shows most promise in this area. QOL assessments and subjective well-being assessments are numerous and often relate specifically to stroke. Table 5–2 lists some that are used more frequently with people with communication disorders, including aphasia, and are appropriate for people with motor speech disorders.

Assessment of Motor Speech Disorder in Context

The context in which the motor speech disorder exists should be considered in assessment and intervention. Fatigue and cognitive impairment, which can co-exist with dysarthria in specific medical conditions (e.g., MS, PD, Huntington's disease, etc.) can impact on performance on motor speech assessments, making it difficult to extrapolate the true impact of the speech disorder itself. In addition, the medical condition, which gave rise to the speech disorder, can present with its own challenges and exacerbate the speech disorder. Fatigue associated with MS can result

Table 5–2. Assessments Used to Evaluate Quality of Life and Well-being in Populations with Communication Impairment

Assessment Measure
Visual Analog Mood Scales (Stern, 1997).
Burden of Stroke Scale (Doyle, McNeil, Mikolic, Prieto, Hula, Lustig, & Elman, 2004).
Stroke and Quality of Life Scale –39 (SAQOL–39) (Hilari, Byng, Lamping, & Smith, 2003).
Aachen Life Quality Scale (Engell, Hutter, Willmes, & Huber, 2003).
WHOQOL Instrument (The WHOQOL Group, 1998).
Quality of Communication Life Scale (ASHA QCL) (Paul, Frattali, Holland, Thompson, Caperton, & Slater, 2004).
Stroke Impact Scale (Duncan, Wallace, Lou, Johnson, Embretson, & Laster, 1999).
Short Form 36 Health Survey (SF–36) (Ware & Sherbourne, 1992).
Ryff Psychological Well-being Scale (Ryff, 1989).
Psychosocial Well-being Index (Lyon, Carisk, Keisler, Rosenbek, Levine, Kampula et al., 1997).
Sickness Impact Profile (Bergner, Bobbitt, Carter, & Gilson, 1981.

in an increase in dysarthric speech (Blaney & Lowe-Strong, 2009; Yorkston et al., 2007). For people with PD, problems with freezing, attention, and fatigue can impact on speech production and communication (Miller, et al. 2006). Cognitive impairment that exists in association with progressive neurological conditions such as MS, PD, and Huntington's disease can add to further problems with communication (Hartelius, Jonsson, Rickeberg, & Laakso, 2009; Miller et al., 2006; Yorkston et al., 2007).

Reports from people with MS who had cognitive, language, speech, and swallowing impairments stated that these impairments were "minor when compared to the other symptoms of MS (e.g., tiredness, eyesight, coordination, depression, frustration, incontinence, and permanent damage done by the condition)" (Klugman & Ross, 2002, p. 216). Walshe (2003a) examined the perceptions of people who had acquired dysarthria arising from a range of progressive and nonprogressive disorders. It was evident from these accounts that although the speech disorder might seem a devastating problem for the individual, this often was not the case.

One way of examining this area is to ask speakers to rate speech relative to other worries and concerns at that point in time (Walshe et al., 2009). This provides the clinician with insight into the importance of speech to the individual and provides a perspective on motivation and commitment to rehabilitation. The importance of speech versus physical function may not stay constant throughout the course of an illness. For example, in Walshe and Miller's study (in press), one of the participants saw speech as being very important, particularly in the past, but at the time of interview, his physical impairment was of greater concern as it was affecting his activities more than speech. This could be more relevant when working with people who have progressive degenerative speech disorders in which the course of medical and physical conditions are unstable and remain in decline.

Considerations for Intervention

A detailed discussion on intervention approaches is beyond the scope of this chapter, and it is clear that before we can make gains in this area, more must be learned about the psychosocial impact on the speaker. Nonetheless, what we know currently can assist in taking some immediate action in the construction and enactment of therapy. For example, focus on impairment alone is not likely to improve psychosocial outcome. Studies conclude that severity of speech impairment does not relate to the person's perception of the severity of the disorder or its impact on the speaker (Ball et al., 2004; Dickson et al. 2008; Hartelius et al., 2008; Walshe, 2003a). Although this relationship needs to be more systematically examined, strategies to tackle negative psychosocial

impact will need to be integrated into therapy programs.

Cant and McCrum's earlier references to speech therapy and self-esteem imply that we must consider our role in the delivery of impairment based therapy. Simmons-Mackie and Damico (1999) eloquently discuss the dynamics that exist between clinician and client suggesting that clinician and client adopt "necessary roles as competent expert and incompetent patient in order for therapy to proceed in an orderly and efficient fashion" (p. 313).

Direct positive experiences, in the clinical setting and beyond, which convince people that they are competent are important to self-esteem. Considering experiences that will help rebuild self-esteem should be integrated into the therapy program.

Moving therapy beyond the clinical environment also is an important consideration. Educating key stakeholders involved in interaction with people with motor speech disorders is an important SLP role. This includes employers, work colleagues, general public, policy makers, etc. Education needs to continue within health-care service providers as speakers report negative attitudes within healthcare settings. This is borne out by Fox and Pring's (2005) findings that medical physicians tended to underestimate the cognitive competence of people with dysarthria.

Specific approaches to psychosocial impact such as Personal Construct Theory (PCT) (Kelly, 1955), life coaching (Worrall, Brown, Cruice, Davidson, Hersh et al., 2010) and Solution Focused Brief Therapy (SFBT) may play a role in directly tackling the psychosocial impact. Worrall et al., report some success with life-coaching to help people with aphasia. Burns (2010) provides an example of the clinical application of SFBT with a client with PD and communication impairment, and Brumfitt (1999) suggests that there is much we can learn from other areas of psychology and sociology. Clearly, more research on efficacy of approaches is required with a warning to SLPs to remain within the scope of practice.

Directions for Research

We need to learn more about the psychosocial impact of motor speech disorders in order to assist the development of appropriate interventions and outcome measures and to assist in policy planning and development. In addition to the questions raised previously, a number of additional central questions remain unanswered. For example, what is the nature and extent of psychological impact of motor speech disorders on the individuals and their caregivers? What role do variables such as severity of impairment, etiology, time postonset, concomitant physical disability, age, gender, financial status, social support, coping mechanisms, etc., play in influencing the psychosocial impact of motor speech disorders? Specifically, do the experiences of people with dysarthria differ from those of people with AOS? How do experiences of people with motor speech disorders differ from those of people with other communication disorders (e.g., aphasia, spasmodic dysphonia, hearing impairment, cognitive impairment, etc.)? Baylor, Yorkston and Eadie's (2005) exploration of the experiences of people with spasmodic

dysphonia suggests that many common themes exist (negative impact on self-concept, self-esteem, avoidance of communication situations). However, Garcia, et al.'s (2002) exploration of factors affecting work integration suggests that people with dysarthria can differ in relation to perceived environmental and attitudinal barriers. Findings of a recent study by Brumfitt (2006), in which 63% of SLPs did not differentiate between the psychosocial effects of dysarthria, dysphagia, and aphasia, suggest that a need exists to delineate among disorders.

Further questions arise regarding differences in the experiences of people with acquired motor speech disorders compared with experiences of developmental motor speech disorders. It is known that older people with cerebral palsy who are AAC users can experience social exclusion, loneliness, and isolation as a result of their communication difficulties (Balandin, Berg, & Waller, 2006). Safilios-Rothschild (1981) and Weinberg (1988) suggest, in the absence of any supporting empirical data, that there may be differences in perception of disability between congenital and acquired conditions. Safilios-Rothschild asserts that people with acquired disability will have experienced at least some years as a nondisabled person and

> . . . *may have their own prejudiced attitudes towards the disabled.* (p. 7)

One could argue that people who have developmental motor speech disorders (e.g., following cerebral palsy) may have accommodated this into their identity, but no evidence supports this hypothesis.

Conclusion

It is safe to conclude that acquired motor speech disorders significantly can impact psychological and social functioning, but there is still much more work to be done in the area, and the literature drawn on here is from a limited selection. It might seem that we are a long way off from having strong robust evidence base for interventions in this area, but there is much that we can build on from similar disciplines. The common strands that link motor speech disorders with other related fields (aphasia, spasmodic dysphonia, hearing impairment, and even fluency) (see Bricker-Katz, Lincoln, & McCabe, 2009; Finn, Howard, & Kubala, 2005) could help clinicians negotiate a clearer pathway in clinical practice. In addition, the chronic illness literature, already well-developed in examining psychosocial impact in conditions that co-exist with motor speech disorders, could provide some additional valuable guidance. Building on the shoulders of this research should ensure that we have a firm footing on which to tackle the many questions posed here, ensuring that this area of motor speech disorders will forge ahead rather than lag behind over the coming years.

References

Antonius, K., Beukelman, D., & Reid, R. (1996). Communication disability of Parkinson's disease: Perceptions of dysarthric speakers and their primary communication partners. In D. A. Robin, K. M. Yorkston, & D. R. Beukelman (Eds.), *Disorders of motor speech: assessment, treatment and clinical characterization* (pp. 275–286). Baltimore, MD: Paul Brookes.

Antonucci T. C., & Akiyama, H. (1987). Social networks in adult life and a preliminary examination of the convoy model. *Journal of Gerontology, 42,* 519–527.

Bakes, T., Kroenke, K., Plue, L., Perkins, S., & Williams, S. (2006). Outcomes among family caregivers of aphasic versus non-aphasic stroke survivors. *Rehabilitation Nursing, 31,* 33–42.

Balandin, S., Berg, N., & Waller, A. (2006). Assessing the loneliness of older people with cerebral palsy. *Disability and Rehabilitation, 28,* 469–479.

Ball, L. J., Beukelman, D. R., & Pattee, G. L. (2004). Communication effectiveness of individuals with amyotrophic lateral sclerosis. *Journal of Communication Disorders, 37,* 197–215

Baumeister, R. (1995). Self and identity: An introduction. In A. Tesser (Ed.), *Advanced social psychology* (pp. 51–97). New York, NY: McGraw Hill.

Baylor, C., Yorkston, K. M., & Eadie, T. (2005). The consequences of spasmodic dysphonia on communication related quality of life: A qualitative study of the insider's experiences. *Journal of Communication Disorders, 38,* 395–419.

Bergner, M., Bobbitt, R., Carter, W., & Gilson, B. (1981). The sickness impact profile: Development and final revision of a health status measure. *Medical Care, 19,* 787–805.

Berry, W. R., & Saunders, S. B. (1983). Environmental education: The universal management approach for adults with dysarthria. In W. R. Berry (Ed.), *Clinical dysarthria* (pp. 203–216). San Diego, CA: College Hill Press.

Beukelman, D. A., Yorkston, K., & Reichle, J. (Eds.) (2000). *Augmentative and alternative communication for adults with acquired communication disorders.* Baltimore, MD: Paul Brookes.

Blackstone, S., & Hunt Berg, M. (2003). *Social networks: A communication inventory for individuals with complex communication needs and their communication partners.* Monterey, CA: Augmentative Communication.

Blaney, B. E., & Lowe-Strong, A. (2009). The impact of fatigue on communication in multiple sclerosis. The insider's perspective. *Disability and Rehabilitation, 31,* 170–180.

Breakwell, G. (1986). *Coping with threatened identities.* London, UK: Methuen.

Bricker-Katz, G., Lincoln, M., & McCabe, P. (2009). A life-time of stuttering: How emotional reactions to stuttering impact activities and participation in older people. *Disability and Rehabilitation, 31,* 1742–1752.

Brumfitt, S. (1993). Losing your sense of self: What aphasia can do. *Aphasiology, 7,* 349–371.

Brumfitt, S. (1999). *The social psychology of communication impairment.* London, UK: Whurr.

Brumfitt, S. (2006). Psychosocial aspects of aphasia: Speech and language therapists' views on professional practice. *Disability and Rehabilitation, 28,* 523–534.

Brumfitt, S. (2010). *Psychological well-being and acquired communication impairments.* Chichester, UK: Wiley-Blackwell.

Brumfitt, S., & Clarke, P. (1983). An application of psychotherapeutic techniques to the management of aphasia. In C. Code & D. Müller (Eds.), *Aphasia therapy* (pp. 89–100). London, UK: Cole and Whurr.

Brumfitt, S., & Sheeran, P. (1999). *VASES: The Visual Analogues Self-Esteem Scale.* Bicester, UK: Winslow Press.

Burns, K. (2010). Solution focused brief therapy for people with acquired communication impairments. In S. Brumfitt (Ed.), *Psychological well-being and acquired communication impairments* (pp. 197–215). Chichester UK: Wiley-Blackwell.

Buschenfeld, K., Morris, R., & Lockwood S. (2009). The experience of partners of young stroke survivors. *Disability and Rehabilitation, 31,* 1643–1651.

Byng, S., Pound, C., & Parr, S. (2000). Living with aphasia: A framework for ther-apy interventions. In I. Papathanasiou (Ed.), *Acquired neurogenic communication disorders: A clinical perspective* (pp. 49–75). London, UK: Whurr.

Cant, R. (1997). Rehabilitation following a stroke: A participant perspective. *Disability and Rehabilitation, 19,* 297–304.

Charmaz, C. (1983). Loss of self: A fundamental form of suffering in the chronically ill. *Sociology of Health and Illness, 5,* 168–195.

Code, C., & Herrmann, M. (2003). The relevance of emotional and psychosocial factors in aphasia to rehabilitation. *Neurological Rehabilitation, 13,* 109–132.

Code, C., & Müller, D. J. (1992). *The Code-Müller Protocols: Assessing perceptions of psychosocial adjustment to aphasia and related disorders.* London, UK: Whurr.

Cooley, C. H. (1902). *Human nature and the social order.* New York, NY: Scribner.

Cruice, M., Worrall, L., & Hickson, L. (2006). Quantifying aphasic people's social networks in the context of non-aphasic peers. *Aphasiology, 20,* 1210–1225.

Dalemans, R., De Witte, L., Wade D. T., & Von den Heuvel, W. (2008). A description of social participation in working age persons with aphasia: A review of the literature. *Aphasiology, 22,* 1071–1091.

Davidson, B., Howe, T., Worrall, L., Hickson, L., & Togher, L. (2008). Social participation for older people with aphasia: The impact of communication disability on friendships. *Topics in Stroke Rehabilitation, 15,* 325–340.

Demo, D. H. (1992). The self-concept over time: Research issues and directions. *Annual Review of Sociology, 18,* 303–326.

Dickson, S., Barbour, R. S., Brady, M., Clark, A. M., & Paton, G. (2008). Patients' experiences of disruptions associated with post-stroke dysarthria. *International Journal of Language and Communication Disorders, 43,* 135–153.

Diener, E. (2009). *The science of well-being.* Netherlands: Springer.

Donovan, N., Velozo, C. A., & Rosenbek, J. (2007). The Communicative effectiveness survey: Investigating its item level psychometric properties. *Journal of Medical Speech Language Pathology, 15,* 433–477.

Doyle, P. J., McNeil, M. R., Mikolic, J. M. Prieto, L., Hula, W. D., Lustig, L. J., & Elman, R. J. (2004). The Burden of Stroke Scale (BOSS) provides valid and reliable score estimates of functioning and well-being in stroke survivors with and without communication disorders. *Journal of Clinical Epidemiology, 57,* 997–1007.

Duchan, J., Maxwell, M., & Kovarsky, D. (1999). Evaluating competence in the course of everyday interaction. In D. Kovarsky, J. Duchan, & M. Maxwell (Eds.), *Constructing (in)competence: Disabling evaluations in clinical and social interaction* (pp. 3–26). Mahwah, NJ: Lawrence Erlbaum.

Duffy, J. R. (2005). *Motor speech disorders: Substrates, differential diagnosis and management.* St. Louis, MO: Elsevier Mosby.

Duncan, P., Wallace, D., Lai, S., Johnson, D., Embretson, S., & Laster, L. (1999). The stroke impact scale version 2.o. Evalustion of reliability, validity and sensitivity to change. *Stroke, 30,* 2131–2140.

Ellis-Hill, C., & Horn, S. (2000). Changes in identity and self-concept: A new theoretical approach to recovery following a stroke. *Clinical Rehabilitation, 14,* 279–287.

Enderby, P., & Emerson, J. (1995). *Does speech and language therapy work?* London, UK: Whurr.

Engell, B., Hutter, B., Willmes, K., & Huber, W. (2003). Quality of life in aphasia: Validation of a pictorial self-rating procedure. *Aphasiology, 17,* 383–396.

Finn, P., Howard, R., & Kubala, R. (2005). Unassisted recovery from stuttering: self-perceptions of current speech behavior, attitudes, and feelings. *Journal of Fluency Disorders, 30,* 281–305.

Fox, A., & Pring, T. (2005). The cognitive competence of speakers with acquired dysarthria: Judgements by doctors and speech and language therapists. *Disability and Rehabilitation, 27,* 1399–1403.

Fransella, F. (1972). *Personal change and reconstruction.* London, UK: Academic Press.

Garcia, L., Laroche, C., & Barrette, J. (2002). Work integration issues go beyond the nature of the communication disorder. *Journal of Communication Disorders, 35,* 187–211.

Gouick, J., & Gentleman, D. (2004). The emotional and behavioural consequences of traumatic brain injury. *Trauma, 6,* 285–292.

Griffin, W. A., & Greene, S. M. (1994). Social interaction and symptom sequences: A case study of orofacial brachykinesia exacerbation in Parkinson's disease during negative marital interaction. *Psychiatry, 57,* 269–274.

Hartelius, L., Elmberg, M., Holm, R., Lövberg, A., & Nikolaidis, S. (2008). Living with dysarthria: Evaluation of a self-report questionnaire. *Folia Phoniatrica et Logopaedica, 60,* 11–19.

Hartelius, L., Jonnson, M., Rickeberg, A., & Laakso, K. (2009). Communication and Huntington's disease: Qualitative interviews and focus groups with persons with Huntington's disease, family members, and carers. *International Journal of Language and Communication Disorders, ifirst,* 1–13.

Herrmann, M. (1997). Studying psychosocial problems in aphasia: some conceptual and methodological considerations. *Aphasiology, 11,* 717–725.

Higginbotham, D. J., & Wilkins, D. P. (1999). Slipping through the timestream: Social issues of time and timing in augmented interactions. In D. Kovarsky, J. Duchan, & M. Maxwell (Eds.), *Constructing (in)competence: Disabling evaluations in clinical and social interaction* (pp. 49–82). Mahwah, NJ: Lawrence Erlbaum.

Hilari, K., Byng, S., Lamping, D. L., & Smith, S. C. (2003). Stroke and quality of life scale-39 (SAQOL-39): Evaluation of acceptability, reliability and validity. *Stroke, 34,* 1944–1950.

Hill, C. (1997). Biographical disruption, narrative and identity in stroke: Personal experience in acquired chronic illness. *Auto/Biography*, *5*, 131–144.

Hunter, M. D., Robinson, I. C., & Neilson, S. (1993). The functional and psychological status of patients with amyotrophic lateral sclerosis: some implications for rehabilitation. *Disability and Rehabilitation*, *15*, 119–126.

Jordan, L., & Kaiser, W. (1996). *Aphasia: A social approach*. London, UK: Chapman & Hall.

Kelly, G. (1955). *The psychology of personal constructs* (Vols. 1 & 2). New York, NY: Norton.

Klugman, T., & Ross, E. (2002). Perceptions of the impact of speech, language, swallowing and hearing difficulties on quality of life of a group of South African persons with multiple sclerosis. *Folia Phoniatrica et Logopaedica*, *54*, 201–221.

Layder, D. (1993). *New strategies in social research: An introduction and guide*. Cambridge, UK: Polity Press.

Lewis, K., Kaufman, J., Gonzales, M., Wimmer, A., & Christakis, N. (2008). Tastes, ties, and time: A new social network dataset using Facebook.com. *Social Networks*, *30*, 330–342.

Long, A., Hesketh, A., & Bowen, A. (2009). Communication outcome after stroke: A new measure of the carer's perspective. *Clinical Rehabilitation*, *23*, 846–856.

Lyon, J. G., Carisk, D., Keisler, L., Rosenbek, J., Levine, R., Kampula, J., Ryff, C., Coyne, S., & Blanc, M. (1997). Communication partners: Enhancing participation in life and communication for adults with aphasia in natural settings. *Aphasiology*, *11*, 693–708.

Markus, H., & Nurius, P. (1987). Possible selves: The interface between motivation and the self-concept. In K. Yardley & T. Honess (Eds.), *Self and identity: Psychosocial perspectives* (pp. 157–172). London, UK: John Wiley and Sons.

McAdams, D. (1993). *The stores we live by: Personal myths and the making of the self*. New York, NY: Morrow.

McCrum, R. (1998). *My year off: Rediscovering life after a stroke*. London, UK: Picador.

Mead, G. H. (1925). The genesis of the self and social control. *International Journal of Ethics*, *35*, 251–273.

Mead, G. H. (1934). *Mind, self and society*. Chicago, IL: University of Chicago Press.

Michallet, B., Tetreault, S., & Le Dorze, G. (2003). The consequences of severe aphasia for the spouses of aphasic people: a description of the adaptation process. *Aphasiology*, *17*, 835–859.

Miller, N., Noble, E., Jones, D., Allcock, L., & Burn, D. J. (2008). How do I sound to me? Perceived changes in communication in Parkinson's disease. *Clinical Rehabilitation*, *22*, 14–22.

Miller, N., Noble, E., Jones, D., & Burn, D. (2006). Life with communication changes in Parkinson's disease. *Age and Ageing*, *35*, 235–239.

Montgomery, G. K., & Erikson, L. M. (1987). Neuropsychological perspectives in amyotrophic lateral sclerosis. In B. R. Brookes (Ed.), *Neurologic clinics* (pp. 61–81). Philadelphia, PA: W. B. Saunders.

Murray, J. B. (1996). Depression in Parkinson's disease. *Journal of Psychology*, *130*, 659–667.

Nettleton, S. (1995). *The sociology of health and illness*. Cambridge, UK: Polity Press.

Papathanasiou, I., Macdonald, L., Whurr, R., Brookes, G. B., & Jahanshahi, M. (1997). Perceived stigma among patients with spasmodic dysphonia. *Journal of Medical Speech-Language Pathology*, *5*, 251–261.

Parr, S. (2001). Psychosocial aspects of aphasia: Whose perspectives? *Folia Phoniatrica et Logopaedica*, *53*, 266–288.

Parr, S. (2007). Living with severe aphasia: tracking social exclusion. *Aphasiology*, *21*, 98-123.

Paul, D. R., Frattali, C., Holland, A. L., Thompson, C. K., Caperton, C. J., & Slater, S. C. (2004). *Quality of communication life scale*. Rockville, MD: The American Speech-Hearing Association.

Remy, P., Doder, M., Lees, A., Turjanski, N., & Brooks D. (2005). Depression in parkinson's disease: Loss of dopamine and noradrenaline innervation in the limbic system. *Brain, 128,* 1314–1322.

Roland, K. P., Jenkins, M. E., & Johnson, A. M. (2010). An exploration of the burden experienced by spousal caregivers of individuals with Parkinson's disease. *Movement Disorders, 25,* 189–193.

Rombough, R., Howse, E. L., & Bartfay, W. (2006). Caregiver strain and caregiver burden of primary caregivers of stroke survivors with and without aphasia. *Rehabilitation Nursing, 31,* 199–209.

Rosenberg, M. (1965). *Society and the adolescent self-image.* Princeton NJ: Princeton University Press.

Rosenberg, M. (1987). depersonalization: The loss of personal identity. In T. Honess & K. Yardley (Eds.), *Self and identity: Perspectives across the lifespan* (pp. 193–206). London, UK: Routledge and Kegan Paul.

Russell, D. W. (1996). UCLA loneliness scale: Reliability, validity and factor structure. *Journal of Personality Assessment, 66,* 20–40.

Ryff, C. (1989). Happiness is everything, or is it? Explorations on the meaning of well-being. *Journal of Personality and Social Psychology, 57,* 1069–1081.

Safilios-Rothschild, C. (1981). Disabled persons' self-definitions and their implications for rehabilitation. In A. Brechin, P. Liddiard, & J. Swain (Eds.), *Handicap in a social world* (pp. 5–13*).* Sevenoaks, UK: Hodder Stoughton/Open University Press.

Sapir, S., & Aronson, A. E. (1990). The relationship between psychopathology and speech and language disorders in neurologic patients. *Journal of Speech and Hearing Disorders, 55,* 503–509.

Shrauger, J. S., & Schoeneman, T. G. (1979). Symbolic interactionist view of self-concept: Through the looking glass darkly. *Psychological Bulletin, 86,* 549–573.

Simmons-Mackie, N., & Damico, J. (1999). Social role negotiation in aphasia therapy: Competence, incompetence and conflict. In D. Kovarsky, J. Duchan, and M. Max-

well (Eds.), *Constructing (in)competence: Disabling evaluations in clinical and social interaction* (pp. 313–341). Mahwah, NJ: Lawrence Erlbaum.

Starkstein, S. E., & Robinson, R. G. (1988). Aphasia and depression. *Aphasiology, 2,* 1–20.

Stern, R. (1997). *Visual analog mood scales manual.* Florida: Psychological Assessment Resources.

Thomas, S. (2010). Evaluation of anxiety and depression in people with acquired communication impairments. In S. Brumfitt (Ed.), *Psychological well-being and acquired communication impairments* (pp. 25–43). Chichester, UK: Wiley-Blackwell.

Turner-Stokes, L., & Hassan, N. (2002). Depression after stroke: A review of the evidence base to inform the development of an integrated care pathway. *Clinical Rehabilitation, 16,* 231–247.

Tyerman, A. D., & Humphrey, M. (1984). Changes in self-concept following head injury. *International Journal of Rehabilitation Research, 7,* 11–23.

U.S. Preventative Services Task Force. (2009). Screening for depression in adults: U.S. preventative services task force recommendation statement. *Annals of Internal Medicine, 151,* 784–792.

Vickery, C., Sepehri, A., & Evans, C. (2008). Self-esteem in an acute stroke rehabilitation sample: a control group comparison. *Clinical Rehabilitation, 22,* 179–187.

Wallin, M., Wilken, J., Turner, A., Williams, R., & Kane, R. (2006). Depression and multiple sclerosis: Review of a lethal combination. *Journal of Rehabilitation Research and Development, 41,* 45–62.

Walshe, M. (2003a). *"You have no idea. You have no idea what it is like . . . not to be able to talk." Exploring the impact and experience of acquired dysarthria from the speaker's perspective.* Unpublished doctoral thesis. Trinity College, Dublin, Ireland.

Walshe, M. (2003b). Impact of acquired neurological dysarthria on the speaker's self-concept. *Journal of Clinical Speech and Language Studies, 12/13,* 9–33.

Walshe, M., & Miller, N. (in press). Living with acquired dysarthria: The speaker's perspective. *Disability and Rehabilitation*.

Walshe, M., Peach, R., & Miller, N. (2009). The dysarthria impact profile: Validation of an instrument to measure psychosocial impact in dysarthria. *International Journal of Language and Communication Disorders, 44,* 693–715.

Wambaugh, J. L, Duffy, J. R., McNeil, M. R., Robin, D. A., & Rogers, M. (2006). Treatment guidelines for acquired apraxia of speech: A synthesis and evaluation of the evidence. *Journal of Medical Speech-Language Pathology, 14,* xv–xxxiii

Ware, J. J., & Sherbourne, C. D. (1992). The MOS 36 item short form survey (SF-36): Conceptual framework and item selection. *Medical Care, 30,* 473–483.

Weinberg, N. (1988). Another perspective: attitudes of people with disabilities. In H. Yuker (Ed.), *Attitudes towards persons with disabilities* (pp. 141–153). New York, NY: Springer.

The WHOQOL Group. (1998). Development of the World Health Organization WHOQOL-BREF quality of life assesment. *Psychological Medicine, 28,* 551–558.

World Health Organization. (2001). *International classification of functioning disability and health (ICF).* Geneva, Switzerland.

World Health Organization Quality of Life Group. (1995). The World Health Organization quality of life assessment: Position paper from the World Health Organization. *Social Science and Medicine, 41,* 1403–1409.

Worrall, L., Brown, K., Cruice, M., Davidson, B., Hersch, D., Howe, T., & Sherratt, S. (2010). The evidence for a life coaching approach to aphasia. *Aphasiology, 24,* 497–514.

Worrall, L., & Hickson L. (2003). *Communication disability in aging: from prevention to intervention.* Clifton Park, NY: Delmar Learning

Yorkston, K. M., Baylor, C. R. ,Klasner, E. R., Deitz, J., Dudgeon, B. J., Eadie, T., . . . Amtmann, D. (2007). Satisfaction with communicative participation as defined by adults with multiple sclerosis. *Journal of Communication Disorders, 40,* 433–451.

Yorkston, K. M., Beukelman, D., Strand, E., & Bell, K. (1999). *Management of motor speech disorders in children and adults* (2nd ed.). Austin TX: Pro-Ed.

Yorkston, K. M., Klasner, E. R., & Swanson, K. M. (2001). Communication in context: A qualitative study of the experiences of individuals with multiple sclerosis. *American Journal of Speech Language Pathology, 10,* 126–137.

6

Measurement of Communicative Participation

KATHRYN M. YORKSTON, PH.D.
CAROLYN R. BAYLOR, PH.D.

Participation within the ICF Framework

Participation, defined simply as "involvement in life situations," is a critical component of the World Health Organization's (WHO) *International Classification of Functioning, Disability, and Health* (ICF) (World Health Organization, 2001 #6710). The construct of participation is valuable for understanding how people engage in various activities in the context of their day-to-day lives to fulfill life roles such as work, caring for family, household management, relationships, and social or community activities. Participation is thought to be influenced by a number of factors including physical function, the ability to perform various activities, and external factors that characterize the circumstances in which a person lives (Cardol, 2002 #4899) (see also Chapter 1, "The ICF Framework and Its Relevance to the Assessment of People with Motor Speech Disorders," by Hartelius and Miller, this book). Disability influences participation in varied and substantial ways. The presence of disability has been found to lead to participation that is less diverse, is restricted more to the home setting, involves fewer social relationships, and includes less active recreation (Law, 2002).

The ability to communicate is a prerequisite for participation in many everyday activities. *Communicative participation* has been defined as "taking part in life situations where knowledge, information, ideas or feelings are exchanged" (Eadie et al., 2006). This definition contains two important ideas. The term "life situation" reflects that communication occurs within a social context of what is being communicated, where, when, why, and with whom. The second critical term, "exchange," reflects the reciprocal nature of communication. When motor speech disorders interfere with participation in life roles, many negative consequences may result, for example, loss of employment, social isolation, and difficulty pursuing services including healthcare. Understanding communicative participation is critical for understanding how well people with motor speech disorders are meeting their communication needs in their daily lives and how intervention might help people to better meet those needs.

In this chapter, we argue that communicative participation is a key outcome measure in motor speech disorders. With the adoption of the ICF framework by the field of speech-language pathology, the need for techniques to measure participation in the clinical setting has become apparent. Measures of communicative participation would not replace those that address physiologic function and/or speech activities (i.e., acoustic measures of voice, accuracy of word production, speech intelligibility), rather they would capture the adequacy of speech in real-life situations. This chapter places motor speech disorders within the framework of the ICF and distinguishes communicative participation from the other constructs, such as quality of life. It also describes the development of a tool to measure communicative participation in community-dwelling adults with motor speech disorders. Finally, some preliminary applications of this tool to examine factors associated with communicative participation is presented.

Distinguishing Communicative Participation from Other Constructs

In order to develop valid, reliable, and useful instruments, constructs must be defined clearly. Understanding the differences between communicative participation and other related constructs

is an important first step in the development process. Although communicative participation is a likely contributor to quality of life (QOL), it is a different construct. QOL is a global, multidimensional indicator of a person's well-being encompassing a wide range of variables including physical, psychological, social, spiritual, and financial well-being. Participation is a more circumscribed construct specifically addressing a person's involvement in various life situations (i.e., fulfilling work roles, family roles, etc.). Communicative participation refers specifically to fulfilling the communication aspects of those roles. When communicative participation changes as a result of a change in the underlying impairment or perhaps because of improvements due to intervention, those changes may not be apparent in a global QOL measure when a myriad of other issues such as physical health, financial stress, or emotional stress might be driving an individual's overall QOL. In contrast, a measure tailored specifically to communicative participation would better capture and document changes in communicative participation in response to intervention programs, time, or other variables.

Since the adoption of the ICF, there has been discussion about the distinctions (or lack thereof) between the activity and participation components of the framework. Without entering into a detailed debate on the topic, we consider the view that activity limitations and participation restrictions may exist at different points along a continuum as opposed to representing completely distinct constructs. In the context of motor speech disorders, activities might be thought of as the execution of speech tasks independent of any context, although participation is the use of speech within a real-life context to meet a real-life need or goal. For example, a person with dysarthria may have an intelligibility level of 80% when performing the *activity* of reading sentences to the clinician in the therapy room. The relevant question for *participation* is whether the person has adequate intelligibility to satisfactorily engage in conversations with friends and family, to successfully communicate with store clerks or other service providers in the community, or to make phone calls to make appointments.

Measurement Challenges

Stewart and colleagues summarized the difficulty in measuring participation as, "The unique nature of individuals' roles and habits, and the relationship of these with equally unique impairments, disabilities and environments, create significant difficulties in developing a 'gold standard' of handicap [sic] useful in a range of settings" (p. 312) (Stewart, Kidd, & Thompson, 1995). Measurement of communicative participation is complicated by a number of issues, which are presented in the following sections.

Measurement of Participation Requires Participation-Focused Instruments

A tempting assumption is that people who have more severe motor speech disorders have more restricted participation than those with less severe speech disorders. However, as discussed previously, participation is distinct from other components of the ICF frame-work such as physical impairments and activity limitations. Adequacy of communication participation cannot be inferred from measures at the level of impairment (changes in bodily function) or activity limitation (inability to execute the task of speaking). For example, two speakers with dysarthria, each with 90% sentence intelligibility on tasks performed in the therapy room (an activity limitation), might have different participation outcomes depending on their unique communication needs and the supports and barriers in their environment. Adequacy of participation is influenced by external factors such as environmental, social, and personal variables (Bickenbach, Chatterji, Badley, & Ustun, 1999; Cardol et al., 1999) as well as the ability to physically perform activities. To measure communicative participation, we must directly ask about communication in real-life contexts instead of making inferences about participation based on the performance of skills within the therapy room.

Communicative Participation Is Complex

As mentioned previously, communicative participation is a complex construct affected by many variables. These variables, and hence the success of participation, may change from one situation to the next. Some examples of variables include features of the physical environment (i.e., background noise), characteristics of communication partners (i.e., patience to engage in slower communication pace), and perspectives of the speakers with dysarthria (i.e., communication priorities and needs). Along with the complexity of factors that may shape participation, there also are many different aspects of participation that could be measured. Some indicators of communicative participation could be tallies of how many different communication situations people engage in and how often, as well as tallies of the number of communication partners in an individual's routine environment (Cruice, Worrall, Hickson, & Murison, 2005). A different understanding of participation might come from assessing how difficult it is for people to participate in various situations, how much assistance they need, or how successfully they accomplish their communication tasks. With all of the possible ways that participation could be measured, one key question is how to reduce this complexity to create manageable instruments that still meaningfully reflect the real-life experiences of people with communication disorders.

Objective and Subjective Indicators of Participation

The preceding paragraph describes the complex set of issues associated with communicative participation, any of which might be interesting to measure. Some of these variables might be considered to be objective, such as tallies of how often or for how long individuals engage in various communication situations. For example, how much time do they spend visiting with family or friends in social situations? How many phone calls do they make in a week? Tallies inform us about what activities people engage in and how often they do so. They provide us with data to describe patterns of participation and to identify different patterns across dif-

ferent groups, such as those with motor speech disorders. The problem with tallies is that they give an incomplete picture of participation. Although tallies might tell us how often someone engages in a situation, tallies do not tell us whether a person's participation is adequate to meet their needs for life roles and goals. Judgments about the success of participation may depend on several variables such as whether or not the task was accomplished, the ease or difficulty of the task, the comfort of the individual in participating in the situation, the importance of the situation to the individual, and many other factors (Yorkston et al., 2007). For example, a person who communicates with dozens of people each day might find participation less satisfactory than one who speaks with a small number of people in valued situations. For these reasons, subjective indicators may be as, or even more, important than objective indicators in determining the adequacy of communicative participation. The adequacy of participation for meeting life roles and goals cannot be inferred from tallies of how often someone performs activities (Brown et al., 2004; Hemmingsson & Jonsson, 2005; Perenboom & Chorus, 2003).

Self-report versus Proxy-report

With the recognition of the importance of subjective measures of participation, the next critical question is who should provide those ratings. The general recommendation is that the person with the disability should provide a self-report of the adequacy of participation because he or she is the only person who experiences living with the disability and understands how the physical impairment interacts with contextual and personal variables to create satisfactory or unsatisfactory participation (Brown et al., 2004; Law, 2002). Self-report measures recognize the autonomy of the person with the communication disorder and promote a more accurate representation of the individual's life experiences than do proxy reports completed by family or health-care providers. The challenge with self-report measures by people with communication disorders, however, is that some may have language or cognitive impairments severe enough to threaten their ability to provide self-report information. When these situations arise, proxy reports may be warranted, although proxy ratings always must be done with the recognition that proxies have limitations in their ability to understand the perspective of the person who lives with the communication disorder. Research has shown widely variable relationships between self-report and proxy reports on a variety of issues, although there does seem to be a trend in that proxy reports more closely resemble self-reports on more "objective" measures (i.e., tallies of activities) as opposed to more subjective measures (QOL or other psychosocial domains) (Cruice, Worrall, Hickson, & Murison, 2005; Van der Linden et al., 2008; Williams et al., 2006).

What Is the Benchmark for Adequate Communicative Participation?

The final measurement challenge to be discussed here is the question of what is adequate or satisfactory communicative participation. One possible option is to compare the communication activities of adults with motor speech disorders to those of "typical" adults with the assumption that the frequency, duration, independence, or ease with which typical adults engage in communication situations is the standard against which the communicative participation of people with communication disorders should be compared. However, research suggests that different groups of stakeholders place different values on the importance of various communication activities (Worrall, McCooey, Davidson, Larkins, & Hickson, 2002). The meaning of adequate participation may vary greatly from one person to another, depending on what they need to be able to do with their speech. For example, some people may have undemanding speech environments with long periods of quiet and infrequent needs to talk for long periods of time. For others, the demands for speech usage are extraordinary with work or personal goals largely dependent on high-quality, expressive speech (Baylor, Yorkston, Eadie, Miller, & Amtmann, 2008).

In addition to varying speech demands, different individuals have different criteria for successful participation. The definition of satisfactory communicative participation was explored in people with Multiple Sclerosis (MS) (Yorkston et al., 2007). The results showed that the definition of satisfactory participation differed depending on how well the communication task was accomplished, how comfortable the communication situation was, and the personal importance or meaning of the communication situation. With these different characterizations of successful participation, a convincing argument can be made that the definition of adequate or satisfactory participation should be made by individual determination and not an external normative standard about what participation "should" be (Brown et al., 2004; Law, 2002). Measuring changes in each person's communicative participation over time as their medical conditions or life situations change may be more meaningful than comparing one person's participation to another's.

In summary, measuring communicative participation is challenging because of the complexity and subjectivity of the construct. There are many possible ways to measure communicative participation, and these multiple perspectives will contribute to our understanding of the impact of motor speech disorders on participation in life situations. However, in pursuing a clinically useful and meaningful instrument, there are several key guiding principles including the importance of considering communication activities in the context of real-life situations, the sampling of a variety of communication environments for a representative view of complex realities, the unique perspective of the person with the communication disorder that might not be captured by proxy raters, and individuality in determining the criteria for successful communicative participation. In short, people with motor speech disorders must be asked directly whether their communicative participation is adequate to meet their needs for their life roles and goals.

Lack of Available Communicative Participation Instruments

In the prior section, we acknowledge that there are many possible ways to measure communicative participation

that would provide useful information, but that the options must include a subjective self-report instrument by which people with motor speech disorders can report whether their communicative participation is adequate to meet their own communication needs. A recent literature review (Eadie et al., 2006) has revealed a lack of participation-focused instruments in the field of communication disorders leaving speech pathologists with few options for measuring the important construct of communicative participation.

Existing instruments have several characteristics that limit their abilities to serve as measures of communicative participation. First, the majority of instruments in speech pathology traditionally have focused on impairment or activity limitation. As discussed earlier, from a theoretical perspective, participation is a distinct construct from impairment or activity limitation and, hence, measures of one cannot be used as indicators of another. Instruments used to assess impairment or activity limitations typically focus on relatively simple communication skills and do not include aspects of the complex communication environments or unique needs and priorities that are central to understanding communicative participation.

In more recent years, several instruments targeting assessment of psychosocial aspects of communication disorders have emerged. The area of voice disorders has generated several examples including the *Voice Handicap Index* (VHI) (Jacobson et al., 1997), the *Voice-Related Quality of Life* scale (V-RQol) (Hogikyan & Sethuraman, 1999), the *Voice Activity and Participation Profile* (VAPP) (Ma & Yiu, 2001), and the *Voice Symptoms Scale* (VoiSS) (Deary,

Wilson, Cardin, & Mackenzie, 2003). Psychosocial scales exist in other areas as well, including dysarthria (Walshe, Peach, & Miller, 2008). These tools have advanced greatly our understanding of the psychosocial consequences of motor speech and voice disorders, and many of them do contain participation-related questions. However, none of these can function as a specific communicative participation instrument because each contains a variety of constructs (Eadie et al., 2006) including physical symptoms, performance of basic speech tasks, and personal emotional coping. Because of the mixed content of the questionnaires and the methods of psychometric development, items related to communicative participation in these instruments cannot be distinguished from other constructs, therefore confounding the measurement of communicative participation. Finally, although recent attention has been given to instruments such as the Communication Effectiveness Survey (Donovan, Kendall, Young, & Rosenbek, 2008), this survey assesses a limited number of communication situations and initially was developed informally without strong psychometric input into its measurement properties.

The Communicative Participation Item Bank

Under funding from the National Institutes of Health (NIH), a multidisciplinary team representing Speech-Language Pathology, Educational Psychology, Occupational Therapy, and Rehabilitation Psychology has begun development of a self-report communicative participation instrument, the Communicative Participation Item Bank. The following describes the work of this team to construct this IRT-based instrument to measure communicative participation in community-dwelling adults across a variety of communication disorders including motor speech, voice, and mild-moderate language or cognitive-communication disorders. The goal for the Communicative Participation Item Bank is that it will provide meaningful data for clinical and research purposes in an efficient and psychometrically sound manner. The development of the Communicative Participation Item Bank was patterned after the methods used by the Patient-Reported Outcomes Measurement Information Systems (NIHpromis.org), which is an NIH roadmap initiative to implement high-quality, self-report health measurement instruments (DeWalt, Rothrock, Yount, & Stone, 2007; Reeve et al., 2007). Several key steps in the PROMIS item bank development process will be outlined as implemented for the Communicative Participation Item Bank later in this chapter.

Defining the Construct

The initial step in developing the Communicative Participation Item Bank was to define the construct that the instrument would measure. According to the definition of communicative participation proposed by Eadie et al. (2006), the items need to address communication that occurs in real-life situations. To this end, the items need to identify aspects of specific communication environments including the communication partner, the purpose of the communication, and the physical and/or social setting. The items also need to reflect an active exchange between communication partners. Items, furthermore, need to represent the variety of communication situations in which community-dwelling adults typically engage.

As part of defining the construct, the Communicative Participation Item Bank was restricted to situations involving communication through speech. Communicative participation actually occurs through many communication modalities—speaking and listening, reading, writing, signing, and augmentative communication. Although communicative participation ultimately should be evaluated through all relevant modalities, the Communicative Participation Item Bank focuses on communication through speech for two reasons. First, unidimensionality of constructs in item banks is critical to measurement using Item Response Theory (IRT) (to be discussed later in this chapter). Prior research has suggested that mixing multiple communication modalities in an item bank may violate the key IRT criterion of essential unidimensionality (Doyle, Hula, McNeil, Mikolic, & Matthews, 2005) and, thus, confound measurement. Second, this item bank is intended for use across diverse populations, not all of whom will have impairments affecting comprehension, reading, or writing (i.e., individuals with degenerative neuromotor diseases affecting motor speech only). We see development of companion item banks addressing other communication modalities as important steps in future research.

After defining the scope of item content, we explored response options. What do we want to know about par-

ticipation? As discussed previously, one of the challenges in measuring communicative participation is the many different aspects of participation that could be measured—each giving a different angle or perspective on participation. The Communicative Participation Item Bank was designed to give a single, overall rating of the adequacy of participation from the viewpoint of the person who lives with the communication disorder. The response format asks people to rate how much their "condition" (meaning the communication disorder and any associated health conditions) interferes with participation in a variety of communication situations. This overall rating does not provide insight into *why* people rate participation as they do. For example, some people may report high levels of interference in participation due to poor speech intelligibility while others may associate interference with unhelpful communication environments. These are questions that need to be explored in more detail through clinical interviews. However, by providing one overall rating, clients and research participants can provide efficiently a summation of their experiences with communicative participation with further details about the participation pursued as needed through interviews or other questionnaires that address other constructs of interest (i.e., fatigue, depression, social support, pain, etc.).

As mentioned previously, the item bank is intended for people with motor speech, voice, and related disorders as well as for those with mild-moderate language or cognitive-communication disorders. This instrument is not intended for those with severe language or cognitive-communication disorders for several reasons. One reason is that people with more severe cognitive or linguistic disorders may not be able to reliably engage in self-report at the language level reflected in the items. Second, those with severe-profound language or cognitive disorders may not necessarily be participating in the types of community situations included in the item bank. Other assessment tools exist for those with more severe cognitive or language disorders (e.g., ASHA Functional Assessment of Communication Skills (ASHA FACS) (Frattali, Thompson, Holland, Wohl, & Ferketic, 1995) or ASHA Quality of Communication Life (QCL) Scale; (Paul et al., 2004). These instruments include response formats that may be more accessible to people with severe cognitive-linguistic impairments (including pictorial response formats), and some are designed to rely on proxy ratings when communication impairments are so severe as to preclude self-report. Furthermore, these questionnaires focus more on basic communication skills that might be relevant for the level of function of someone with severe cognitive or language disorders but would not capture the complex experiences of higher functioning people. Current research is underway using IRT to develop instruments that may address some of the concerns that are more specific to people with aphasia (Doyle, McNeil, Le, Hula, & Ventura, 2008).

Constructing Candidate Items

After defining the construct, a large pool of candidate items was created by the research team. The items were derived from a review of the literature and mea-surement principles for participation as discussed previously. Items were constructed to represent a variety of life domains including household management, occupation, community involvement, social and leisure activities, and relationships. The items were intended to reflect a range of communication situations including addressing more basic needs (i.e., telling someone at home what you would like to eat; making a phone call to schedule an appointment) to more complex and abstract communication (i.e., negotiating; discussing current events). The items were written to meet the following criteria: (1) simple, universally understood wording; (2) one attribution (idea) per item; (3) brief (<10 words); (4) free of age, gender, and social class biases; (5) free of double or implicit negatives; and (6) avoidance of items likely to be endorsed by everyone or no one. See Figure 6–1 for a sample of candidate items.

Qualitative Review of Items

After an initial pool of candidate items was generated, the process of item refinement and selection for a final core item bank began. This involves both qualitative and quantitative analyses of the items with decisions about item retention, removal, or modification based on the results of both types of analyses. The first step is qualitative item review through a process called cognitive interviewing (Willis, 2005). In cognitive interviewing, also called think-out-loud techniques, participants with communication disorders are interviewed as they answer the candidate items in the item bank. This technique is useful in identifying ambiguous, unclear, or

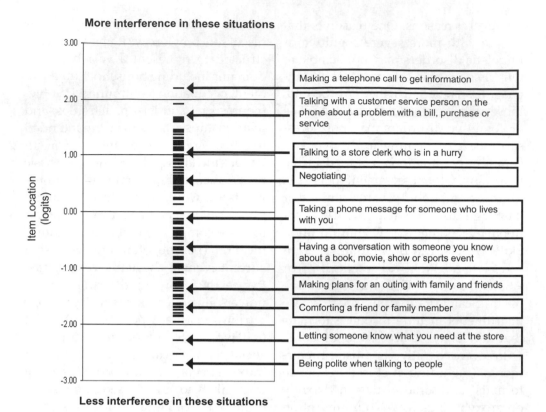

Figure 6–1. This presents a sample of results from Baylor et al. (2009) showing item difficulty values of the Communicative Participation Item Bank for a sample of individuals (*n* = 208) with spasmodic dysphonia. The vertical scale is logits, which is an interval scale generated in IRT analyses and represents the likelihood of a participant responding to items in a particular manner. The typical desired logit range for an item bank targeting a wide range of latent trait levels is from –3.0 to +3.0 logits. Each of the 131 items is represented by a horizontal tic mark along the scale. The text of 10 of the items is presented in this figure to illustrate the types of communication situations represented at different points along the scale. The items at the high end of the range (i.e., making a telephone call to get information) are items about which participants were more likely to report interference, whereas items at the lower end of the range are items about which participants are less likely to report interference.

inappropriate items. The process of item selection was an iterative one in which items were reviewed by participants, modified based on participant responses, and then reviewed again by new participants. Approximately 35 individuals have participated in cognitive interviews to review the items.

These individuals represent a range of medical conditions associated with communication disorders including spasmodic dysphonia (SD) (Yorkston et al., 2008), Multiple Sclerosis (MS), Amyotrophic Lateral Sclerosis (ALS), Parkinson's Disease (PD), stuttering, and communication disorders related to stroke including aphasia, apraxia, and dysarthria. Cognitive interviews continue until the point of saturation, which is the point at which additional interviews yield no further notable changes in item content or format.

Results of the interviews suggested that for item content, participants' ratings of interference in participation depend heavily on the communication context such as the familiarity of the communication partner, the physical surroundings (i.e., background noise), and the purpose of the conversation (i.e., casual interaction versus a high priority or "high stakes" situations). In terms of response options, prior qualitative interviews with people with MS suggested that participants were able to provide an overall indication of the adequacy of their participation in that they talked about their "satisfaction" with participation (Yorkston et al., 2007). The cognitive interviews supported the use of an overall rating, but participants preferred response options that asked them to rate "interference" rather than other dimensions such as satisfaction. Participants felt that being asked about satisfaction did not allow them to convey how their motor speech disorder "got in the way" and how it had impacted their lives, many times in negative or undesirable ways (Yorkston et al., 2008).

Psychometric Analysis of Items and Creation of an Item Bank

After completion of the cognitive interviews, item bank construction continues with psychometric analyses. These analyses help researchers determine the most appropriate items to retain in a final item bank for an optimally valid and reliable instrument. Advances in modern psychometric methods, including the use of IRT, have made it possible to develop a new generation of self-report instruments using protocols that can yield highly precise estimates of latent traits (Cella et al., 2007; Reeve et al., 2007). IRT has been used in other fields, such as education for decades, and now is becoming more prevalent in the field of speech pathology with several studies using IRT to evaluate existing instruments (Bogaardt, Hakkestreegt, Grolman, & Lindeboom, 2007; Donovan, Rosenbek, Ketterson, & Velozo, 2006; Donovan, Velozo, & Rosenbek, 2007; Hula, Doyle, McNeil, & Mikolic, 2006) and to compile item sets using items from different existing instruments (Doyle et al., 2005). The following paragraphs provide a very brief overview of the use of IRT for developing item banks and short-form administration formats. For more detailed information, readers are referred to introductory textbooks on IRT (Bond & Fox, 2001; Embretson & Reise, 2000) as well as manuscripts that describe the use of IRT in the full context of item bank development (Baylor et al., 2009; Reeve et al., 2007).

Model-based Measurement of Latent Traits

Latent traits are constructs that cannot be directly observed but can be inferred only from measurements of observed variables. Many examples of latent traits range from an individual's knowledge about a topic (can be observed only by that person's response to questions about the topic) to psychosocial constructs such as QOL (determined by how the person reports QOL). The degree to which a person's experiences interference in communicative participation also is regarded as a latent trait because it is the person's internal judgment about the impact of the communication disorder on life participation. When inferring latent traits from observed variables such as questionnaires, one of the key questions is to what extent does the questionnaire accurately represent the latent trait? IRT addresses this concern through model-based measurement. IRT is based on a mathematical model of the relationship between how individuals respond to items on a questionnaire and the underlying latent trait that the questionnaire is intended to represent. In conceptual terms, for the Communicative Participation Item Bank, the model states that individuals who experience more interference with communicative participation (latent trait) are expected to rate higher interference on items in the item bank. Essentially, participants' responses to the items should reflect their underlying level of the latent trait without significant confounding factors. According to IRT, items that preserve this relationship provide more precise measurement of the latent trait, and these items should be included in the final core item bank. Items that do not retain these measurement properties should be revised or removed from the item bank.

Selecting Items for Core Item Bank

Selecting items for the core item bank requires multiple analyses. Exploratory and confirmatory factor analyses are completed prior to IRT analyses to determine the factor structure of the candidate item set. Most IRT models, including the Rasch model, which is most commonly used in speech pathology, require essential unidimensionality in an item bank. This means that all of the items should measure a single construct or latent trait in order to avoid confounding variables. Additional analyses within IRT are used to select the items for the core item bank. These analyses address issues related to how well participants' responses to items fit the mathematical model (item fit), the range of the latent trait covered by the items (item difficulty and information function), the presence of bias in items (differential item function), and the appropriate number of response categories when using Likert-scale items.

At this time, the Communicative Participation Item Bank has undergone IRT analysis in one population, persons with SD (Baylor et al., 2009). The results are favorable in that they suggest essential unidimensionality of the items, a large core of items with good item fit, and a wide measurement range. An example of selected items with good model fit is presented in Figure 6–1. In this figure, the items are presented along a logit scale. Logits is short for "log odds units" and is an underlying interval scale representing the odds of responding to items in a particular way. The logit scale is used to measure both item difficulty and person ability in IRT. The typical desirable logit range in items is −3 to +3. In Figure 6–1, items with higher logit values represent more difficult communicative participation situations (participants are more likely to report interference in participation). Further testing in populations with other communication disorders is underway with support from the NIH (PI: Baylor) to determine whether the psychometric parameters of the candidate items are invariant across communication disorder populations (e.g., ALS, MS, and head & neck cancer), and to begin validity testing by comparing the instrument to other measures of disease severity.

Administration of IRT-based Item Banks

IRT presents several advantages for assessment. One advantage is that it provides an underlying interval-level measurement scale for latent traits (the logit scale). Interval scale measurement provides several advantages for statistical analyses compared to Likert response formats in ordinal level scaling. For example, true means and standard deviations can be computed for interval scales but not for ordinal scales. A second key advantage of IRT is the use of item banks. Item banks serve as reservoirs containing a large number of items, but the entire item set is not administered as a whole. Instead, subsets of items are drawn from the item bank for each assessment, with the items selected to be most relevant, or to provide the most precise measurement for each individual assessment. The optimal method of administering item banks is through computerized adaptive testing (CAT) (Cook, O'Mallery, & Roddey, 2005; Ware, Sinclair, Gandek, & Bjorner, 2005). In CAT, computerized algorithms are used to select items from the item bank for individuals based on their responses as they progress through the assessment. High levels of measurement precision (reliability) often can be reached in as few as 5–10 CAT-administered items. This provides "measurement efficiency" in that similarly precise measurement as available with traditional non-IRT instruments can be obtained with many fewer items and hence lower respondent burden in CAT (Cook et al., 2005). When CAT technology is not available, targeted short forms can be constructed by extracting items from the item bank that are most relevant to the individual assessment situation. Because the unit of measurement in IRT is the individual item (and not the entire test or form as it is with traditional instruments), items can be interchanged for different participants or for the same participant across time while retaining the ability to compare the scores on the underlying logit scale across people or situations.

Applications of the Communicative Participation Item Bank and Future Directions

Much work remains to be done both in developing high-quality measurement tools for communicative participation as well as using those tools to gain a better understanding of this important construct. Many essential questions remain. Does communicative participation vary across different types of communication disorders? How reliable is self-report of communicative participation in individuals with more severe language or cognitive disorders? How valid are proxy ratings when proxy raters are needed? Can we track changes in communicative participation over time as health status or other conditions change? How can we improve communicative participation for individuals with motor speech disorders? In addition to these questions, it is important to acknowledge cross-cultural difference that may exist (Hwa-Froelich & Vigil, 2004; Pickering & McAllister, 2000). Issues such as familiarity with the testing situation, effects of formal education, and language issues have been discussed in terms of assessment of children with communication problems (Carter et al., 2005). Procedures outlining good practices in translation and cultural adaptation of self-report instruments are available (Wild et al., 2005).

In an early example of this research, a subset of items from the Communicative Participation Item Bank was administered to 498 adults with MS. Results of a regression analysis suggested communicative participation is associated significantly with multiple variables, only some of which reflect speech or cognitive-communication disorders. Other variables significantly associated with communicative participation included fatigue, depression, employment status, and social support. This study suggests that if the goal of intervention is to improve communicative participation, intervention may need to extend beyond traditional speech pathology boundaries to include other health symptoms as well as personal, social, and physical environments (Baylor, Yorkston, Bamer, Britton, & Amtmann, 2010). Future research such as utilizing the Communicative Participation Item Bank and other participation-related instruments will guide clinicians and researchers in helping individuals with motor speech disorders meet their communication

needs. The item bank currently is being tested in various populations and intended for clinical use when psychometric testing has been completed.

Acknowledgement. This project was funded in part by NIH Planning Grant # 1R21 HD 45882-01 and NIDRR grant number H133B031129, with additional technical support from personnel funded by the NIH PROMIS grant at the University of Washington Center on Outcomes Research in Rehabilitation (Grant #5U01AR052171-03).

References

Baylor, C. R., Yorkston, K., Bamer, A., Britton, D., & Amtmann, D. (2010). Variables associated with communicative participation in people with Multiple Sclerosis: A regression analysis. *American Journal of Speech-Language Pathology, 19*, 143–153

Baylor, C. R., Yorkston, K. M., Eadie, T., Miller, R. M., & Amtmann, D. (2008). The levels of speech usage: A self-report scale for describing how people use speech. *Journal of Medical Speech-Language Pathology, 16*(4), 191–198.

Baylor, C. R., Yorkston, K. M., Eadie, T., Miller, R. M., & Amtmann, D. (2009). Developing the communication participation item bank: Rasch analysis results from a spasmodic dysphonia sample. *Journal of Speech Language and Hearing Research, 52*(5), 1302-1320.

Bickenbach, J. E., Chatterji, S., Badley, E. M., & Ustun, T. B. (1999). Models of disablement, universalism and international classification of impairments, disabilities and handicaps. *Social Science and Medicine, 48*, 1173–1187.

Bogaardt, H. C. A., Hakkestreegt, M. M., Grolman, W., & Lindeboom, R. (2007).

Validation of the Voice Handicap Index using Rasch analysis. *Journal of Voice, 21*(3), 337–344.

Bond, T. G., & Fox, C. M. (2001). *Applying the Rasch model: Fundamental measurement in the human sciences.* Mahwah, NJ: Lawrence Erlbaum Associates.

Brown, M., Dijkers, M. P. J. M., Gordon, W. A., Ashman, T., Charatz, H., & Cheng, Z. (2004). Participation objective, participation subjective: A measure of participation combining outsider and insider perspectives. *Journal of Head Trauma Rehabilitation, 19*(6), 459–481.

Cardol, M., Brandsma, J. W., de Groot, I. J. M., van den Bos, G. A. M., de Haan, R. J., & de Jong, B. A. (1999). Handicap questionnaires: What do they assess? *Disability and Rehabilitation, 21*(3), 97–105.

Cardol, M., de Jong, B. A., van den Bos, G. A. M., Bellen, A., de Groot, I. J. M., & de Haan, R. J. (2002). Beyond disability: Perceived participation in people with a chronic disabling condition. *Clinical Rehabilitation, 16*, 27–35.

Carter, J. A., Lees, J. A., Murira, G. M., Gona, J., Neville, B. G. R., & Newton, C. R. J. (2005). Issues in the development of cross-cultural assessments of speech and language for children. *International Journal of Language & Communication Disorders, 40*(4), 385–401.

Cella, D., Yount, S., Rothrock, N., Cershon, R., Cook, K., Reeve, B., . . . Rose, M. (2007). The Patient-Reported Outcome Measurement Information System (PROMIS). *Medical Care, 45*(5 Suppl 1), S3–S11.

Cook, K. F., O'Mallery, K. J., & Roddey, T. S. (2005). Dynamic assessment of health outcomes: Time to let the CAT out of the bag? *Health Services Research, 40*(5), 1694–1711.

Cruice, M., Worrall, L., Hickson, L., & Murison, R. (2005). Measuring quality of life: Comparing family members' and friends' ratings with those of their aphasic partners. *Aphasiology, 19*(2), 111–129.

Deary, I. J., Wilson, J. A., Cardin, P. N., & Mackenzie, K. (2003). VoiSS: A patient-derived voice symptom scale. *Journal of Psychosomatic Research, 54*, 483–489.

DeWalt, D. A., Rothrock, N., Yount, S., & Stone, A. A. (2007). Evaluation of item candidates: The PROMIS qualitative item review. *Medical Care, 45*(5 Suppl 1), S12–S21.

Donovan, N. J., Kendall, D. L., Young, M. E., & Rosenbek, J. (2008). The communicative effectiveness survey: Preliminary evidence of construct validity. *American Journal of Speech-Language Pathology, 17*, 335–347.

Donovan, N. J., Rosenbek, J. C., Ketterson, T. U., & Velozo, C. A. (2006). Adding meaning to measurement: Initial Rasch analysis of the ASHA FACS Social Communication Subtest. *Aphasiology,* (2–4), 362–373.

Donovan, N. J., Velozo, C. A., & Rosenbek, J. C. (2007). The communicative effectiveness survey: Investigating its item-level psychometrics. *Journal of Medical Speech-Language Pathology, 15*(4), 433–447.

Doyle, P., Hula, W. D., McNeil, M. R., Mikolic, J. M., & Matthews, C. (2005). An application of Rasch analysis to the measurement of communicative functioning. *Journal of Speech, Language, and Hearing Research, 48*, 1412–1428.

Doyle, P., McNeil, M., Le, K., Hula, W., & Ventura, M. (2008). Measuring communicative functioning in community-dwelling stroke survivors: Conceptual foundation and item development. *Aphasiology, 22*(7), 718–728.

Eadie, T. L., Yorkston, K. M., Klasner, E. R., Dudgeon, B. J., Deitz, J., Baylor, C. R., . . . Amtmann, D. A. (2006). Measuring communicative participation: A review of self-report instruments in speech-language pathology. *American Journal of Speech-Language Pathology, 15*, 307–320.

Embretson, S. E., & Reise, S. P. (2000). *Item response theory for psychologists.* Mahwah, NJ: Lawrence Erlbarum Associates.

Frattali, C. M., Thompson, C. K., Holland, A. L., Wohl, C. B., & Ferketic, M. M. (1995). *The American Speech-Language-Hearing Association Functional Assessment of Communication Skills for Adults (ASHA FACS)*. Rockville, MD: ASHA.

Hemmingsson, H., & Jonsson, H. (2005). An occupational perspective on the concept of participation in the *International Classification of Functioning, Disability and Health*—Some critical remarks. *American Journal of Occupational Therapy, 59,* 569–576.

Hogikyan, N. D., & Sethuraman, G. (1999). Validation of an instrument to measure voice-related quality of life (V-RQOL). *Journal of Voice, 13*(4), 557–569.

Hula, W., Doyle, P., McNeil, M. R., & Mikolic, J. M. (2006). Rasch modeling of Revised Token Test performance: Validity and sensitivity to change. *Journal of Speech Language and Hearing Research, 49,* 27–46.

Hwa-Froelich, D., & Vigil, D. C. (2004). Three aspects of cultural influence of communication. *Communication Disorders Quarterly, 25*(3), 107–118.

Jacobson, B. H., Johnson, A., Grywalski, C., Silbergleit, A., Jacobson, G., Benninger, M. S., et al. (1997). The Voice Handicap Index (VHI): Development and validation. *American Journal of Speech-Language Pathology, 6*(3), 66–70.

Law, M. (2002). Participation in the occupations of everyday life. *American Journal of Occupational Therapy, 56,* 640–649.

Ma, E. P., & Yiu, E. M. (2001). Voice activity and participation profile: Assessing the impact of voice disorders on daily activities. *Journal of Speech, Language, and Hearing Research, 44*(3), 511–524.

Paul, D., Frattali, C., Holland, A. L., Thompson, C. K., Caperton, C. J., & Slater, S. C. (2004). *ASHA Quality of Communication Life Scale*. Rockville, MD: ASHA.

Perenboom, R. J. M., & Chorus, A. M. J. (2003). Measuring participation according to the International Classification of Functioning, Disability and Health (ICF). *Disability and Rehabilitation, 25*(11–12), 577–585.

Pickering, M., & McAllister, L. (2000). A conceptual framework for linking and guiding domestic cross-cultural and international practice in speech-language pathology. *Advances in Speech Language Pathology, 2*(2), 93–106.

Reeve, B. B., Hays, R. D., Bjorner, J. B., Cook, K. F., Crane, P. K., Teresi, J. A., . . . Cella, D (2007). Psychometric evaluation and calibration of health-related quality of life item banks. *Medical Care, 45*(5 Suppl 1), S22–S31.

Stewart, G., Kidd, D., & Thompson, A. J. (1995). The assessment of handicap and evaluation of the Environmental Status Scale. *Disability and Rehabilitation, 17,* 312–316.

Van der Linden, F. A. H., Kragt, J. J., van Bon, M., Klein, M., Thompson, A. J., Van der Ploeg, H., . . . Uitdehaag, B. M (2008). Longitudinal proxy measurement in multiple sclerosis: Patient-proxy agreement on the impact of MS on daily life over a period of two years. *BMC Neurology, 8*(2), 1–9.

Walshe, M., Peach, R. K., & Miller, N. (2008). Dysarthria Impact Profile: Development of a scale to measure psychosocial effects. *International Journal of Language & Communication Disorders* (epub), 1–23.

Ware, J. E., Jr., Sinclair, S. J., Gandek, B., & Bjorner, J. B. (2005). Item response theory and computerized adaptive testing: Implications for outcomes measurement in rehabilitation. *Rehabilitation Psychology, 50*(1), 71–78.

Wild, D., Grove, A., Martin, M., Eremenco, S., McElroy, S., Verjee-Lorenz, A., & Erikson, P. (2005). Principles of good practice for the translation and cultural adaptation process for patient-reported outcomes (PRO) measures: Report of the ISPOR task force for translation and cultural adaptation. *Value in Health, 8*(2), 94–104.

Williams, L. S., Bakas, T., Brixendine, E., Plue, L., Tu, W., Hendrie, H., & Kroenke, K. (2006). How valid are family proxy assessments of stroke patients' health-related quality of life? *Stroke, 37,* 2081–2085.

Willis, G. B. (2005). *Cognitive interviewing: A tool for improving questionnaire design.* Thousand Oaks, CA: Sage.

World Health Organization. (2001). *International Classification of Functioning, Disability and Health (ICF).* Geneva, Switzerland: Author.

Worrall, L., McCooey, R., Davidson, B., Larkins, B., & Hickson, L. (2002). The validity of functional assessments of communication and the activity/participation components of the ICIHD-2: Do they reflect what really happens in real-life? *Journal of Communication Disorders, 35,* 107–137.

Yorkston, K. M., Baylor, C. R., Deitz, J., Dudgeon, B. J., Eadie, T., Miller, R. M., & Amtman, D. A. (2008). Developing a scale of communicative participation: A cognitive interviewing study. *Disability and Rehabilitation, 30*(6), 425–433.

Yorkston, K. M., Baylor, C. R., Klasner, E. R., Deitz, J., Dudgeon, B. J., Eadie, T., . . . Amtmann, D. A (2007). Satisfaction with communicative participation as defined by adults with multiple sclerosis: A qualitative study. *Journal of Communication Disorders, 40,* 433–451.

7

Cognition and Its Assessment in Motor Speech Disorders

CATHERINE MACKENZIE, PH.D.

Introduction

Motor speech disorder (MSD) rarely occurs as an isolated sequel to or sign of neurological damage. The causative injury in dysarthria and apraxia of speech commonly results in a variety of impairments, and resultant limitations in activity and participation, relating to physical, sensory, psychological, and cognitive domains. These impairments may impact negatively on individual presentation, prognosis for maximization of communication status, and speech management. For a high proportion of the MSD population, ability and performance are compromised further by natural aging or concomitant diseases, including dementia. Surgical and pharmaceutical interventions and the potential of the latter to interact with neuropathology also may affect individual status. The focus of this chapter is the cognitive status of the person with MSD, with reference to some common pathologies, and its relevance to motor speech assessment.

Cognitive assessment also is considered, with particular attention to published tools, which may inform the speech-language pathologist (SLP) about the cognitive status of the individual with MSD.

Cognitive Processes

Cognition refers to all the processes by which sensory input is transformed, reduced, elaborated, stored, recovered, and used (Neisser, 1967). Models of cognition vary, but included normally within the construct are perception, attention, memory, and executive function (reasoning, judgment, planning, problem solving). Social cognition encompasses the use of these processes in social situations, including self-awareness and the ability to interpret interactions. Language may be regarded as a cognitive process or as a higher cortical skill in its own right, which, though influenced by cognitive status, may be affected independently.

Cognitive Impairment and Speech Assessment

Assessment is defined here as the process of collecting data for evaluation, interpretation, and diagnosis. The gathering of valid, representative data, which reflects the individual's motor speech ability, may be compromised by cognitive deficit. The client's capacity to provide relevant background information, including an accurate history of difficulty from his/her perspective and self-evaluation of speech changes, effects, and limitations, may be affected likewise. Decisions about management and intervention, which are reached following assessment, may be influenced by the individual's cognitive status.

Social Cognition and Insight

In motor speech assessment, the insight of the client into the speech difficulty, its effects, and the purposes of assessment is an important parameter. Brain damage, especially involving the right hemisphere, may be associated with limitation in insight, leading to discrepancy between the clinician's and client's evaluation of speech difficulties, their severity, and implications. The assessment process is facilitated by the relationship established, in which both clinician and client adopt a "theory of mind," permitting interpretation of emotional and motivational states and knowledge of the communication partner. Theory of mind deficits may contribute to pragmatic communication difficulties in traumatic brain injury (TBI) and lesions affecting the right hemisphere, such as in stroke, both

causes of MSD. Kawamura & Koyama (2007) also demonstrated poor performance on theory of mind assessments in a Parkinson's disease (PD) group who had strong Mini-Mental State Examination (MMSE) scores (Folstein, Folstein, & McHugh, 1975). In the same three neurological groups, TBI, stroke, and PD, there is evidence also of difficulties in interpretation of facial expression and emotional prosody, which have the potential to affect interpretation of the assessor's approach and response to the client.

Perception

Visual processing requirements in assessment may be high, especially for the word or sentence stimuli of intelligibility testing and for picture material used to elicit more spontaneous data, including discourse. Data may be rendered invalid if the presented stimuli are not recognized. Many cortical areas contribute to visual processing, but marked difficulties often are associated with parietal and occipital damage, particularly to the right hemisphere. It is standard practice for clinicians carrying out language testing to conduct visual perceptual screening; in motor speech assessment, perception should not be assumed to be intact, especially where there is cortical damage. The extent to which a visual processing deficit may affect perception of modeled movements of the speech organs is unknown. Auditory perceptual deficit may affect temporal processing, prosodic perception, and, therefore, the meaning derived from language, but also the execution of tasks that involve repetition of prosodic patterns.

Attention

Assessment requires that attention first be aroused and focused. Second, attention must be maintained throughout task instruction; stimulus presentation, with its associated perception and information processing; retrieval of information from memory; and then responding. Third, attention must be selective, in that competing background noise or speech does not cause attention to be diverted from the task in hand. Self-monitoring, important throughout assessment, is reliant on the ability to maintain attention through a task. The mental fatigue and difficulty in concentration, which are common complaints in brain damage and observed frequently in assessment and other clinical activities, are linked closely to deficits in sustaining attention (van Zomeren & Spikman, 2005). Assessment data should be monitored for performance deterioration, evident in negative changes in accuracy and rate, and maintenance of focus. Neglect, which is associated especially with right hemisphere parietal lesions, may limit the information derived from the contralateral side, including the face, which is very relevant to speech and nonspeech oral activities.

Memory

It is impossible to divorce memory from any task in which language is used in instruction, stimulus, or response. In imitative tasks, immediate memory of the model is required. Discourse tasks, including conversation, necessitate working memory of the intention and what already has been said, in addition to declarative and semantic memory, and possibly also procedural memory, and its related event ordering. Throughout test administration, it is expected that information, explanation, and instruction, perhaps given only once, will be recalled, and elements or principles carried forward to a succeeding task. Tasks may be novel and unfamiliar, thus involving new skill acquisition. Memory limitations have been described across a wide range of neurological disorders that cause MSD.

Executive Function

Executive function depends on the basic cognitive processes of perception, attention, and memory. It is wide in scope, encompassing planning, scheduling, strategy use, and rule adherence; generation, fluency, and initiation; shifting and suppression; and concept formation and abstract reasoning (Keil & Kaszniak, 2002). Executive function allows us to conceive an appropriate response; plan, initiate, and order response; anticipate; shift to a new task and requirements; relinquish what is no longer relevant; see the task through to completion, without diversion; solve any problem that arises; and monitor the response for accuracy and appropriateness. Executive function skills, thus, are highly relevant throughout speech assessment; deficit appears to be inevitably present where there is any cognitive process loss.

Decreased Speed

Response slowness is common in people who have MSD, subsequent to various lesion locations. Decreased processing efficiency may underlie much poor task performance, explained as both a consequence and a cause, across a range of cognitive domains (Salthouse, 2000). Low motivation, fatigue, medication, and physical limitation also may be the basis of slowness. Additional time for processing of instructions and stimuli and for response planning, including during conversational interaction, may be needed during assessment. Timed tests are used frequently in motor speech assessment, for example, movement and syllable repetitions. In evaluating responses, it may be necessary to take into account decreased speed explanations, which are additional to MSD. Response should be examined across an entire task, looking not only at mean performance speed, but also at variability.

Cognitive deficits are dependent on the nature and extent of the pathological insult and are commonly multiple and interacting (Halligan & Wade, 2005). In the assessment of a given cognitive process, minimization of confounding factors is possible to a very limited extent. Attention is a prerequisite for memory, and overloading working memory negatively impacts on attention. Failure on a memory task may result from perception deficit. Working memory limitation may affect any task in which adhering to instructions is required. Language task performance may be compromised by visual perceptual impairment. Perception, attention, memory, and language deficits will all influence the completion of executive function tasks. The capacity for language deficit to impact on assessments of cognition and motor speech is of particular importance.

Language

Language is the medium of motor speech assessment. Throughout, the assessor uses spoken, and perhaps also written language, which must be perceived, processed, and understood, with central points committed to memory, and acted on, through response activity and speech output. The language used by the assessor may comprise conversational contribution, question inviting a spoken response, explanation of the purpose of a task, instruction as to the response requirement, or stimuli for imitation or reading. Even in nonspeech activity, such as tongue protrusion or lip rounding, or quasi-speech activity, such as the production of repetitive syllables, important information must be understood, such as the number of movements or the requirement to execute the task at speed or with maximal effort. The expected response may be verbal, involving the selection of words and grammar and sequencing of sentences, in situations where, for example, background information is requested or discourse data are collected as part of the assessment of the person with MSD. Specific words or sentences may be required, perhaps read aloud, within assessment of articulatory accuracy or intelligibility.

The understanding of language used, and any associated verbal responding, may be affected by aphasia and dementia, which may coexist with dysarthria and apraxia of speech. Even without such specific additional disorders, the ability to understand and use language effectively and efficiently during assessment may be decreased by deficits in the cognitive processes, which underpin language, that may be either the result of normal aging or a component of the causative neurological disease. Such effects may be additional to lifelong learning disabilities, present at moderate to severe level in 3–4 people per 1,000 in the general population, and a more difficult to establish prevalence at milder level (Gates, 2003). The increased prevalence of learning difficulty in the TBI population should be noted.

Establishing Cognitive Involvement in Neurological Disorders

Cognitive impairment, and its related activity and participation limitations, is associated with many neurological disorders and diseases that cause MSD. Its presence is firmly established in stroke, TBI, PD, Huntington's disease, hereditary ataxias, and multiple sclerosis. In motor neurone disease, previously thought to be characterized by intact cognition, now some evidence of deficit exists. In considering the cognitive dimension in neurological diseases, the prevalence of both MSD and cognitive impairment are relevant. Statistics given must be taken as indicative only, as prevalence figures are influenced by many research design factors, relating to participant sample and the nature of assessment.

Participant variables that affect prevalence statistics include the number of cases sampled, the extent to which these are representative of the disease population, severity and duration of disease, exclusion criteria, recruitment method, and the appropriateness of normative data. Assessment variables include instrument psychometrics, such as reliability and validity, task sensitivity and specificity, practice effects on repeated testing, and content comprehensiveness. Also relevant are the knowledge, experience, and acumen of the person who diagnoses that the deficit in question is present or not. Diagnosis may be based simply on performance below a cut-off score, but in other instances, it is more subjective, and data must be evaluated in relation to and integrated with, information from other sources. Where definitive diagnostic criteria are lacking, diagnosis is much influenced by the assessor's interpretation of the data.

The views of the individual being assessed, and of others who knew him/her before neurological diagnosis, as to competence and limitations, also may be considered in diagnosis, but may be at odds with the clinician's evaluation. Should memory be judged unimpaired because test performance is within normal limits, although the client reports difficulties? Is diagnosis of word finding difficulty appropriate when the client's score is close to the normal range and the relative comments that before stroke he/she would not have been able to name certain stimuli? Such dilemmas are also familiar in motor speech assessment. Is a diagnosis of dysarthria appropriate when the clinician considers speech to be normal but the client is convinced that it is less clear or strong or melodic than before? According to Sbordone, Saul, & Purisch (2007), neuropsychological test results are often inconsistent with the client's subjective complaints. Although the individual has a unique perspective on his/her difficulties, they caution that limited awareness is common in brain injury. Self-reports are further complicated by aging, and changes noted by the client or others may be unrelated to the neurological disease, but rather a manifestation of the aging process. The verbal means of much cognitive testing, especially in dementia assessment, poses additional obstacles for reliably gauging the extent of impairment in MSD populations, whose responses may be slow, not intelligible, and misconstrued. Overestimation of cognitive involvement is, therefore, possible, but so is underestimation, as people with poor speech are sometimes excluded from cognitive investigations.

Cognitive Deficit in Neurological Disorders

Cognitive deficits associated with five neurological conditions, in which MSD is common, now are considered: stroke, traumatic brain injury, Parkinson's disease, multiple sclerosis, and motor neurone disease. As it is beyond the scope of this chapter to include all diseases whose symptomotalogy includes both MSD and cognitive loss, those with lower disease incidence and prevalence are excluded.

Stroke

In Duffy's (2005) audit data, 22% of 1276 dysarthria cases were vascular. According to the same author, stroke is the major cause of apraxia of speech. Cognitive impairments are frequent in right and especially left stroke populations, including those with lacunar stroke (Fure, Bruun, Engedal, & Thommessen, 2006). Deficits across the full range of cognitive processes have been demonstrated. Estimates of dementia prevalence in stroke vary greatly, influenced by the diagnostic criteria used, including whether depression, cognitive deficit, and aphasia are discriminated satisfactorily from dementia, and the time poststroke. At three months after stroke, Pohjasvaara et al. (1998) diagnosed dementia subsequent to first stroke in 29%, whereas Madureira, Guerreiro, & Ferro (2001) found only 6% to have dementia. Aphasia is present acutely in 33% of people with stroke (Laska, Hellblom, Murray, Kahan, & Von Arbin, 2001). Poor language test performance is common in stroke, not only in those with dementia or aphasia diagnoses. Regardless of the debate as to the extent to which aphasia is influenced by other cognitive effects, many stroke clients with MSD will have cognitive and language impairments. This is especially relevant in upper motor neurone system lesions, cortical or subcortical. However, the role of the cerebellum as a cognitive modulator is recognized increasingly (Paquier & Marien, 2005), including for both script and spatial sequencing(Leggio et al., 2008). Cognitive and linguistic deficits are common in participants who have isolated cerebellar infarcts (Kalashnikova, Zueva, Pugacheva, & Korsakova, 2005).

Traumatic Brain Injury (TBI)

The MSD prevalence in TBI is not well established. Dysarthria has been reported as 10–60%, depending on time postinjury (Yorkston, Honsinger, Mitsuda, & Hammen, 1989). TBI is recognized as a cause also of apraxia of speech (Duffy, 2005). Impairments in attention, memory, and particularly executive function are common, but comprehensive assessment shows more global deficit, strongly associated with severity measures, such as the duration of altered consciousness (Dikmen, Machamer, Winn, & Temkin, 1995). A meta-analysis of Schretlen & Shapiro (2003) showed that for moderate-severe TBI patients tested more than two years after injury, the average cognitive performance was around the 20th percentile of matched controls. For mild injury, by 30 days after lesion, the average performance was indistinguishable from the control performance. The interdependence of language and other aspects of cognitive function is well accepted in TBI, although the use of "cognitive-communication disorder" to signify that impairments in underlying cognitive processes are manifested in listening, speaking, reading, and writing difficulties (Turkstra, Coelho, & Ylvisaker, 2005). Classical aphasia syndromes are rare (Ylvisaker, Szekeres, & Feeney, 2008). Disruption to pragmatic aspects of communication, such as topic management, was found in 86% of a severely brain injured sample (McLennan, Cornis-Pop, Picon-Nieto, & Sigford, 2002). The high prevalence of cognitive and communication deficits in TBI is linked to the typically diffuse nature of the brain damage and the frequent involvement of the frontal lobe, a key site for cognitive ability. When assessing MSD in TBI, especially where severity of injury is classed as moderate or severe, the clinician should anticipate the presence of additional deficits in cognition and communication.

Parkinson's Disease (PD)

Hypokinetic dysarthria is linked firmly with PD and other Parkinsonian syn-dromes, with prevalence as high as 60–80% noted (Adams & Dykstra, 2009). Cognitive decline is usually slowly progressive, although dementia is well documented, with a risk six times higher than in the general population (Aarsland et al., 2001). Twenty years after PD diagnosis, Hely, Reid, Adena, Halliday. & Morris (2008) found dementia to be present in 83% and moderate dysarthria in 81%. Establishing dementia prevalence in PD is hindered by the inconsistency in diagnostic criteria, including reliable differentiation from milder cognitive deficit, depression, motor limitation, the confounding factors of medication that may affect cognition, and the age-related risk of Alzheimer's disease. Foltynie, Brayne, Robbins, & Barker (2004) found some cognitive impairment in 36% of a recently diagnosed PD sample, which may be increased further by inclusion of people with Parkinsonism. Cummings (1995) reports that 30–40% of people with PD have isolated executive function deficit. Memory is spared in some cases (Marti, Tolosa, & Andres, 2007). However, the full range of cognitive impairments occur, encompassing memory, attention, visuospatial abilities, executive function, and language (Nazem et al., 2009). Language deficits, involving, for example, word finding, sentence formulation, and complex sentence comprehension usually are interpreted as manifestations of cognitive impairment. McKinlay, Dalrymple-Alford, Grace, & Roger (2009) showed a strong association between aspects of pragmatic comprehension, for example, inference and metaphor, and performance on tests of processing speed and working memory, all of which were impaired relative to a control group. Emotional processing impairments have been demonstrated in some PD studies, and Kawamura & Koyama (2007) hypothesize that social cognition may be affected at an early stage, limiting the ability to make appropriate decisions, recognize facial expression, and interpret intentions. McNamara & Durso (2003) found a PD group to be impaired on the Prutting & Kirchner (1987) Pragmatic Protocol. Given the dysarthria frequency, it may be concluded that many PD patients, especially with advanced or long-standing disease, will have cognitive deficits, which may or may not fulfill dementia diagnostic criteria. Limitations in pragmatic communication and ability to discern another's perspective also may be present.

Multiple Sclerosis (MS)

Motor speech involvement, most often in the form of mixed ataxic-spastic dysarthria, is present in 40–50% of people with MS (Theodoros, Murdoch, & Ward, 2000). Unlike stroke and PD, because of the typically younger adult group, age-related changes in cognition are not expected in MS. Cognitive deficit is estimated at 40–65% (Amato, Zipoli, & Portaccio, 2008). Impairments are present in measures of general intelligence, verbal skills, memory attention/concentration, cognitive flexibility, and abstraction and are generally more pronounced in chronic progressive than in relapsing-remitting form (Zakzanis, 2000). Discrete process deficits may be observed, but with progression of the disease, cognitive involvement tends to become widespread. Severe dementia (subcortical or combined cortical/subcortical) has been reported in 20–30% of cognitively

impaired people (Rao, Hammeke, McQuillen, Khatri, & Lloyd, 1984), but without assessment that incorporates personality and behavioral features, dementia diagnosis is often questionable. Classical aphasia is unlikely, but performance decrements have been demonstrated in many language measures such as naming, word definition, word fluency, sentence repetition, verbal explanation, verbal reasoning, and high-level comprehension (Murdoch & Lethlean, 2000). Strong associations have been established between dysarthria and cognitive-linguistic task performance (Smith & Arnett, 2007; Mackenzie & Green, 2009), highlighting the need for cognitive and language performance to be monitored in dysarthria resulting from MS.

Motor Neurone Disease (MND)

Traditionally, MND, also known as amyotrophic lateral sclerosis, has been classed as a motor disorder with cognitive function remaining intact. However, several studies have challenged this view, demonstrating both dementia, and "subclinical" cognitive impairment. The dementia in MND is considered a form of fronto-temporal dementia, characterized by impaired new learning, poor working memory and planning, slowness in information processing, and rigidity of thinking and may affect more than 20% of cases (Barson, Kinsella, Ong, & Mathers, 2000). Hanagasi et al. (2002) showed a nondemented group to be impaired significantly relative to control participants in working memory, sustained attention, response inhibition, naming, verbal fluency, and complex visuospatial processing tests.

Apraxia of speech is observed in a small number of people with neurodegenerative diseases, including MND (Duffy, 2006). Dysarthria, usually mixed spastic-flaccid, is virtually inevitable and is associated moderately with cognitive impairment (Sterling et al., 2009). 95% of MND patients are reported to develop severe dysarthria, or inability to speak, therefore requiring augmentative and alternative communication (Ball, Beukelman, & Pattee, 2004). Motor speech assessment, therefore, includes evaluation of the potential for effective AAC use. This and the future system modifications which likely are to be required, are influenced much by cognitive status.

Assessment of Cognitive Skills in People with Motor Speech Disorder

Assessment of cognitive skills should be in the context of a comprehensive view of the patient's medical, behavioral, and environmental status and related managements and may contribute to medical diagnosis. The SLP's motivation for assessment of cognitive skills in a client with MSD may arise from knowledge that cognitive deficit is associated with the causative neurological disease or from informal observation of behavior and responses. In the clinical situation, difficulties in gaining and maintaining the client's attention, understanding or remembering instructions, task shifting, strategy generalization, recalling advice, or finding words may prompt a closer look at cognitive skills. The SLP may carry out cognitive screening to show whether performance has altered from a previous assessment or is within the range of normal for the individual's age and education level. However, many commonly used tests are limited in control of education effects and do not include normative data relevant to elderly people, thus presenting a challenge to interpretation. Furthermore, many of the tools available to the SLP have been standardized on U.S. populations, with unknown application to other countries and cultures.

Heterogeneity is a feature of any group, but especially the elderly population. Mean scores mask the gulf between the very able, whose performance matches that of much younger people, and those whose scores overlap with early dementia. The results of screening measures may indicate the need for more detailed, comprehensive assessment by a neuropsychologist. Many neuropsychological tests are available, most of which are impairment oriented (see Lezak, Howieson, & Loring, 2004; Strauss, Sherman, & Spreen, 2006, for overviews of measures for discrete cognitive processes). This chapter considers mainly instruments in which SLPs are a target user population.

Assessment by the Speech-Language Pathologist

In some neurological diseases, for example stroke, language screening is a standard procedure for people with MSD. In other conditions, such as MS, language assessment is unusual. Many tools and protocols are available to assess language impairment, and to a lesser extent, activity and participation.

Depending on the clinician's purpose, these may include Comprehensive Diagnostic Batteries (e.g., Boston Diagnostic Aphasia Examination (BDAE-3); Goodglass, Kaplan, & Barresi, 2001); Screening (Bedside) Tests (e.g., Aphasia Screening Test; Whurr, 1996); detailed testing of specific aspects of language processing (e.g., Psycholinguistic Assessments of Language Processing (PALPA); Kay, Lesser, & Coltheart, 1992); functional assessments (e.g., American Speech-Language Hearing Association Functional Assessment of Communication Skills for Adults (ASHA FACS; Frattali, Thompson, Holland, Wohl, & Ferketic, 1995); pragmatic profiling (e.g., Pragmatic Protocol; Prutting & Kirchner, 1987), and analysis of discourse, including conversation (e.g., Conversation Analysis Profile for People with Aphasia (CAPPA); Whitworth, Perkins, & Lesser, 1997). The reader is referred to Patterson & Chapey (2008) for details of these and other assessments.

Nonlinguistic cognitive tests also are included in several aphasia batteries. Supplementary to BDAE-3 (Goodglass, et al. 2001) are tests for constructional apraxia, finger agnosia, aculculia, and right-left confusion. The Western Aphasia Battery–Revised (Kertesz, 2007) includes supplemental constructional, visuospatial, and calculation tests, incorporating the Raven's Colored Progressive Matrices. Within a cognitive screen, the Comprehensive Aphasia Test (Swinburn, Porter, & Howard, 2004) includes subtests for visual neglect, semantic memory, word fluency, recognition memory, apraxia, and arithmetic.

The Mini Mental State Examination (MMSE; Folstein et al., 1975) is readily available, simple and quick (average 10 minutes) to administer and score. It commonly is used by health and social care professionals and in research to provide a general indication of cognitive status. MMSE includes tasks for orientation to time and place, recall, design copying, attention, and language (naming, sentence repetition, command execution, reading comprehension, and writing). Processing speed and executive function are not tested. General guidelines are that a normal performance is a score of 24–30 and 20–23, 10–19 and 0–9 are respectively indicative of mild, moderate, and severe cognitive impairment. However, the MMSE lacks sensitivity to mild and early dementia, especially in well-educated people, and may be over-sensitive for some elderly and poorly educated groups (Tombaugh & McIntyre, 1992). The MMSE had been subject to adaptations to suit various populations and circumstances. It is incorporated in the Addenbrooke's Cognitive Examination (ACE: Mathurunath, Nestor, Berrios, Rakowicz, & Hodges, 2005), which is recommended as a more comprehensive tool for cognitive testing (Scottish Intercollegiate Guidelines Network, 2006).

The Cognitive Linguistic Quick Test (CLQT; Helm-Estabrooks, 2001) is designed for SLPs and other appropriately qualified professionals to use with adults who have, or are suspected to have, acquired neurological dysfunction. To maximize the suitability of CLQT for people with language difficulty, including aphasia, language demands have been minimized in several tasks. A Spanish version is available. Administration time is 15–30 minutes. CLQT comprises 10 tasks, which evaluate various combinations of attention, memory, executive function, visuospatial skills, and language. Scores in each of these five domains are translated into severity ratings, for age groups 18–69 and 70–89, within normal limits, mild, moderate, and severe, facilitating comparison across cognitive areas. A composite severity rating is calculated. The clock drawing task, requiring all five cognitive processes, is scored separately as an independent mini-screen for cognitive dysfunction.

The Arizona Battery for Communication Disorders of Dementia (ABCD; Bayles & Tomoeda, 1993) primarily is intended for identification and quantification of the linguistic communication deficits associated with Alzheimer's disease and has been used widely in dementia research. It is a useful tool for profiling linguistic and cognitive skills with other populations also, including multiple sclerosis (Mackenzie & Green, 2009). Response requirements allow for its use with nonambulatory patients. The ABCD comprises four screening tasks and 14 subtests (mental status, story retelling immediate, following commands, word learning, comparative questions, repetition, object description, reading comprehension words, reading comprehension sentences, generative naming, semantic category, confrontation naming, concept definition, generative drawing, figure copying, and story retelling delayed). Selected subtests may be used. Subtest scores are used to calculate construct scores in mental status, episodic memory, linguistic expression, linguistic comprehension, and visuospatial construction, thus permitting cross-construct comparison and a total overall score. Administration time is 45–90 minutes. Normative data are given for Alzheimer's disease, nondemented Parkinson's disease, elderly (mean age 70) and young

(mean age 20) normal groups. Some data from a small group with Parkinson's disease with dementia also are included. Armstrong, Bayles, Borthwick & Tomoeda (1996) reported excellent correspondence between UK and U.S. populations, using a few alterations appropriate to the UK, and concluded the ABCD could be used with confidence in the UK.

The Burns Brief Inventory of Communication and Cognition (Burns, 1997) comprises three test inventories: left hemisphere, right hemisphere, and complex neuropathology (intended for multiple lesion, early dementia, closed head injury), each taking around 30 minutes to administer. Its purpose is to assist SLPs in identification of communication and cognitive deficits in adults with neurological impairment, and treatment planning. The left hemisphere, right hemisphere, and complex neuropathology inventories comprise, respectively, 16 tests for auditory comprehension, verbal expression, reading, writing, and numerical reasoning, 12 tests for visual scanning and tracking, visuospatial skills, prosody, and abstract language, and 15 tests for orientation, factual memory, auditory attention, and memory, visual perception, visual attention, and memory. Performance in the areas assessed is categorized within three severity levels, so facilitating profiling of strengths and weaknesses and prioritization of treatment goals.

The Ross Information Processing Assessment (RIPA-2; Ross-Swain, 1996) is designed primarily for SLPs to examine cognitive-linguistic skills in TBI, aged 15–90, but has application to other diagnostic groups. Ten subtests assess immediate memory, recent memory, temporal orientation, spatial orientation,

orientation to environment, recall of general information, problem solving, abstract reasoning, organization, and auditory processing and retention. Subtest raw scores are converted into percentiles and standard scores, equated to mild, moderate, marked and severe ratings.

The Mini Inventory of Right Brain Injury (MIRBI-2; Pimental & Knight, 2000) includes tasks and observations for attention, ability to explain incongruities, absurdities, figurative language and similarities, affective language, emotions and affect processing, understanding humor, praxis, and expressive ability. MIRBI-2 is intended for use by SLPs and other health professionals. Testing time is 15–30 minutes. Raw scores are converted to percentiles and stanines. A severity index and deficit profile for ages 20–80 is provided, based on underlying disorders of processing. A right-left hemisphere differential subscale is included.

Interpretation of Test Results

Cognitive assessment results must be interpreted with care, as low scores may result from variables other than cognitive deficit. Depression is common in brain damaged and elderly populations and may mimic (pseudodementia), or coexist with dementia, especially in the early stages. Many tests necessitate verbal responses or comprehension of instructions and questions. Some dementia screening measures are entirely language based, such as that of Kilada et al. (2005), which consists of a sentence repetition and animal name generation, reported to have higher

sensitivity for early dementia than MMSE. The potential for misdiagnosis by inexperienced testers is high, when such measures are used with people who have aphasia or other language deficits. Using a language modified MMSE, Pashek (2008) found an average 10-points score increase in people with aphasia, relative to MMSE scores.

Additional problems, relevant to the MSD population, which may affect cognitive and linguistic assessment, include fatigue, pain, absence attacks, sleep deprivation, visual disturbances (including agnosia), motor disturbances (including apraxia), hearing loss, effects of medication, alcohol, recreational drugs, anxiety, task unfamiliarity, poor rapport with the assessor, and cultural divergence. Responding may be affected further by initiation difficulty, slow speaking rate, intelligibility limitation, and micrographia.

Assessment of cognitive processes remains generally impairment focused, and much concern exists about the ecological validity of typically used measures. According to the principle of verisimilitude (Franzen & Wilhelm, 1996), the cognitive demands of the individual patient's functional settings should determine the tests used. Examples of cognitive tests that aim to take account of everyday demands are the Rivermead Behavioral Memory Test (Wilson, Cockburn, & Baddeley, 1985) and the Test of Everyday Attention (Robertson, Ward, Ridgeway, & Nimmo-Smith, 1994). The clinician working with the patient who has dysarthria or apraxia of speech may question the extent to which performance on a decontextualized cognitive test or battery reflects capacity to co-operate in motor speech assessment or derive benefit from intervention. Although appropriate cognitive assessment will provide useful information, the value of the experienced clinician's informal observation of the client's functioning in clinical situations, combined with a knowledge of cognition and its deficit in the causative neurological disorders, should not be overlooked.

Conclusion

Cognitive deficit occurs in many neurological disorders, with the potential to compromise motor speech assessment, affecting the relevance of selected procedures or tools, the conduct of the data-collecting exercise, and subsequent interpretation, treatment planning, and conclusions. The ability to follow instruction, recall information, and learn and apply new skills may be affected. Information, advice, and practice material may require adaptation. Where dysarthria or apraxia of speech is the presenting symptom, assessment often should extend beyond motor speech. Many tools are available that will provide a view of strengths and weaknesses across the cognitive processes, which may affect everyday life in social situations and in education and employment contexts. Cognitive status is likely to be an important variable influencing the outcome of motor speech intervention.

References

Aarsland, D., Andersen, K., Larsen, J. P., Lolk, A., Nielsen, H., & Kragh-Sorensen, P. (2001). Risk of dementia in Parkinson's disease: A community-based, prospective study. *Neurology, 56,* 730–736.

Adams, S. G., & Dykstra, A. (2009). Hypokinetic dysarthria. In M. R. McNeil (Ed.), *Clinical management of sensorimotor speech Disorders* (2nd ed., pp. 166–186). New York, NY: Thieme.

Amato, M. P., Zipoli, V., & Portaccio, E. (2008) Cognitive changes in multiple sclerosis. *Expert Review of Neurotherapeutics, 8,* 1585–1596.

Armstrong, L., Bayles, K. A., Borthwick, S. E., & Tomoeda, C. K. (1996). Use of the Arizona Battery for Communication Disorders of Dementia in the UK. *European Journal of Disorders of Communication, 31,* 171–180.

Ball, L., Beukelman, D., & Pattee, G. (2004). Augmentative and alternative communication acceptance by persons with amyotrophic lateral sclerosis. *Augmentative and Alternative Communication, 20,* 113–123.

Barson, F. P., Kinsella, G. J., Ong, B., & Mathers, S. E. (2000). A neuropsychological investigation of dementia in motor neurone disease (MND). *Journal of the Neurological Sciences, 180,* 117–113.

Bayles, K. A. & Tomoeda, C. K. (1993). *Arizona Battery for Communication Disorders of Dementia.* Tucson, AZ: Canyonlands.

Burns, M. S. (1997) *Burns Brief Inventory of Communication and Cognition.* San Antonio, TX: Psychological Corporation.

Cummings, J. L. (1995). *The neuropsychiatry of Alzheimer's disease and related dementias.* London, UK: Dunitz.

Dikmen, S. S., Machamer, J. E., Winn, R., & Temkin, N. R. (1995). Neuropsychological outcome at 1-year post head injury. *Neuropsychology, 9,* 80–90.

Duffy, J. R. (2005). *Motor speech disorders: Substrates, differential diagnosis and Management* (2nd ed.). St Louis, MO: Elsevier Mosby.

Duffy, J. R. (2006). Apraxia of speech in degenerative neurologic disease. *Aphasiology, 20,* 511–527.

Folstein, M. F., Folstein, S. E., & McHugh, P. R. (1975). 'Mini-Mental State': A practical method of grading the cognitive state of patients for the clinician. *Journal of Psychiatric Research, 12,* 189–198.

Foltynie, T., Brayne, C. E. G., Robbins, T. W., & Barker, R. A. (2004). The cognitive ability of an incident cohort of Parkinson's patients in the UK. The CamPaIGN study. *Brain, 127,* 550–560.

Franzen, M. D., & Wilhelm, K. L. (1996). Conceptual foundations of ecological validity in neuropsychology. In R. J. Sbordone & C. J. Long (Eds.), *The ecological validity of neuropsychological testing* (pp. 51–69). Orlando, FL: St Lucie Press.

Frattali, C., Thompson, C. K., Holland, A. L., Wohl, C. B., & Ferketic, M. K. (1995). *American Speech-Language Hearing Association Functional Assessment of Communication Skills for Adults (ASHA FACS).* Rockville, MD: ASHLA.

Fure, B., Bruun, W. T., Engedal, K., & Thommessen, B. (2006). Cognitive impairments in acute lacunar stroke. *Acta Neurologica Scandinavica, 114,* 17–22.

Gates, B. (2003). *Learning disabilities: Toward inclusion.* New York, NY: Churchill Livingstone.

Goodglass, H., Kaplan, E., & Barresi, B. (2001). *The Boston Diagnostic Aphasia Examination (BDAE-3).* Baltimore, MD: Lippincott, Williams, and Wilkins.

Hanagasi, H. A., Gurvit, I. H., Ermutlu, N., Kaptanoglu, G., Idrisoglu, H. A., Emre, M., & Demiralp, T. (2002). Cognitive impairment in amyotrophic lateral sclerosis: Evidence from neuropsychological investigation and event-related potentials. *Cognitive Brain Research, 14,* 234–244.

Halligan, P. W., & Wade, D. T. (2005). Introduction. Is rehabilitation of deficits effective? In P. W. Halligan & D. T. Wade (Eds.), *Effectiveness of rehabilitation for cognitive deficits* (pp. xi–xv). Oxford, UK: Oxford University Press.

Helm-Estabrooks, N. (2001). *Cognitive Linguistic Quick Test.* San Antonio, TX: Psychological Corporation.

Hely, M. A., Reid, W. G. J., Adena, M. A., Halliday, G. M., & Morris, J. G. L. (2008). The Sydney multicenter study of Parkinson's disease: The inevitability of dementia at 20 years. *Movement Disorders, 23,* 837–844.

Kalashnikova, L., Zueva, Y., Pugacheva, O., & Korsakova, N. (2005). Cognitive impairments in cerebellar infarcts. *Neuroscience and Behavioral Physiology, 35,* 773–779.

Kawamura, M., & Koyama, S. (2007). Social cognitive impairment in Parkinson's disease. *Journal of Neurology, 254* (Suppl 4), IV/49-IV/53.

Kay, J., Lesser, R., & Coltheart, M. (1992). *Psycholinguistic Assessments of Language Processing (PALPA).* Hove, UK: Erlbaum.

Keil, K., & Kaszniak, A. (2002). Examining cognitive function in individuals with brain injury: A review. *Aphasiology, 16,* 305–335.

Kertesz, A. (2007). *Western aphasia battery—Revised.* San Antonio, TX: Harcourt.

Kilada, S., Gamaldo, A., Grant, E. A., Moghekar, A., Morris, J. C., & O'Brien, R. J. (2005). Brief screening test for the diagnosis of dementia: Comparison with the Mini-Mental State Exam. *Alzheimer Disease and Associated Disorders, 19,* 8–16.

Laska, A. C., Hellblom, A., Murray, V., Kahan, T., & Von Arbin, M. (2001). Aphasia in acute stroke and relation to outcome. *Journal of Internal Medicine, 249,* 413–422.

Leggio, M. G., Tedesco, A. M., Chiricozzi, F. R., Clausi, S., Orsini, A., & Molinari, M. (2008). Cognitive sequencing impairment in patients with focal and atrophic cerebellar damage. *Brain, 131,* 1332–1343.

Lezak, M. D., Howieson, D. B., & Loring, D.,M. (2004). *Neuropsychological assessment* (4th ed.). New York, NY: Oxford University Press.

Mackenzie, C., & Green, J. (2009). Cognitive-linguistic deficit and speech intelligibility in chronic progressive multiple sclerosis. *International Journal of Language and Communication Disorders, 44,* 401–420.

Madureira, S., Guerreiro, M., & Ferro, J. M. (2001). Dementia and cognitive impairment three months after stroke. *European Journal of Neurology, 8,* 621–627.

Mathurunath, P. S., Nestor, P. J., Berrios, G. E., Rakowicz, W., & Hodges, J. R. (2005). A brief cognitive test battery to differentiate Alzheimer's disease and frontotemporal dementia. *Neurology, 55,* 1613–1620.

Marti, M., Tolosa, E., & Andres, C. (2007). Dementia in Parkinson's disease. *Journal of Neurology, 254,* suppl. 1, 41–48.

McKinlay, A., Dalrymple-Alford, J. C., Grace, R. C., & Roger, D. (2009). The effect of attentional set-shifting, working memory, and processing speed on pragmatic language functioning in Parkinson's disease. *European Journal of Cognitive Psychology, 21,* 330–346.

McLennan, D. L., Cornis-Pop, M., Picon-Nieto, L., & Sigford, B. (2002). The prevalence of pragmatic communication impairments in traumatic brain injury. *Premier Outlook, 3,* 1–8.

McNamara, P., & Durso, R. (2003). Pragmatic communication skills in patients with Parkinson's disease. *Brain and Language, 84,* 414–423.

Murdoch, B. E., & Lethlean, J. B. (2000). Language disorders in multiple sclerosis. In B. E. Murdoch and D. Theodoros (Eds.), *Speech and language disorders in multiple sclerosis* (pp. 155–194). London, UK: Whurr.

Nazem, S., Siderowf, A. D., Duda, J. E., Ten Have, T., Colcher, A., Horn, S. S., . . . Weintraub, D. (2009). Montreal Cognitive Assessment performance in patients with Parkinson's disease with normal global cognition according to Mini-Mental State Examination score. *Journal of the American Geriatrics Society, 57,* 304–308.

Neisser, U. (1967). *Cognitive psychology.* New York, NY: Appleton-Century-Crofts.

Paquier, P. F., & Marien, P. (2005). A synthesis of the role of the cerebellum in cognition. *Aphasiology, 19,* 3–19.

Pashek, G. V. (2008). Screening mental status is adults with aphasia using a language-modified form of the Mini-Mental State Examination: A preliminary investigation. *Journal of Medical Speech-Language Pathology, 16,* 1–19.

Patterson, J. P., & Chapey, R. (2008). Assessment of language disorders in adults. In R. Chapey (Ed.), *Language intervention strategies in aphasia and related neurogenic communication disorders* (pp. 64–162). Philadelphia, PA: Lipincott Williams and Wilkins.

Pimental, P. A., & Knight, J. A. (2000). *Mini Inventory of Right Brain Injury* (MIRBI-2). Austin, TX: Pro-Ed.

Pohjasvaara, T., Erkinjuntti, T., Ylikoski, R., Hietanen, M., Vataja, R., & Kaste, M. (1998). Clinical determinants of poststroke dementia. *Stroke, 29,* 75–81.

Prutting, C., & Kirchner, D. (1987). A clinical appraisal of the pragmatic aspects of language. *Journal of Speech and Hearing Disorders, 52,* 105–119.

Rao, S. M., Hammeke, T. A., McQuillen, M. P., Khatri, B. O., & Lloyd, D. (1984). Memory disturbance in chronic progressive multiple sclerosis. *Archives of Neurology, 41,* 625–631.

Robertson, I. H., Ward, T., Ridgeway, V., & Nimmo-Smith, I. (1994). *The test of everyday attention.* Bury, UK: Thames Valley.

Ross-Swain, D. (1996). *Ross Information Processing Assessment–2.* Austin, YX: Pro-Ed.

Salthouse, T. A. (2000). Steps towards the explanation of adult age differences in cognition. In T. J. Perfect & E. A. Maylor (Eds.), *Models of cognitive aging* (pp. 19–49). Oxford, UK: Oxford University Press.

Sbordone, R. J., Saul, R. E., & Purisch, A. D. (2007). *Neuropsychology for psychologists, health care professionals and attorneys.* London, UK: CRC Press.

Schretlen, D. J., & Shapiro, A. M. (2003). A quantitative review of the effects of traumatic brain injury on cognitive functioning. *International Review of Psychiatry, 15,* 341–349.

Scottish Intercollegiate Guidelines Network (2006). SIGN 86, *Management of patients with dementia.* Edinburgh, UK: SIGN.

Smith, M., & Arnett, P. (2007). Dysarthria predicts poorer performance on cognitive task requiring a speeded oral response in an MS population. *Journal of Clinical and Experimental Neuropsychology, 29,* 804–812.

Sterling, L. E., Jawaid, A., Salamone, A. R., Murthy, S. B., Mosnik, D. M., Mcdowell, E., . . . Schulz, P. E. (2010). Association between dysarthria and cognitive impairment in ALS: A prospective study. *Amyotrophic Lateral Sclerosis, 11,* 46–52.

Strauss, E., Sherman, E. M. S., & Spreen, O. (2006). *A compendium of neuropsychological tests* (3rd ed.). New York, NY: Oxford Press.

Swinburn, K., Porter, G., & Howard, D. (2004). *Comprehensive aphasia test.* Hove, UK: Psychology Press.

Theodoros, D. G., Murdoch, B. E., & Ward, E. C. (2000). Perceptual features of dysarthria in multiple sclerosis. In B. E. Murdoch and D. Theodoros (Eds.), *Speech and language disorders in multiple sclerosis* (pp. 30–46). London, UK: Whurr.

Tombaugh, T. N., & McIntyre, N. J. (1992). The Mini-Mental State Exam: A comprehensive review. *Journal of the American Geriatrics Society, 40,* 922–935.

Turkstra, L. S., Coelho, C., & Ylvisaker, M. (2005). The use of standardized tests for individuals with cognitive-communication disorders. *Seminars in Speech and Language, 26,* 215–222.

van Zomeren, A. H., & Spikman, J. M. (2005). Testing speed and control: The assessment of attentional impairments. In P. W. Halligan & D. T. Wade (Eds.), *Effectiveness of rehabilitation for cognitive deficit* (pp. 71–80). Oxford, UK: Oxford University Press.

Whitworth, A., Perkins, L., & Lesser, R. (1997). *Conversation Analysis Profile for People with Aphasia (CAPPA).* London, UK: Whurr.

Whurr, R. (1996). *Aphasia screening test.* London, UK: Whurr.

Wilson, B. A., Cockburn, J., & Baddeley, A. (1985). *The Rivermead Behavioural Memory Test.* Bury, UK: Thames Valley.

Ylvisaker, M., Szekeres, S. F., & Feeney, T. (2008) Communication disorders associated with traumatic brain injury. In R. Chapey (Ed.), *Language intervention strategies in aphasia and related neurogenic communication disorders* (pp. 879–962). Philadelphia, PA: Lippincott Williams and Wilkins.

Yorkston, K. M., Honsinger, M. J., Mitsuda, P. M., & Hammen, V. (1989). The relationship between speech and swallowing disorders in head-injured patients. *Journal of Head Trauma Rehabilitation, 4,* 1–16.

Zakzanis, K. K. (2000). Distinct neurocognitive profiles in multiple sclerosis subtypes. *Archives of Clinical Neuropsychology, 15,* 115–136.

8

Conversation Analysis and Acquired Motor Speech Disorders in Everyday Interaction

STEVEN BLOCH, PH.D.
RAY WILKINSON, PH.D.

Introduction

This chapter presents Conversation Analysis (CA) as a rigorous and systematic approach to the assessment of naturally occurring conversational talk. Its relevance to the assessment of motor speech disorders (MSDs) is explored through a review of CA principles and an analysis of extracts featuring an adult with acquired dysarthria engaged in everyday conversation. Although conversation traditionally has not been a major area of MSD assessment, it can be seen to be a phenomenon of central importance in understanding the impact of dysarthria on everyday life. Conversation is the main environment for speech in daily living. As such, it is the place where the problems created by

dysarthria can be seen to be most manifest and consequential for people with MSDs and their everyday conversation partners.

A contemporary history of motor speech disorders highlights the importance of auditory-perceptual, acoustic, and physiologic features, particularly in the diagnosis and measurement of acquired dysarthria (Duffy, 2007). For the degenerative dysarthrias, this importance is reflected in the predominance of research addressing acoustic/perceptual and neurophysiological features of MSDs (Yorkston, 2007). Descriptive tools most commonly used in UK clinical practice (Enderby & Palmer, 2007; Robertson, 1982) have evolved from the pioneering work of Darley, Aronson, and Brown (1969a, 1969b). Such tools have enabled clinicians to profile speech features and describe systematically the deviation of individual speech components from acceptable norms. They also provide a framework for treatment planning and outcome measure baselines.

Recent research also has begun to look beyond speech examination and perception in isolation in order to place MSDs within a communicative and participative context. The work of Hustad on intelligibility and comprehensibility, for example, demonstrates the significance of visual, alphabetic, and semantic cues for judgments of intelligibility (Hustad, Jones, & Dailey, 2003; Hustad, 2006; Hustad, 2007; Hustad & Lee, 2008). Hustad (2008) also highlights an important distinction between listener comprehension and ratings of intelligibility. These findings indicate that intelligibility and comprehension ratings together provide a more accurate picture of dysarthric speech comprehension than single word measures alone.

Existing MSD assessment tools typically utilize single or multiple-word reading stimuli, but attempts have been made to incorporate extended narrative and/or conversation samples (Lowit-Leuschel & Docherty, 2001). Enderby and Palmer's (2007) Frenchay Dysarthria Assessment, for example, includes a judgment of conversation within its "intelligibility" subsection. Assessors are instructed to engage the patient in conversation for five minutes before rating their intelligibility. Such approaches recognize the importance of conversation, but the analysis of such data remains underspecified in comparison with more rigorous speech analysis methods. The main difficulty here is that experimental methods developed for understanding MSDs cannot be adapted easily to the analysis of those same problems in everyday conversation.

A complementary way in which MSDs in conversation can be addressed is by using an analytical framework within which individual turns and the larger sequences in which they occur, rather than phonemes, words, or sentences in isolation, are the focus of enquiry. This framework focuses attention on how actions are accomplished through conversation and the practices used to accomplish these actions. Conversation Analysis (CA) is perhaps the most developed method available for the investigation of naturally occurring conversation, with more than 40 years of accumulated findings on the nature of "normal" (nondisordered) conversation. As such, CA provides a method and a set of findings that can now be applied to conversations involving speakers with dysarthria. The aim here is to investigate the ways in which dysarthria can create problems for participants in daily life, and the methods participants may use to try to compensate for the effects of dysarthria in conversation.

An Overview of Conversation Analysis

CA is the qualitative data-driven study of naturally occurring conversation. It takes conversation as the primary means of human interaction and attempts to describe the management of interaction between speakers. Rather than focusing on speech or language in isolation, CA directs attention to turns in conversation—how they are designed, ordered, understood, and, importantly, what they achieve (their *actions*). Action here refers to whatever a turn or series of turns is being used to do by the participants, such as story telling, evaluating, asking, and answering questions, and so on (Schegloff, 2007).

Pioneered through the work of Sacks and Schegloff during the 1960s and 1970s, CA evolved within an environment of more traditional forms of sociological and linguistic enquiry. At that time, linguistic research was influenced heavily by the work of Chomsky (1965), generating an idealized view of language competence, with theoretical examples used to demonstrate theories of language and a focus on the structure of language grammar in isolation. With minimal reference to functional language use in conversation, there was little opportunity to examine how naturally occurring conversational talk might display orderly properties and how the orderliness of that talk might be the result of the participants in conversation producing talk in certain socially conventional ways (Schegloff & Sacks, 1973). It is the description and explication of this orderliness that forms the basis of CA enquiry.

Key Principles of Conversation Analysis

CA is informed by a number of principles and assumptions. Four of these are summarized as follows:

1. *The importance of everyday and naturally occurring talk*. Everyday conversation is the most fundamental and common medium through which humans conduct their everyday lives (Schegloff, 1982, 1992) and yet, surprisingly, it has largely remained on the fringe of formal linguistics and speech analysis research. CA takes naturally occurring talk (as opposed to the elicitation of speech through tasks or experimentally controlled dialogue) as its starting point of enquiry.

2. *Order in conversation*. There is an assumption within CA that order in conversation is created through, and maintained by, participants themselves (Schegloff & Sacks, 1973). This order manifests itself through the turn-taking system (Sacks, Schegloff, & Jefferson, 1974). The existence of order at all points of conversation is fundamental to CA's philosophy, and its motivation is to identify the order that participants create (Sacks, 1984).

3. *Turns in interaction are contextually oriented*. Importantly, there is a double-context in play at all points in conversation (Heritage, 1984: p. 242). Each turn is *context-shaped* by its predecessor. That is, most turns in a sequence will be conditional on what has occurred immediately prior. Second, each turn is *context-renewing*. In this sense, a current turn will form a context for what is to be done at the next turn in any sequence.

4. *The ongoing display of understanding*. Through each next turn, a participant displays some analysis, understanding, or appreciation of the prior turn (Heritage, 1984). It is through this public display that another participant may judge

how to proceed in their own next turn at talk—particularly if there has been a problem in understanding. Further, as Sacks et al. (1974: p. 729) state, "since it is the parties' understandings of prior turns' talk that is relevant to their construction of next turns, it is THEIR understandings that are wanted for analysis." This latter point is of particular importance in understanding the distinction between CA and more traditional methods of enquiry in speech and language; namely, CA research addresses how participants themselves make sense of each other's talk.

Readers interested in exploring the relationship between CA and the more diverse approach known as discourse analysis (DA) are encouraged to refer to Woofitt's (2005) text. Important distinctions include CA's focus on participant management of interaction, its descriptive precision, and the use of audio/video recordings to justify its empirical claims.

CA Data Collection and Analysis

CA methods are shaped by the preceding principles, particularly with reference to data sources and subsequent analysis. First, there is the importance of naturally occurring conversation. The talk itself may be from any setting or context (e.g., domestic or institutional); the relevant point being that what is produced should not be scripted or styled in order to produce a specific conversation outcome.

Second, there is the importance of data collection methods. The method of data collection in CA is directed by both the need to acquire as naturally occurring talk as possible *and* by the need to have data in a form that may be examined at length. Audio/visual recordings of interaction have the advantage of being in a format that can be played repeatedly and transcribed. Much CA work now utilizes video collection techniques. This has afforded the opportunity to examine and describe a wider range of behaviors, especially nonverbal features of talk and how they combine with verbal features. Specifically, the nonverbal action can be treated as action in its own right and not simply as "back-up" for verbal activity (Heath, 1998).

Third, analysis of data in CA is based on a notion of data-driven enquiry. This differs from analyst-driven methods in that potential findings are not presupposed but rather emerge through thorough investigation of the raw data supported by and presented through written transcriptions. Practically, this means that the use of precoded categories of behavior are viewed as being less satisfactory than an analysis of the particular behaviors being used in the conversation under investigation. The rationale is that researchers cannot judge what is a relevant feature of action through talk unless the procedures used by conversational participants themselves are first examined.

The process of CA itself is based on repeated viewings/listenings of recorded conversations and continual refinement of the transcriptions. These transcriptions are based commonly on conventions formulated by Jefferson (1984); see the appendix for details.

Notable practices and patterns of action emerge from this process. Pomerantz and Fehr (1997) and Hutchby and Woofit (1998) provide further details on the tools of analysis.

As these patterns of interaction are identified (e.g., the ways in which problems with speech are noted by the recipient of a turn), collections of extracts are made. These collections then are refined and recategorized as necessary.

Applying CA to the Study of MSDs in Conversation

CA established itself over the past 40 years by primarily addressing everyday talk between people engaged in mundane conversation. Its main motivation always has been to understand how people use talk to manage the activity of being social and how they maintain social order through conversation.

In more recent years, CA has been extended beyond mundane conversation to include the analysis of institutional talk, in which one or more of the participants can be seen to be designing their talk in relation to their work-based activities (Drew & Heritage, 1992) as well as the study of talk of people with communication impairments, particularly people with aphasia (see collections of papers in Hesketh & Sage [1999] and Goodwin [2003]), and traumatic brain injury (Body & Parker, 2005). The use of CA methods in the study of MSDs emerged in the 1990s with work by Collins and colleagues (Collins & Markova, 1995; Collins, Markova, & Murphy, 1997; Collins & Markova, 1999) addressing adults with developmental MSDs. This has developed with research involving children with developmental disorders in conversation with their peers (Clarke & Wilkinson, 2007, 2008), adults with acquired neurogenic conditions including amyotrophic lateral sclerosis/motor neurone disease (ALS/MND) (Bloch & Wilkinson, 2004; Bloch, 2005; Bloch & Beeke, 2008; Bloch & Wilkinson, 2009, Bloch, in press) and multiple sclerosis (Rutter, 2009). One unifying theme of these CA-informed MSD research studies is the examination of multimodality in interaction, particularly the ways in which augmentative and alternative (AAC) system use is integrated with natural speech and/or gesture (Wilkinson, Bloch, & Clarke, in press).

Exploring Troubles and Repair in Conversations of People with MSD

This section focuses on one area of talk pertinent to MSDs in interaction, namely the occurrence and management of problems. In observing nonimpaired talk in everyday conversation, it becomes clear that speech and language rarely are produced perfectly. Typically, there are troubles in speaking, hearing, or understanding talk in conversation (Schegloff, 1997). These troubles are apparent through false starts, repeats of words, overlaps, requests for clarity, and so on. Thus, although interaction through conversation clearly works, outstanding features of what might be considered imperfection need to be understood in terms of how they arise, where they occur, and how they are dealt with.

CA literature uses the term *repair* to describe the practices used by participants to highlight and manage problems or troubles within interaction. The case can be made for distinguishing between a trouble in talk and the practices employed to deal with it (Schegloff, 1987). Within speech pathology, for example, Schegloff (1987) states that the focus has been largely on theories of error/trouble production and not on the ways in which such troubles are managed. Thus, CA draws attention to *how* troubles are highlighted as such by the participants and how they are dealt with. Often in the analysis, it is also possible to see which aspect of the turn is being treated by the participants as the trouble source.

The practices of repair are presented by Schegloff, Jefferson, and Sacks (1977). A central finding of this work is the recognition that repair can, and often does, take place in two distinct stages:

1. Initiation of repair: The displaying of something as a trouble
2. Completion of repair: What may be called the "repair" itself on a particular trouble source

Repair can involve the self or other. In this context, *self* refers to the person whose turn contains the trouble and *other* to a person in the interaction other than the one whose talk contained the trouble. In addition, Schegloff (1979) notes that the practice of repair is designed for success, and usually a single repair effort resolves the trouble it addresses. However, it is clear that all not all repairs are resolved with one effort or attempt (Schegloff, 1979). This can be particularly the case with the talk of a speaker with dysarthria (SWD) (Bloch, 2006).

Schegloff et al. (1977) identify a clear preference within the organization of conversation for *self-repair*—that is, for the speaker of a trouble source to repair his or her own trouble. This may occur within the same turn in the form of self-initiated self-repair (e.g., restating a word produced incorrectly) or in another turn following the identification of a problem by someone else, that is, other-initiated self-repair (e.g., a conversation partner saying "what?"). Thus, a typical way in which a turn may be shown to be difficult to understand is that the recipient initiates repair on it in the following turn.

An Exploration of Trouble Sources and Repair in MSD Talk

Previous work has shown that other-initiation of repair (OI) is one way in which the problematic talk of people with acquired MSDs is addressed regularly (Bloch & Wilkinson, 2004; Rutter, 2009). It also has been shown that participants can find the nature of trouble sources more complex than they appear initially (Bloch & Wilkinson, 2009). Work to date demonstrates that there is more to disordered speech in interaction than simply intelligibility, and that a number of issues can affect the *understandability* (Bloch & Wilkinson, 2004, 2009) of a turn. By understandability, we mean how a turn is understood by a recipient in relation to immediately prior turn(s). This differs from *comprehensibility* (Barefoot, Bochner, Johnson, & Eigen, 1993;, Yorkston, Strand, & Kennedy, 1996) insofar as it addresses sequential context and not just semantic/linguistic context.

In the following paragraphs, we exemplify the practice of other initiated self-repair by providing two extracts of talk with associated analysis. The participants featured in these extracts are identified by the pseudonyms Mary and Stan (a married couple). Mary, 65, had been diagnosed with amyotrophic lateral sclerosis/motor neurone disease approximately 12 months prior to the recording. At the time of recording for video 1, she presented with moderately hypernasal speech with reduced respiratory support and variable precision of tongue function for sound production. Her voice had a strangled quality, and her pitch range was reduced. Stan (72) reported mild hearing difficulties of his own, but no other communication disorders were reported or observed.

Figure 8–1, Extract 1 (Bloch & Wilkinson, 2004) demonstrates other-initiated self-repair, with the speaker without dysarthria displaying a problem (→b) by locating the trouble source in the prior turn of the SWD (→a). The repair then is attempted by the SWD (→c).

In this example, Mary and Stan are talking about a journey the previous day. Mary has just indicated that the day was a success, and she proceeds to talk about her ability to access the family car (line 01). In line 04 Stan produces an other-initiation of repair, which treats line 01 as problematic. This is followed by Mary's completion of the repair (line 06). The completion then is repeated and acknowledged by Stan in line 09. A key to the Jefferson (1984) transcription conventions used here can be found in the appendix.

Following a 0.9 second pause, Stan displays some form of difficulty in line 04. His repair initiation locates Mary's prior turn in line 01 as problematic. In this way, Mary's turn in line 01 can be

---

Extract 1 (Bloch and Wilkinson 2004: extract 1)


```
01  →  a  Mary    and my getting in (0.6) the ⌈(↓car.)                          ⌉
02                                            ⌊((drops hand & looks to Stan))   ⌋
03                (0.9)
04  →  b  Stan    getting in what?
05                (0.5)
06  →  c  Mary    the ⌈↓car:                        ⌉
07                    ⌊((drops hand & looks to Stan)) ⌋
08                (0.8)
09         Stan    the car (.) oh yeah.
10                (1.0)
11         Mary    was ⌈very good          ⌉
12         Stan        ⌊that's a that's a  ⌋ (.) that's a huge improvement (.) ⌈isn't it⌉
13         Mary                                                                ⌊mm     ⌋
```

See Appendix for transcript conventions.

Figure 8–1.

described as the "trouble source" turn. In addition, Stan shows that he has understood partially Mary's turn by locating the specific point at which the trouble is located. Thus, by specifying "getting in what?" (rather than, for example, "what?" or "pardon?"), Stan initiates an action that not only informs Mary of which part of her turn he is having a problem with, but also which parts of her turn he is treating as unproblematic and understandable. Thus, Stan's display of understanding is of particular significance in seeing how the trouble is made explicit and subsequently managed. The expectation following this initiation of repair is that some form of self-repair action by Mary will now follow, and that it will deal with at least that part of her turn that Stan has signalled as being problematic for him. Thus, Mary's next action at line 06, "the car," is an attempt to repair that part of her prior turn specified by Stan in his repair initiation as problematic. In this instance, "car" is produced with slightly more emphasis with an extended vowel sound.

The repair sequence concludes with Stan's display of understanding via a redoing of Mary's prior turn followed by a recognition and agreement. By saying "the car" himself, Stan is showing to Mary exactly what he has understood. Observations from the full data set from which this extract is selected indicate that other repetitions of self-repaired trouble sources feature strongly in conversations of this type and may be doing important work in concluding the repair sequence. Mary's next turn (line 11) adds further information to her first utterance, and by doing so, acknowledges Stan's interpretation of her repaired turn.

In the second extract in Figure 8–2, Stan again identifies a turn by Mary as problematic to understand, but here it can be seen that the way in which he presents what he has understood and not understood of Mary's turn is itself problematic. Prior to the talk in Extract 2, Mary and Stan have been talking about a woman (Carol) who has been diagnosed with cancer and attends a hospice at which Mary also uses for day care. Stan begins by asking who told Mary that Carol had cancer.

In his talk at line 14, Stan produces a question turn, specifying a body area option for the cancer. This makes relevant a next turn answer by Mary. She begins her next turn with an extended "mm" sound followed by a lifting of her finger and the production of "(↓mine mm)" (line 17). Following this, Mary looks at Stan (line 18). Her gaze in this case may function both to signal that she has completed her turn and also to look for signs of whether Stan has understood her or not. As seen in Extract 1, Stan displays that he is having trouble understanding what Mary has said in line 17.

Of particular interest here is the form of Stan's other-initiation of repair. Stan begins by repeating back what he thinks he has heard ("mind the") as part of a query about what Mary has said ("mind the what?"). It becomes clear from Mary's self-repair in line 22, however, that what she had been trying to say in line 17 was "spine." Following her self-repair attempt, Stan then offers a trial understanding ("spine?"). This turn is designed for acceptance or rejection by Mary who proceeds to show her acceptance through an affirming head nod (line 26). The talk then continues with both speakers going on to offer

Extract 2 (Bloch and Wilkinson, 2009: extract 3)

001		Stan:	who told you Carol was er had cancer.
002			(0.7)
003		Mary:	well she did.
004			(0.8)
005		Stan:	((*raises eyebrows*)) who?
006			(0.5)
007		Mary:	h (0.2) <u>she</u> did
008			(0.2)
009		Stan:	SHE did
010			(0.2)
011		Mary:	(*nods*)=
012		Stan:	=°yeah°
013			(0.8)
014		Stan:	⌈cancer of the sp ⌉ine was it no cancer of the (1.0) the hip was it
015		Mary:	⌊ (unintelligible) ⌋
016			(0.5)
017	a →	Mary:	mm: ((*points finger*)) ⌈ (↓mine mm) ⌉
018			⌊((*drops finger*)) ⌋ ((*looks to Stan*))
019			(2.0)
020	b →	Stan:	mind the what?
021			(0.6)
022	c →	Mary:	((*breathes in*)) °s°↓pine
023			(1.0)
024		Stan:	spine?
025			(0.3)
026		Mary:	((*nods*)) na⌈sty ⌉
027		Stan:	⌊↓°ah: ⌋ (.) °m:°
028			(1.2)
029		Stan:	I suppose that's a bad place to get treated really innit

Figure 8–2.

evaluations of the fact that Carol has cancer of the spine (lines 26 and 29).

In this extract, it can be seen that while Stan realizes he is having problems understanding Mary's turn, he does not fully grasp what it might be about the turn that is making it problematic. First, it can be seen that Stan here is on the wrong track as to which part of Mary's turn he is treating as having understood ("mind the"), and, linked to this, what the nature of the trouble here is. In fact, we can see in retrospect that Stan has a problem in interpreting both what the *word* is that Mary is attempting to say (i.e., "spine") and what the *social action* is (i.e., a correction) that Mary is attempting to produce with that word (see Wilkinson, 1999, for a somewhat similar misinterpretation by a hearer of an aphasic speaker's attempt at correction).

In comparing both extracts, note that the recipient follows the SWD's turn with a silence, often lasting for a significant period of time. In this context, the silence is treated as a withholding of an other-initiation of repair (Schegloff et al., 1977). In normal conversation, this withholding has been shown to provide the prior speaker with an opportunity to carry out the preferred activity of self-repair (Schegloff, et al. 1977). In the two examples here, however, it is notable that the opportunity for self-initiation of repair is not taken up by the SWD. In our data, this lack of an attempt at self-repair by the SWD, even when an opportunity is provided by a withholding of other-initiation of repair, appears to be common (Bloch & Wilkinson, 2009).

The analysis of these examples here is necessarily limited by the space available, but we have aimed to show the scope of a detailed investigation using CA principles. With this type of approach in mind, it is now possible to consider its application to the assessment of MSDs.

Developing a CA-Influenced Approach to MSD Assessment

The preceding analysis has explored repair initiation by other enabling us to consider the part MSDs play within a natural communication context. Specifically, it places the functional consequence of MSDs (namely unintelligibility) under closer scrutiny than normally possible through a listener perception task. By drawing on CA principles and primary CA research on repair, we can see

where trouble sources occur, how they are encountered, and, crucially, how they are dealt with by participants. Again, it is not so much speech errors that are important here but rather the ways in which the effects of MSDs, including speech errors brought about by MSDs, may be treated as trouble sources by the participants themselves and managed by them. Additionally, this analysis brings to our attention the very practical accomplishment of understanding and how this is achieved. It is not simply the case that understanding happens as an all or nothing event, rather, as shown in the preceding extracts, understanding and the checking of understanding (especially in an environment of MSDs) can become explicit activities in their own right.

Here, as in previous work (Bloch & Wilkinson, 2004, 2009) we suggest complementing existing MSD assessments with a refined analysis of conversation using CA principles. Three main reasons for this suggestion are as follows:

1. Acknowledging the status of both participants.
   In existing MSD experimental work, participants typically are classified into specific roles of speaker, most commonly the person with an MSD, and listener, a person required to judge or rate the activity of the speaker (Liss, 2007). CA takes a different perspective by attending to the activities of *both* (or more) participants in a conversation. This is achieved through consideration of each participant's turn design and the larger sequences they construct. Whether and how the effects of an MSD might be significant to the

participants is something that will be observed from the data itself. This presents a notable departure from current clinical assessment approaches in which the independently rated speech qualities of the SWD are at the heart of the assessment process. As demonstrated in the preceding extracts, the management of troubles, for example, is one very salient area in which the conversational partner has an equally relevant role as the SWD in both the identification of trouble sources as well as their repair. In these terms, a conversation partner is not just a listener who judges the relative competence of a speaker with reference to (un)intelligibility but rather an equal player in whatever activity is being pursued currently within the talk. As such, with this approach, we move from the monadic focus, which is the main traditional approach within MSD research, to a dyadic one, in which a main focus of assessment and management becomes how two or more participants construct the conversation together.

2. Understanding the impact of MSDs on conversation.
One of the outcomes of a clinical dysarthria assessment will be to establish the level of impact on a speaker's life and the lives of their significant others. There is little value in offering to treat a problem if it is only of interest to the clinician. An assumption that might be drawn from a perceptual speech assessment is the degree to which a deviation from the norm

influences communicative ability. In contrast, evidence suggests that a severe MSD does not necessarily result in severe communication disability. Bloch (2005) and Bloch and Beeke (2008) provide an analysis of an interaction between a man with severe progressive dysarthria in conversation with his mother. The dyads use a system of multiturn utterances in which single/paired words and letter names are produced one by one, effectively spelling aloud, and then repeated. Each turn by the son is redone by the coparticipant until the whole intended utterance is complete. In this way, inherent problems with unintelligibility are minimized, and even where problems occur, their resolution is relatively efficient. On any perceptual or intelligibility rating scale, the speech of this man is judged to be severe, but in interaction, it is possible to see how he and his interlocutor have developed methods of talking together that allow them to have relatively successful conversations using talk. A similar conclusion could be drawn from a more general observation of this couple in conversation, but it is argued here that a CA-informed approach facilitates a much finer level of insight into how dysarthria-in-interaction operates. This in turn provides motivation for the development of tailored clinical intervention approaches that draw on an individual couple's own interaction system irrespective of its correspondence with "normal" conversation patterns.

Thus, for the mother-son dyad mentioned previously, one could summarize their turn pattern as single/paired letter name or word followed by listener repetition. However, it also is observed that the repetitions do not result in unnecessary next-turn confirmations. This offers an insight into how ordinary turn exchanges can be produced under quite extraordinary conditions.

3. Measuring change in progressive dysarthria.
   One potential benefit of CA is in measuring change. The approach originally was developed as a tool for sociological, not clinical, enquiry and has begun only recently to be used to look at change over time within clinical populations (Wilkinson, Gower, Beeke, & Maxim, 2007). It may not be desirable (or even possible) to standardize natural conversation for comparison purposes, but with repeated within-case measures, it is possible to identify features of interaction that alter over time. Such features may provide important insights in to how interaction skills are preserved/deteriorate, adapt to accommodate physical change, or improve as a result of treatment. Importantly, potential changes in both the SWD *and* their conversation partner(s) would be of interest here.

In summary, the principles of CA enable us to focus on what issues in the talk the participants themselves treat as relevant and to consider the impact of the MSD on how actions are accomplished in conversation despite the motor speech problems. This enables us to appreciate that an MSD may not be problematic to participants *all* of the time and that participants may well develop their own strategies for overcoming the likely consequences of increasingly unintelligible speech.

Future Directions

CA's methods and underlying philosophy provide a strong foundation on which to build an applied approach to MSD interaction assessment/profiling and to generate new ideas for intervention. It is likely that most clinicians do not have the time to transcribe large amounts of data (Armstrong, Brady, Mackenzie, & Norrie, 2007) but the identification and description of strategic interaction features in conversations featuring individual speakers with dysarthria is certainly viable (see similar applied approaches for people with aphasia and cognitive problems). Work already has identified some of the features that regularly occur in MSD related interaction, namely the management of troubles (Bloch & Wilkinson, 2009; Collins & Markova, 1995) and adaptations to change (Bloch, 2005; Bloch & Beeke, 2008). There also have been developments in the understanding of AAC use in interaction involving children (Clarke & Wilkinson, 2007, 2008) and adults (Bloch & Wilkinson, 2004; Bloch, in press). There is still a need for further research into interaction between people with MSDs in conversation with others. The effects of different coparticipants also may prove to be important with respect to possible differences between familiar and unfamiliar partners and between different health/social care professional groups.

With reference to a user-friendly MSD-in-interaction assessment tool, the first author currently is developing a CA-based clinical profiling system for dysarthria in conversation. This will draw on existing tools using CA principles for people with cognitive problems (Perkins, Whitworth, & Lesser, 1997) and those with aphasia (Whitworth, Perkins, & Lesser, 1997). It will enable clinicians to explore interaction with clients in a more systematic way, focusing on the interactive behavior of individual dyads. The need for long and detailed transcriptions for clinical use may not necessarily be required, providing the clinician understands the fundamental principles of applied CA and is able to identify key interaction practices.

Future work aims to develop and evaluate intervention programs that target interaction for dyads in a more meaningful way. Central to this work is the recognition of heterogeneity within the main diagnostic groups. Individuals with the same neurodegenerative diseases may share similar speech pathologies but may well differ in interaction patterns both within and across different coparticipants. A CA-informed approach to MSD assessment and intervention is unlikely to be suitable for every client, but it is likely that some will benefit from a more rigorous and structured approach to interaction. Evidence for those most likely to benefit has yet to be produced.

It has been proposed in this chapter that the clinical assessment of MSDs in interaction using CA principles is both desirable and feasible. Existing findings show how people with MSDs manage trouble sources and adapt their talk to minimize anticipated problems. Future work will develop these themes and offer ways in which results from traditional assessment tools can be enhanced through the understanding of MSDs in conversation.

References

Armstrong, L., Brady, M., Mackenzie, C., & Norrie, J. (2007). Transcription-less analysis of aphasic discourse: A clinician's dream or a possibility? *Aphasiology* 21, 355–374.

Barefoot, S. M., Bochner, J. H., Johnson, B. A., & Eigen, B. A. v. (1993). Rating deaf speakers' comprehensibility: An exploratory investigation. *American Journal of Speech-Language Pathology, 2,* 31–35.

Bloch, S. (2005). Co-constructing meaning in dysarthria: Word and letter repetition in the construction of turns. In K. Richards & P. Seedhouse (Eds.), *Applying conversation analysis* (pp. 38–55). Basingstoke, UK: Palgrave Macmillan.

Bloch, S. (2006). *Trouble sources and repair in acquired dysarthria and communication aid use: A conversation analysis study.* Unpublished doctoral dissertation. University of London, London, UK: PhD.

Bloch, S. (in press). Anticipatory other-completion of augmentative and alternative communication (AAC) talk: A conversation analysis study. *Disability & Rehabilitation.*

Bloch, S., & Beeke, S. (2008). Co-constructed talk in the conversations of people with dysarthria and aphasia [Dec]. *Clinical Linguistics & Phonetics, 22,* 974–990.

Bloch, S., & Wilkinson, R. (2004). The understandability of AAC: A conversation analysis study of acquired dysarthria.

Augmentative and Alternative Communication, 20, 272–282.

Bloch, S., & Wilkinson, R. (2009). Acquired dysarthria in conversation: Identifying sources of understandability problems. *International Journal of Language & Communication Disorders, 44,* 769–783.

Body, R. & Parker, M. (2005). Topic repetitiveness after traumatic brain injury: An emergent, jointly managed behavior. *Clinical Linguistics and Phonetics, 19,* 379–392.

Chomsky, N. (1965). *Aspects of the theory of syntax.* Cambridge, MA: MIT Press.

Clarke, M., & Wilkinson, R. (2007). Interaction between children with cerebral palsy and their peers 1: Organizing and understanding VOCA use. *Augmentative and Alternative Communication, 23,* 336–348.

Clarke, M., & Wilkinson, R. (2008). Interaction between children with cerebral palsy and their peers 2: Understanding initiated VOCA-mediated turns. *Augmentative and Alternative Communication, 24,* 3–15.

Collins, S., & Markova, I. (1995). Complementarity in the construction of a problematic utterance in conversation. In I. Markova, C. F. Graumann, & K. Foppa (Eds.), *Mutualities in dialogue* (pp. 238–263). Cambridge, UK: Cambridge University Press.

Collins, S., & Markova, I. (1999). Interaction between impaired and unimpaired speakers: Inter-subjectivity and the interplay of culturally shared and situation specific knowledge. *British Journal of Social Psychology, 38,* 339–368.

Collins, S., Markova, I., & Murphy, J. (1997). Bringing conversations to a close: The management of closings in interactions between AAC users and "natural" speakers. *Clinical Linguistics & Phonetics, 11,* 467–493.

Darley, F. L., Aronson, A. E., & Brown, J. R. (1969a). Differential diagnostic patterns of dysarthria. *Journal of Speech and Hearing Research, 12,* 246–269.

Darley, F. L., Aronson, A. E., & Brown, J. R. (1969b). Clusters of deviant speech dimensions in the dysarthrias. *Journal of Speech and Hearing Research, 12,* 462–496.

Drew, P., & Heritage, J. (Eds.) (1992). *Talk at work.* Cambridge, UK: Cambridge University Press.

Duffy, J. R. (2007). History, current practice, and future trends and goals. In G. Weismer (Ed.), *Motor speech disorders: Essays for Ray Kent* (pp. 7–56). San Diego, CA: Plural.

Enderby, P., & Palmer, R. (2007). *Frenchay dysarthria assessment* (2nd ed.). Austin, TX: Pro-Ed.

Goodwin, C. (Ed.). (2003). *Conversation and brain damage.* New York, NY: Oxford University Press.

Heath, C. (1998). The analysis of activities in face-to-face interaction using video. In D. Silverman (Ed.), *Qualitative research: Theory, method and practice,* 183–200. London, UK: Sage.

Heritage, J. (1984). *Garfinkel and ethnomethodology.* Cambridge, UK: Polity Press.

Hesketh, A., Sage, K. E. (1999). Special issue: Conversation analysis—Overview. *APHASIOLOGY, 13,* 4–5.

Hustad, K. C. (2006). Estimating the intelligibility of speakers with dysarthria. *Folia Phoniatrica et Logopeadica, 58,* 217–228.

Hustad, K. C. (2007). Effects of speech stimuli and dysarthria severity on intelligibility scores and listener confidence ratings for speakers with cerebral palsy. *Folia Phoniatrica et Logopeadica, 59,* 306–317.

Hustad, K. C. (2008). The relationship between listener comprehension and intelligibility scores for speakers with dysarthria [Jun]. *Journal of Speech, Language, and Hearing Research, 51,* 562–573.

Hustad, K., Jones, T., & Dailey, S. (2003). Implementing speech supplementation strategies: Effects on intelligibility and speech rate of individuals with chronic severe dysarthria. *Journal of Speech, Language, and Hearing Research, 46,* 462–474.

Hustad, K. C., & Lee, J. (2008). Changes in speech production associated with alphabet supplementation [Dec]. *Journal of Speech, Language, and Hearing Research, 51*, 1438–1450.

Hutchby, I., & Woofitt, R. (1998). *Conversation analysis*. Cambridge, UK: Polity Press.

Jefferson, G. (1984). Transcript notation. In J. M. Atkinson & J. Heritage (Eds.), Structures of social action (pp. ix–xvi). Cambridge, UK: Cambridge University Press.

Liss, J. M. (2007). The role of speech perception in motor speech disorders. In G. Weismer (Ed.), *Motor speech disorders*, 187–219. San Diego, CA: Plural.

Lowit-Leuschel, A., & Docherty, G. J. (2001). Prosodic variation across sampling tasks in normal and dysarthric speakers. *Logopedics Phoniatrics Vocology, 26*, 151–164.

Perkins, L., Whitworth, A., & Lesser, R. (1997). *Conversation analysis profile for people with cognitive impairment*. London, UK: Whurr.

Pomerantz, A., & Fehr, B.J. (1997). Conversation analysis: an approach to the study of social action as sense making practices. In T. A. v. Dijk (Ed.), *Discourse studies: A multidisciplinary introduction* (pp. 64–91). London, UK: Sage.

Robertson, S. J. (1982). *Dysarthria profile*. London, UK: Robertson.

Rutter, B. (2009). Repair sequences in dysarthric conversational speech: A study in interactional phonetics. *Clinical Linguistics & Phonetics, 23*, 887–900.

Sacks, H. (1984). Notes on methodology. In J. M. Atkinson and J. Heritage (Eds.), *Structures of social action: Studies in conversation analysis* (pp. 21–27). Cambridge, UK: Cambridge University Press.

Sacks, H., Schegloff, E., & Jefferson, G. (1974). A simplest systematics for the organization of turn-taking for conversation. *Language, 50*, 696–735.

Schegloff, E. (1979). The relevance of repair to syntax-for-conversation. *Syntax and Semantics, 12*, 261–286.

Schegloff, E. (1982). Discourse as an interactional achievement: Some uses of "uh huh" and other things that come between sentences. *Analyzing Discourse: Text and Talk*, 71–93.

Schegloff, E. (1987). Some sources of misunderstandings in talk-in-interaction. *Linguistics, 25*, 201–218.

Schegloff, E. (1992). Repair after next turn: The last structurally provided defense of intersubjectivity in conversation. *American Journal of Sociology, 97*, 1295–1345.

Schegloff, E. (1997). Practices and actions: Boundary cases of other-initiated repair. *Discourse Processes, 23*, 499–545.

Schegloff, E. (2007). *Sequence organization in interaction: A primer in conversation analysis* (Vol. 1). New York, NY: Cambridge University Press.

Schegloff, E., Jefferson, G. and Sacks, H. (1977). The preference for self-correction in the organization of repair in conversation. *Language, 53*(2), 361–382.

Schegloff, E., & Sacks, H. (1973). Opening up closings. *Semiotica, 7*, 289–327.

Whitworth, A., Perkins, L., & Lesser, R. (1997). Conversation analysis profile for people with aphasia (CAPPA). London, UK: Whurr.

Wilkinson, R. (1999). Sequentiality as a problem and resource for intersubjectivity in aphasic conversation: Analysis and implications for therapy. *Aphasiology, 13*, 327–343.

Wilkinson, R., Bloch, S., & Clarke, M. T. (in press). On the use of graphic resources by people with communication disorders in the construction of turns-in-interaction. In C. Goodwin, C. LeBaron, & J. Streek (Eds.), *Multimodality and human activity: Research on behavior, action and communication*. Cambridge, UK: Cambridge University Press.

Wilkinson, R., Gower, M., Beeke, S., & Maxim, J. (2007). Adapting to conversation as a language-impaired speaker: Changes to aphasic turn construction over time. *Communication & Medicine, 4*, 79–97.

Woofitt, R. (2005). *Conversation analysis and discourse analysis: A comparative and critical introduction*. London, UK: Sage.

Yorkston, K. (2007). The degenerative dysarthrias: A window into critical clinical and research issues. *Folia Phoniatricia Logopaedica, 59,* 107–117.

Yorkston, K., Strand, E., & Kennedy, M. (1996). Comprehensibility of dysarthric speech: Implications for assessment and treatment planning. *American Journal of Speech-Language Pathology, 5,* 55–66.

Appendix

Key to Transcription Symbols

[	A large left-hand bracket links an ongoing utterance with an overlapping utterance or nonverbal action point where the overlap/simultaneous nonverbal action begins.
]	A large right-hand bracket marks where overlapping utterances/ simultaneous nonverbal action stops overlapping.
=	An equal sign marks where there is no interval between adjacent utterances.
(.)	A full stop in single parens indicates an interval of less than one-tenth of a second in the stream of talk.
(0.6)	A number in single parens indicates the length, in tenths of a second, of a pause in the talk.
oh:	A colon indicates an extension of the sound or syllable it follows (more colons prolong the stretch).
.	A full stop indicates a stopping fall in tone, *not necessarily the end of a sentence.*
,	A comma indicates a continuing intonation.
?	A question mark indicates a rising inflection, *not necessarily a question.*
!	An exclamation mark indicates an animated tone, *not necessarily an exclamation.*
-	A single dash indicates a halting, abrupt cut-off to a word or part of a word.
↑↓	Marked rising and falling shifts in intonation are indicated by upward and downward pointing arrows immediately *prior* to the rise or fall.
stress	Underlining indicates emphasis.
((*nods*))	Italicized text between double parens describes nonverbal behavior.
°no°	Degree signs indicate a passage of talk that is *quieter* than surrounding talk.
TALK	Capital letters indicate talk delivered at a *louder volume* than surrounding talk.
heh	Indicates discernible aspiration or laughter (the more hehs, the longer the aspiration/laughter).

fu(h)n   An h in single parens marks discernible aspiration or laughter *within* a word in an utterance.

°h   Discernible inhalation (the more h's, the longer the inhalation).

>talk<   Lesser than/greater than signs indicate sections of an utterance delivered at a *greater speed* than the surrounding talk.

⌈yes
⌊*((nods))*   Italicized text in double parens represents a gloss or description of some nonverbal aspect of the talk and is linked to simultaneous talk with large brackets (see previous).

(dog)   Single parens containing either a word, phrase, or syllable count (if utterance is very unclear) mark where target item(s) is/are in doubt.

9

Telerehabilitation and the Assessment of Motor Speech Disorders

DEBORAH THEODOROS, PH.D.

Introduction

The assessment of motor speech disorders (MSDs) is a complex process requiring a range of strategies designed to explore the neurological impairment of the speech mechanism, the individual's communicative ability, and the capacity and opportunity for the person to participate in everyday life. Assessment requires a face-to-face interaction between the speech-language pathologist (SLP) and the client, involving primarily perceptual and observational techniques. Although the conventional method of face-to-face assessment is considered the gold standard, the ubiquity of such an approach clearly is at odds with ever-increasing health-care costs, changes in models of health care, the increasing demand for rehabilitation services, and the rapid developments in telecommunication technologies.

Telerehabilitation, which involves the delivery of rehabilitation services via information and communication technologies (Rosen, 1999), has the potential to address some of these issues and provide clinicians with an alternate and/or supplementary mode of service delivery. It encompasses assessment and therapeutic intervention; education and training to clients, their families, and other health professionals; monitoring of progress; specialist consultation; and a means by which people with a disability may network with others (Rosen, 1999; Savard, Borstad, Tkachuck, Lauderdale, & Conroy, 2003). As the assessment of motor speech disorders is based primarily on an auditory-visual interaction between the patient and clinician, this process is readily applicable to the online environment. Telerehabilitation has evolved from the broader areas of telemedicine and telehealth, which have been stimulated by a number of worldwide health, economic, and societal changes.

The Benefits of Telerehabilitation

The development of telerehabilitation and other telehealth services has been inspired primarily by the need to provide greater and more equitable access to health services (Craig & Patterson, 2006; Demiris, Shigaki, & Schopp, 2005; Hjelm, 2006; Rosen, 1999; Torsney, 2003; Winters, 2002). Although health service equity has been the initial driver, telerehabilitation also has been encouraged as a means of reducing health-care costs, meeting the increasing demand for services, and providing a method of service delivery that supports a community-based model for rehabilitation. The rapid and sophisticated advances in telecommunication technologies in recent years have led simultaneously to increasing consumer expectation and demand for greater health-care information and interaction.

One of the major issues for many people with an acquired MSD is achieving optimal and timely access to rehabilitation services. For some, such access may be difficult, if not impossible, due to their geographical location, their associated mobility issues, the availability of transport, and the need for a care giver to accompany them (Rosen, 1999). Furthermore, the costs involved in traveling to and from the nearest health facility may be prohibitive for many people living in these areas. Access to speech-language pathology services in rural and remote areas is affected particularly by difficulties in the recruitment, retention, and ongoing professional development of speech clinicians in these locations (Bashshur, 1995; Picker-

ing et al., 1998; Rosen, 1999). As a result of these issues, it is probable that both the quality and quantity of speech rehabilitation services will be affected in rural and remote communities. Although it is not difficult to comprehend the access problems for people who live in rural environments, several of these issues also are pertinent to individuals living in urban areas. It is quite possible for persons with an MSD to live close to a health facility but be unable to attend for assessment and treatment due to their physical impairment, transport difficulties, or care giver requirements. As such, these individuals require an alternate means for accessing rehabilitation services.

Compounding the issues of mobility and distance for people with neurological speech impairment is the change in health-care models from an inpatient focus to a more community-based rehabilitation and outpatient model of care (Rosen, 2004; Schopp, Hales, Brown, & Quetsch, 2003; Winters & Winters, 2004). Although this model reflects a broader and more positive perspective of disability and health as advocated by the World Health Organization (World Health Organization, 2001), clients now experience earlier discharge from inpatient rehabilitation facilities and greater use of outpatient services. The availability and/or accessibility of these services may vary in a client's local community. Within this model, telerehabilitation may play a valuable role in providing speech rehabilitation services that are more client-centered and community-based as opposed to a center-based medical model of care (Rosen, 2004; Schopp et al., 2003).

An increasing demand for speech-language pathology services is inevi-

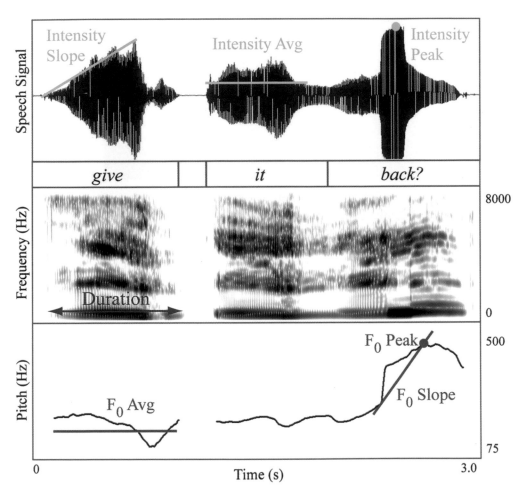

Color Plate 1. Composite Praat screenshot displaying the acoustic waveform (*top panel*), spectrogram (*middle panel*), and F0 contour (*bottom panel*). A subset of possible quantitative measures are illustrated in the overlay.

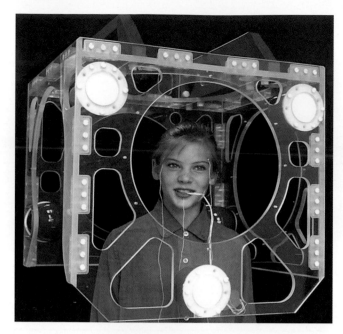

Color Plate 2. Carstens Articulograph AG500 for 3-D recording of facial and intra-oral movements. Transduction and subject interface is shown including the EMA Cube and small sensor coils positioned on and in the speaker's mouth. The fixed transmitters are attached to the acrylic case. Reprinted with permission granted by Brigitta Carstens, Carstens Medizinelektronik GmbH, D37120 Lenglern (Germany).

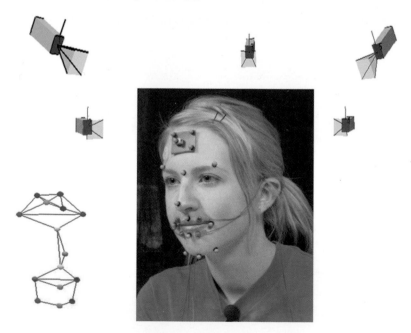

Color Plate 3. A 5-camera (Eagle 4MP, Motion Analysis Corporation) configuration for sampling 4-mm diameter reflective markers on the face simultaneously with two channels of perioral EMG and voice audio. (Courtesy of the Communication Neuroscience Laboratories, University of Kansas, 2010.)

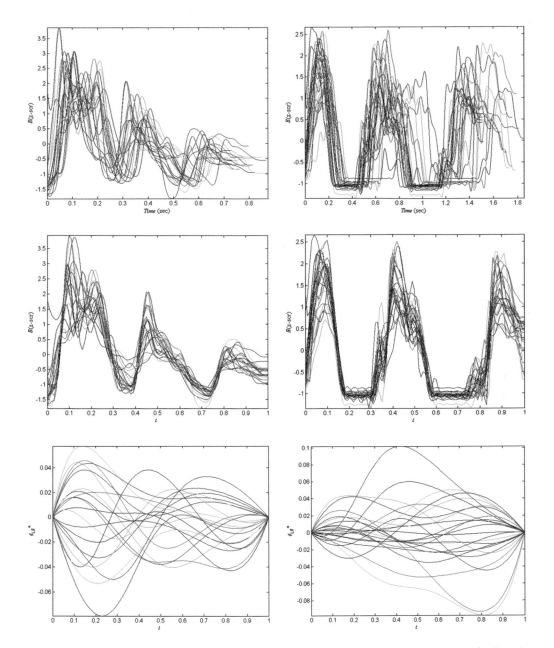

Color Plate 4. Example results comparing variability in a healthy speaker (*left column*) and an ataxic speaker (*right column*) for repetitions of "Well we'll will." The first row is low pass filtered speech energy (20 Hz cut-off) transformed to z-scores. The second row shows the data registered using Functional Data Analysis. The bottom row plots the phase error, i.e., the distortion to the relative time line used to bring the records into alignment (*as seen in the middle row*). Negative values correspond to relatively early occurrences of speech events and vice versa. Variability in relative timing can be indexed by averaging the standard deviation of phase errors in a similar manner to the STI. For further examples of these data see Anderson et al. (2008).

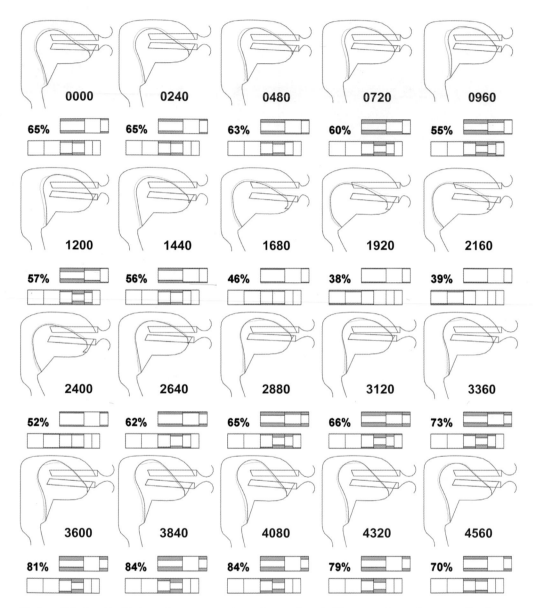

Color Plate 5. Trial and error groping of speaker 1. The speaker tries to articulate a realization of /u/. Time is indicated in ms. Degree of similarity of current somatosensory state with respect to somatosensory state of the /u/ realization is given in percent. The shaded areas in the tactile contact pattern indicate contact of vocal tract organs or articulators (*adjacent to the percentage; from left to right*: contact area of tongue body, tongue tip, lips) with regions of the vocal tract wall (*below; from left to right*: lower pharyngeal, upper pharyngeal, velar, palatal, post-alveolar, and alveolar region).

table with the rapidly developing aging population worldwide. The United Nations Organization reports that by 2050, one in every five persons will be 60 years or older, compared to the current statistic of one in every ten persons (United Nations Program on Ageing, 2007). The number of people requiring speech rehabilitation services following acquired neurological impairment will be expected to rise as a consequence of this demographic shift. Telerehabilitation has the potential to assist in the management of this increased demand by enabling timely and cost-effective rehabilitation services to a greater number of people. Faster and more efficient clinician contact with a client may be achieved through telerehabilitation, enabling a greater number of consultations (Bashshur, 1995; Torsney, 2003). Furthermore, the capacity of the SLP to engage in regular and timely monitoring of a client's progress from a distance has the potential to facilitate greater client self-management, and possibly, the increased use of health practitioner assistants and family members to implement treatment programs otherwise conducted by speech clinicians.

The universal and ongoing need to contain health-care costs has highlighted an additional benefit of telerehabilitation as a method of service delivery. Costs to the health care system and to private individuals when accessing rehabilitation services may include client travel to and from a health facility and/or the costs associated with an outreach service provided by a center (e.g., clinician travel costs and time spent away from regular caseload) (Bashshur, 1995). In some health-care systems, these expenses may preclude

many people from receiving effective rehabilitation (Bashshur, 1995). Telerehabilitation has the potential to reduce such costs by providing speech services within the home or local community. Future research is needed, however, in order to establish clearly the cost-benefit relationship of telerehabilitation in its various forms.

Although telerehabilitation clearly has the potential to improve access to speech-language services, the capacity to optimize the rehabilitation process should be considered as an important benefit of this mode of service delivery. Both assessment and treatment of the speech disorder may be enhanced by this approach. The assessment of a motor speech disorder may be improved by the clinician's ability to perform multiple baseline assessments of the person's speech as well as post-treatment evaluations without requiring the client to attend a clinic several times. Home-based assessment via telerehabilitation and the use of mobile technologies to record speech have the added benefit of allowing the clinician to assess the client's everyday communication within a natural, rather than clinical environment, thus providing a more realistic assessment of treatment outcome (Temkin, Ulicny, & Vesmarovich, 1996). Furthermore, records of client performance can be compiled easily and efficiently via telerehabilitation through the use of store-and-forward technology. Such technology enables real-time audio and video recordings and provides a permanent digital record of speaker performance over time (Constantinescu, et al., In press a; Hill et al., 2006; Hill, Theodoros, Russell, & Ward, 2009a).

With respect to the treatment of motor speech disorders, current theory and evidence from the neuroscience literature suggest that intensive and long-term neurorehabilitation following brain impairment is critical to recovery and to maintenance of a skill (Kleim & Jones, 2008; Ludlow et al., 2008). Telerehabilitation has the potential to enable an appropriate level of intensity and duration of treatment; enhance motivation, compliance, and self-management; improve continuity of care by monitoring progress from a distance; and enable timely adjustments to management plans (Bashshur, 1995; Torsney, 2003; Winters & Winters, 2004).

Telerehabilitation Research

The development of telerehabilitation applications for the management of communication and swallowing disorders has gained momentum in recent years with an increasing worldwide interest in telehealth services and the rapid growth in telecommunication technologies. The types and levels of sophistication of the technology used in these applications have varied from simple telephones to customized Internet-based video-conferencing systems incorporating dedicated assessment and treatment software tools.

Current telerehabilitation research has focused largely on the validation of assessment and treatment protocols in order to support this mode of service delivery. To date, studies have reported on the assessment and/or treatment of acquired neurogenic motor speech and language disorders, swallowing dys-

function, stuttering, speech, and swallowing disorders associated with laryngectomy; voice disorders; and speech, language, and literacy disorders in children (see Table 9–1). Overall, these studies have demonstrated comparability between online and FTF assessments, as well as positive clinical outcomes following online treatment.

Assessing Motor Speech Disorders via Telerehabilitation

The earliest attempts to assess motor speech disorders at a distance were reported by Wertz et al. (1987) and Duffy, Werven, & Aronson (1997) in their studies on the diagnoses of neurogenic communication disorders. Wertz et al. (1987) reported the use of video, computer technology, and the telephone to assess and diagnose 36 participants with suspected neurogenic communication disorder. The research comprised three simulated interaction conditions: Traditional face-to-face; closed circuit television; and computer controlled video laserdisc over the telephone. A comparison of the results of standardized assessments across the three conditions revealed an average of 92% agreement in diagnosis. The authors claimed that an accurate diagnosis of neurogenic communication disorders was possible using these technologies within a simulated setting.

Similarly, Duffy et al. (1997) found that a diagnosis of a neurogenic communication disorder could be made with confidence via a satellite video-conferencing link from a rural area.

Table 9–1. Telerehabilitation Research in Speech-Language Pathology

Communication Disorders and Dysphagia	Research Studies
Acquired neurogenic speech and language disorders (aphasia, dysarthria, apraxia of speech)	Brennan, Georgeadis, Baron, & Barker, 2004
	Constantinescu, Theodoros, Russell, Ward, Wilson, & Wootton, 2010
	Constantinescu et al., in press a, in press b
	Duffy, Werven, & Aronson, 1997
	Georgeadis, Brennan, Barker, & Baron, 2004
	Hill, Theodoros, Russell, Cahill, Ward, & Clark, 2006
	Hill, Theodoros, Russell, & Ward, 2009a, 2009b
	Hill, Theodoros, Russell, Ward, & Wootton, 2009
	Palsbo, 2007
	Theodoros, Hill, Russell, Ward, & Wootton, R, 2008
	Theodoros, Constantinescu, Russell, Ward, Wilson, & Wootton, 2006
	Vestal, Smith-Olinde, Hick, Hutton, & Hart, 2006
	Wertz et al., 1987
Dysphagia	Perlman & Witthawaskul, 2002
Stuttering	Harrison, Wilson, & Onslow, 1999
	Kully, 2000
	Lewis, Packman, Onslow, Simpson, & Jones, 2008
	O'Brian, Packman, & Onslow, 2008
	Sicotte, Lehoux, Fortier-Blanc, & Leblanc, 2003
	Wilson, Onslow, & Lincoln, 2004
Head and neck oncology	Myers, 2005
	Ward et al., 2007
	Ward, Crombie, Trickey, Hill, Theodoros, & Russell, 2009
Voice disorders	Mashima, Birkmire-Peters, Holtel, & Syms, 1999
	Mashima, Birkmire-Peters, Syms, Holtel, Burgess, & Peters, 2003
Speech, language, and literacy disorders in children	McCullough, 2001
	Waite, Cahill, Theodoros, Russell, & Busuttin, 2006
	Waite, Theodoros, Russell, & Cahill, in press a, 2010 b

A very high level of agreement (96%) for diagnosis was found to exist between the clinician who viewed 24 video-recorded speech samples via a satellite and the rural clinician. Following examination of additional retrospective data, Duffy et al. (1997) indicated that although some uncertainties of diagnosis occurred for a small percentage of participants, this number was not grossly disproportionate to the frequency of uncertainty that occurs in routine clinical practice. These investigators concluded that this mode of service delivery represented a viable alternative to face-to-face consultation in circumstances in which distance prevented a timely and cost-effective service or specialized expertise was unavailable.

Current research involving the assessment of motor speech disorders via telerehabilitation has been designed to not only establish the validity and reliability of diagnosis, but also for the assessment of specific components of the speech mechanism and speech production processes. Studies have included both informal and standardized assessments of motor speech in order to provide a comprehensive evaluation consistent with traditional clinical protocols. Although it is well-recognized that valid and reliable assessments are critical to the development of an evidence base for the management of motor speech disorders via telerehabilitation, research in this area is only just beginning.

Comprehensive validation studies of motor speech assessment have been conducted recently by Australian researchers in the Telerehabilitation Research Unit at the University of Queensland. These studies evaluating the validity and reliability of the assessment of dysarthria

(Constantinescu et al., In press a; Hill et al., 2006; Hill et al., 2009a) and apraxia of speech (Hill, Theodoros, Russell, & Ward, 2009b) were conducted using custom-built software that enabled real-time video-conferencing between two computers situated at two different sites. The software was designed specifically for operation using a low bandwidth (128 kbits/s) via an Internet Protocol (IP) connection. The bandwidth used in these studies was consistent with the minimum bandwidth available at the time in public health facilities. Web cameras on the participant computer enabled real-time video-conferencing and the recording of high-quality video and audio files of the participant's performance during assessment tasks. Using store-and-forward technology, these files were forwarded from the participant's computer to the clinician for viewing and analyses as required. In addition, the system enabled the display of assessment stimuli on the participant's computer in the form of images and written materials.

In a pilot study involving 19 participants with dysarthric speech associated with traumatic brain injury, stroke, and PD, Hill et al. (2006) explored the feasibility and effectiveness of this telerehabilitation system in assessing the motor speech mechanism, speech intelligibility, perceptual speech features, and the level of severity of the dysarthric speech disturbance. In this particular study, one assessment was conducted face-to-face in the traditional manner, and a second assessment was conducted online on a different day. Agreement statistics comparing two assessment methods showed that measures of dysarthria severity, speech intelligibility in sentences, and most perceptual ratings fell within clinically acceptable criteria. Several ratings on the Frenchay Dysarthria Assessment (Enderby, 1983), however were not found to be comparable between assessment environments. The investigators concluded that the online assessment of dysarthria was feasible, although further refinement of the research design and technology was required in order to confirm the reliability of assessment via the Internet.

In response to the findings of this pilot study, Hill et al., (2009a) redesigned the telerehabilitation system and research methodology and embarked on a reevaluation of online assessment of dysarthric speech. Enhancements to the system and test environment included improved store-and-forward software, remotely controlled web cameras on the participant computer, and improved room lighting. Methodological adjustments included the introduction of simultaneous face-to-face and online assessment in order to reduce participant and rater variability, and the inclusion of an informal motor speech assessment, a diagnostic category for the type of dysarthria, and a participant satisfaction questionnaire. Assessment results for a further 24 participants revealed that a valid and reliable evaluation of dysarthria in adults was achievable on both standardized and informal assessments. Good to very good strength of agreement between the two assessment modes was determined overall. Comparable intra-rater and inter-rater reliability was found in both the telerehabilitation and face-to-face assessment environments on all measures. Despite the strong overall agreement between the assessment methods, the percentage level of

agreement between clinicians for the diagnosis of type of dysarthria was low (54%). In view of the fact that the diagnosis of milder forms of dysarthria based on perceptual assessment is inherently problematic (Kreiman, Gerratt, Kempster, Erman, & Berke, 1993), it is likely that this level of agreement reflected more the inadequacy of perceptual evaluation as opposed to the assessment environment. All of the 11 participants who were assessed online completed the participant satisfaction questionnaire and reported that they were more than satisfied or very satisfied with assessment via telerehabilitation.

As part of a larger study to investigate the feasibility and effectiveness of delivering the Lee Silverman Voice Treatment (LSVT®) online, Constantinescu et al. (In press a) reported on the assessment of hypokinetic dysarthria in 61 people with PD. The simultaneous assessment protocol included perceptual analysis of voice, articulatory precision, and speech intelligibility, an informal oromotor examination, and acoustic measures of vocal sound pressure level (SPL), phonation time, and fundamental frequency (Fo) range. Although the same telerehabilitation system as described in Hill et al. (2009a) was used in this study, additional hardware (acoustic speech processor) was developed specifically for this project for the measurement of vocal SPL and Fo, in keeping with the standard clinical measurements taken during a pre-LSVT® assessment session (Ramig, Countryman, Thompson, & Horii, 1995). Agreement statistics revealed comparable levels of agreement between the two assessment environments for the majority of perceptual and acoustic measures. Similarly, intra- and inter-rater reliability of the assessors was found to be consistent across both assessment environments. Participant satisfaction with online assessment was high with 80% of 30 participants indicating that they were either more than satisfied or very satisfied. The findings of this study suggested that assessment of the hypokinetic dysarthria associated with PD can be validly and reliably assessed via a customized telerehabilitation system.

In order to explore the capacity of telerehabilitation to validly and reliably assess other types of motor speech disorders, Hill et al. (2009b) evaluated the simultaneous assessment of 11 participants with acquired apraxia of speech using the Apraxia Battery for Adults-2 (ABA-2) (Dabul, 2000). Results revealed no significant differences between the subtest scores obtained in either the online or face-to-face assessment environments, as well as moderate to very good agreement between assessors. Intra- and inter-rater reliability was noted to be reasonable, although not confirmed statistically. Participant overall satisfaction with the online assessment was found to be high in the five cases assessed primarily by this method. However, it was evident that online assessment was more difficult, and less satisfying, for one participant with severe apraxia of speech due to the inadequacy of the telerehabilitation system in transmitting written responses from the participant. Despite these limitations, which require further technological improvements and investigation with a larger sample size, the findings of the study suggested that a valid standardized assessment of apraxia of speech was feasible.

Assessment Technology

To ensure the validity and reliability of telerehabilitation for clients with disordered speech and to establish this mode of service delivery within mainstream healthcare, online applications must replicate traditional face-to-face procedures as closely as possible. The nature of some rehabilitation interventions is such that certain procedures would be difficult, if not impossible to perform (e.g., observation of soft palate movement or laryngeal elevation), without physical contact with the client. Telerehabilitation applications must, therefore, incorporate the technology to facilitate these measures or procedures and ensure that the technology is user-friendly and intuitive to the clinician. Rapidly increasing advances in digital compression, human-technology interface design, connectivity, and the capacity to embed measurement tools into a telerehabilitation application suggest that clinicians should remain open-minded and optimistic that the more complex interactions with their clients may be facilitated within the online environment (Feng & Winters, 2007; Russell, 2004; Winters, 2002; Winters & Winters, 2004). Indeed, it is possible that telerehabilitation technology may enhance clinical consultations by providing sophisticated software tools for data collection and analysis.

Speech rehabilitation readily lends itself to the online environment due to the predominantly audio-visual interaction between the client and the clinician. Compared to counterparts in other rehabilitation specialties, such as physiotherapy and occupational therapy, SLPs assess and treat their clients with considerably less physical contact. However, a number of essential tools are required to facilitate SLP consultations via telerehabilitation, to ensure valid and reliable assessments. These include an environment in which an audio-visual interaction can occur with the client, a mechanism to present auditory and visual (images, text, demonstrations) stimuli, and the capacity to record high-quality audio and video files of client performance. In most clinical consultations, measurement of the acoustic parameters of speech also will form an integral part of assessment, and where possible, should be incorporated into the design of a telerehabilitation system. In order to facilitate communication exchange between the clinician and a client with limited speech intelligibility, a means by which written responses can be transmitted to the clinician at the remote site is advantageous. Furthermore, appropriate measures must be taken to ensure the security of the telecommunication connection in the telerehabiltation system, in order to protect client confidentiality.

Many of these technological features have been embedded in recent telerehabilitation applications designed to assess clients with motor speech and language disorders. Real-time video-conferencing using either an Integrated Services Digital Network (ISDN) or Internet Protocol (IP) connection has become a standard medium for interaction between two participants. The audio and visual quality of the video-conferencing is dependent at any one time on available bandwidth and the stability of the connection. In order to overcome any degradation of the audio and visual quality of the video-conference due to connection problems, store-and-forward technology often is incorporated into a telerehabilitation system. Such technology was included in the system developed at the University of Queensland to enable the clinician to view the client's speech performance during assessment in real-time, despite any alterations in video-conference quality (Constantinescu et al., In press a; Hill et al., 2006; Hill et al., 2009a, 2009b). In this particular system, the store-and-forward software utilized a second web camera on the client's computer to record high quality audio data and video images in real-time. These files were stored on the client's computer, compressed, and forwarded via an IP connection to the clinician's computer where they could be readily retrieved and analyzed. For example, this process ensured that oromotor function could be adequately assessed, particularly in relation to speed of movement, a parameter significantly affected by latency in the videoconference signal.

As a consequence of store-and-forward technology, high-quality audio and video files can be obtained throughout assessment sessions, providing a permanent digital record of client performance. Although such files may be recorded by conventional audio and digital recording devices in a traditional face-to-face consultation, the integration of the recording software within the telerehabilitation system improves the ease with which this data may be obtained and, therefore, constitutes an advantage of online assessment.

Another essential requirement of a telerehabilitation system for the assessment of motor speech disorders is the capacity of the clinician to display various audio and visual stimuli. Data sharing software may be used to send audio or video demonstrations of each assessment task to the client in situations where the video-conference quality compromised the task instruction and real-time demonstration (Constantinescu et al., In press a; Hill et al., 2006; Hill et al., 2009a). In these studies, images and/or text were transmitted similarly to the client's computer screen, and the font size was adjusted remotely by the clinician as required.

Objective measurement of acoustic parameters of speech and voice commonly is used in clinical assessment and in research studies of dysarthria

(Kent, Weismer, Kent, Vorperian, & Duffy, 1999). For example, measures such as vocal SPL and Fo are core components of the assessment battery for people with hypokinetic dysarthria and should be considered for inclusion in telerehabilitation applications. Constantinescu et al., (In press a) in their study of the assessment of people with PD, developed an acoustic processor that displayed measures of vocal SPL and Fo and integrated this into their telerehabilitation system (Figure 9–1). Similarly, the duration of phonation and speech may be recorded automatically by timing software rather than hand-held stopwatches, thus increasing the accuracy (Constantinescu et al.,

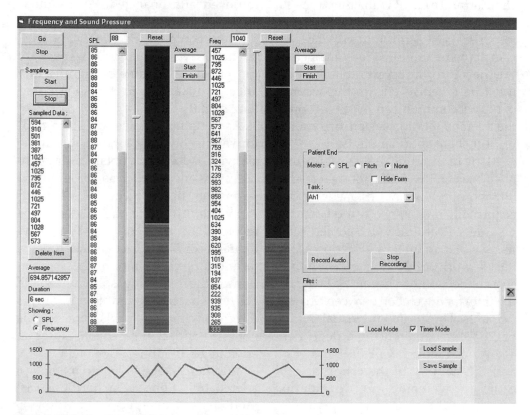

Figure 9–1. Sound pressure level (SPL) and fundamental frequency (F0) output display from the acoustic processor.

In press a; Hill et al., 2006; Hill et al., 2009a). It is conceivable that other software tools designed to measure physiological parameters of the speech mechanism (e.g., facial symmetry) may be developed and incorporated into telerehabilitation systems in the future.

Barriers to the Use of Telerehabilitation

Although successful telerehabilitation systems for delivering speech pathology services are beginning to emerge, several obstacles must be overcome before this mode of service delivery will be seen as integral to speech pathology practice. These barriers include professional fear; client characteristics; the paucity of clinical outcome and economic data; the limited availability of online assessment and treatment tools that can replicate face-to-face practice; and reimbursement, ethical, and legal issues.

One of the main barriers to the uptake of telerehabilitation is clinician misperception and fear due to lack of information about the benefits of this method of service delivery (Winters & Winters, 2004). Some clinicians feel that telerehabilitation may threaten their traditional role and expertise and fail to see how this method of service delivery can replace conventional face-to-face intervention (Winters & Winters, 2004). A critical factor underpinning the advancement of telerehabilitation is the notion that it is not intended to replace traditional rehabilitation methods, but rather to enhance them, and in doing so enable a greater number of clients to access more effective and efficient services. Ongoing clinician and SLP student edu-

cation regarding the various ways in which telerehabilitation may be utilized to provide such services will be important in the establishment of telerehabilitation (Theodoros & Russell, 2008).

Clinician reticence in the use of telerehabilitation also may be linked to the fear of technology (Winters & Winters, 2004). Although it is anticipated that such fear may begin to dissipate over successive generations of SLPs who are becoming increasingly computer-literate, the introduction of telerehabilitation to any service requires initial training and ongoing support to ensure clinician usage (Theodoros & Russell, 2008; Winters & Winters, 2004).

An awareness of the shortcomings of telerehabilitation for every client with a communication disability is another important precept underpinning this method of service delivery. It is certainly the case that some assessment and treatment procedures are not amenable to the telerehabilitation environment (e.g., physical examination or manipulation of the larynx). Similarly, not all clients are suited to this environment due to the severity and nature of their physical, communicative, and cognitive disabilities. Hill et al. (2009b) reported some degree of difficulty in the online assessment of clients with severe apraxia of speech in which an alternate means of communication (writing) was required, and the system was unable to provide this alternative effectively at the time of assessment. Similarly, Theodoros et al. (2008) found that the assessment of conversational speech, naming, and paraphasia in clients with more severe forms of aphasia could be problematic via telerehabilitation due to the effects of intermittent audio break up in the videoconference, affecting client-clinician interaction and cueing for naming tasks. Ultimately, the clinician must determine the suitability of each client for this mode of service delivery and be responsible for ensuring that the telerehabilitation system will meet their client's assessment and treatment needs. Consideration of human factors in the design of telerehabilitation applications is paramount to successful implementation (Krupinski et al., 2006; Stronge, Rogers, & Fisk, 2007) and particularly relevant to those clients with significant physical and cognitive disability.

One of the major barriers to the uptake of telerehabilitation is the paucity of a robust evidence base to support clinical and economic outcomes. Although telerehabilitation research is accumulating steadily, few large-scale assessment and treatment studies are reported in the literature (Mashima & Doarn, 2008; Theodoros & Russell, 2008). In concert with this research is the need to establish reliable and valid outcome measures that provide a holistic view of the client's communicative function in various environments pre- and postintervention. To date, most of the telerehabilitation research remains laboratory-based, and as such, lacks ecological validity. Krupinski et al. (2006) indicated the need for community-based research in order to demonstrate ecological validity. These authors also stressed the importance of examining features common, and unique, to different communities, that may influence the implementation and acceptance of a telehealth service.

Although ecological validity of a telerehabilitation service is an important factor to establish, the economical attributes of the service are critical to its sustainability in today's health-care systems worldwide. Economic analysis of any telerehabilitation service involves examination of the benefits and/or costs to the recipient and the health-care provider. It requires detailed information concerning the costs of technology, facilities, personnel, time expended by client and service provider, client and provider travel expenses, as well as the effects on quality of life (Armstrong, Dorer, Lugn, & Kvedar, 2007; Krupinski et al., 2006; Loane et al., 2001; Muennig, 2002). Studies of the economic outcomes of telerehabilitation for speech pathology services may need to include both cost-minimization (Ellis, Reiter, Wheeler, & Fendrick, 2002) and cost-utility analyses (Muennig, 2002). Cost-minimization analyses compares the cost of two or more interventions that provide similar outcomes in order to identify the lowest-cost intervention (Ellis et al., 2002), whereas cost-utility analyses examine health-related quality-of-life measures (Muennig, 2002). Both of these analyses will inform clinicians and administrators as to the economic benefits of telerehabilitation in the management of their clients and potentially support the introduction of this mode of service delivery into mainstream health care.

The successful implementation of telerehabilitation services in speech-language pathology undoubtedly will depend on the capacity of the applications to simulate face-to-face practice and demonstrate enhanced client management (e.g., improved access to services not previously available) and convenient ongoing monitoring. Indeed, recent research has focused mainly on converting conventional assessment and treatment protocols into a telerehabilitation environment and then comparing these to the usual face-to-face procedures (Hill et al., 2006; Hill et al., 2009a, 2009b; Theodoros et al., 2008; Winters & Winters, 2004). The ability to create new and innovative applications incorporating assessment and treatment tools and sophisticated data analyses will continue to increase with rapid advances in technology.

The limited reimbursement currently available for speech-language pathology services via telerehabilitation has had a significant negative impact on the implementation of these services in some countries. A survey of Medicaid programs in the United States conducted by Palsbo (2004) revealed that only 10 out of 51 American states and districts (Hawaii, Minnesota, Nebraska, Arizona, Colorado, Georgia, Iowa, Montana, South Dakota, and Utah) were reimbursed for telerehabilitation or telemedicine. A major barrier to reimbursement is the paucity of strong evidence to support this method of service delivery and the need to develop specific telerehabilitation reimbursement codes (Theodoros & Russell, 2008). Reimbursement for telerehabilitation is being pursued actively by organizations such as the American Telemedicine Association (http://www.americantelemed.org) and the American Speech-Language-Hearing Association (ASHA, http://www.asha.org). Despite reimbursement issues, it is likely that telerehabilitation will be integrated into public health-care systems in many countries where reimbursement from private health insurers will not determine the use of this service.

Although telerehabilitation has the potential to provide access to speech pathology services at considerable distances from a clinician, a number of ethical and legal barriers need to be over-

come in order for this to be achieved. Clinician licensure has the potential to be problematic in some countries where providers are required to not only be licensed in their state/region of practice but also in the area where the client resides (Denton & Gladstone, 2005). These cross-border requirements have further legal and insurance implications with respect to malpractice (Denton, 2003). Insurance for telerehabilitation services may need to be obtained in both states/regions in which the clinician practices (Denton, 2003). Speech-language pathology services delivered via telerehabilitation also raise the ethical issue of informed consent that must be obtained from clients prior to a consultation (Denton, 2003; Denton & Gladstone, 2005). Clients must be made aware of the benefits, risks, limitations, and privacy standards of this type of service prior to giving consent to participate. The need for some clients to have another person present during the session as an assistant must be addressed with respect to privacy and confidentiality. Organizations such as ASHA (www.asha.org/telepractice/) and the Canadian Association for Speech Language Pathologists and Audiologists (CASLPA) (http://www. caslpa .ca/PDF/position%20papers/teleprac-tice.pdf) have developed professional guidelines and position papers for SLPs on the use of telerehabilitation in order to inform this process and overcome some of these ethical and legal issues.

Despite a number of barriers to the use of telerehabilitation in speech-language pathology, its potential value in providing equitable and cost-effective access to services to people with chronic communication disorders such as dysarthria and apraxia of speech cannot be ignored. The uptake of telerehabilitation within speech-language pathology practice will increase as these barriers are addressed systematically through research, education, and technological advances.

Conclusion

Telerehabilitation has the potential to have a significant impact on speech-language pathology practice as an alternate means of service delivery. It may not only provide equitable access to services, but also enhance the quality of care for people with chronic communication disorders such as dysarthria and apraxia of speech. The development of new and innovative applications for delivering speech-language pathology services has only just begun. Establishing the validity and reliability of online assessment of motor speech disorders has been an initial step in this process. Further investigation of the clinical and cost-effectiveness of various telerehabilitation applications for the management of motor speech disorders is critical to the integration of this mode of service delivery into mainstream health care.

Future research will involve ongoing development of multimedia video-conferencing systems, the use of mobile technologies, and the creation of interactive websites that will provide even greater ubiquity of service and facilitate client self-management of their communication disorder. The challenge to the speech-language pathology profession is to engage in this research, confront the barriers to implementation, and embrace an advancing mode of service delivery designed to address the impending demands of health care.

References

American Speech-Language-Hearing Association (2005). *Speech-language pathologists providing clinical services via telepractice: Position statement* [Position Statement]. Available from www.asha.org/policy. Retrieved January 28, 2010.

Armstrong, A. W., Dorer, D. J., Lugn, N. E, & Kvedar, J. C. (2007). Economic evaluation of interactive teledermatology compared with conventional care. *Telemedicine and e-Health*, 13, 91–99.

Bashshur, R. L. (1995). Telemedicine effects: Cost, quality, and access. *Journal of Medical Systems*, 19, 81–91.

Brennan, D. M., Georgeadis, A. C., Baron, C. R., & Barker, L. M. (2004). The effect of video-conference-based telerehabilitation on story retelling performance by brain-injured subjects and its implications for remote speech-language therapy. *Telemedicine and e-Health*, 10, 147–154.

Canadian Association for Speech-Language Pathologists and Audiologists (CASLPA) (2006). *CASLPA—Position paper on the use of telepractice for CASLPA speech-language pathologists and audiologists.* Retrieved January 28, 2010 from , http://www.caslpa .ca/PDF/position%20papers/teleprac tice.pdf

Constantinescu, G., Theodoros, D. G., Russell, T., Ward, E. C., Wilson, S. J., & Wootton, R. (2010). Home-based speech treatment for Parkinson's Disease delivered remotely: A case report. *Journal of Telemedicine and Telecare.* 16, 100–104.

Constantinescu, G., Theodoros, D. G., Russell, T., Ward, E. C., Wilson, S. J., & Wootton, R. (In press a). Assessing disordered speech and voice in Parkinson's disease: A telerehabilitation application. *International Journal of Language and Communication Disorders.*

Constantinescu, G., Theodoros, D. G., Russell, T., Ward, E. C., Wilson, S., & Wootton, R. (In press b). Treating disordered speech and voice in Parkinson's Disease online: A randomized controlled noninferiority trial. *International Journal of Language and Communication Disorders.*

Craig, J., & Patterson, V. (2006). Introduction to the practice of telemedicine. In R. Wootton, J. Craig, & V. Patterson (Eds.), *Introduction to telemedicine* (2nd ed., pp. 3–14). London, UK: Royal Society of Medicine Press.

Dabul, B. (2000). *Apraxia battery for adults* (2nd ed.). Austin, TX: Pro-Ed.

Demiris, G., Shigaki, C. L., & Schopp, L. H. (2005). An evaluation framework for a rural home-based telerehabilitation network. *Journal of Medical Systems, 29,* 595–603.

Denton, D. R. (2003). Ethical and legal issues related to telepractice. *Seminars in Speech and Language, 24,* 313–322.

Denton, D. R., & Gladstone, V. S. (2005). Ethical and legal issues related to Telepractice. *Seminars in Hearing, 26,* 43–52.

Duffy, J. R., Werven, G. W., & Aronson, A. E. (1997). Telemedicine and diagnosis of speech and language disorders. *Mayo Clinic Proceedings, 72,* 1116–1122.

Ellis, C. N., Reiter, K. L., Wheeler, J. R., & Fendrick, A. M. (2002). Economic analysis in dermatology. *Journal American Academy of Dermatology, 46,* 271–283.

Enderby, P. (1983). *Frenchay dysarthria assessment.* San Diego, CA: College-Hill Press.

Feng, X., & Winters, J. M. (2007). An interactive framework for personalized computer-assisted neurorehabilitation. *IEEE Transactions on Information Technology in Biomedicine, 11,* 518–526.

Georgeadis, A. C, Brennan, D. M., Barker, L. N., & Baron C. R. (2004). Telerehabilitation and its effect on story retelling by adults with neurogenic communication disorders. *Aphasiology, 18,* 639–652.

Harrison, E., Wilson, L., Onslow, M. (1999). Distance intervention for early stuttering with the Lidcombe Programme. *Advances in Speech Language Pathology, 1,* 31–36.

Hill, A. J., Theodoros, D. G., Russell, T. G., Cahill, L. M., Ward, E. C., & Clark, K.

(2006). An Internet-based telerehabilitation system for the assessment of motor speech disorders: A pilot study. *American Journal of Speech Language Pathology, 15,* 1–12.

Hill, A. J., Theodoros, D. G., Russell, T. G., & Ward, E. C. (2009a). The redesign and re-evaluation of an Internet-based telerehabilitation system for the assessment of dysarthria in adults. *Telemedicine and e-Health, 15,* 840–850.

Hill, A., Theodoros, D. G., Russell, T. G., & Ward, E. C. (2009b). Using telerehabilitation to assess apraxia of speech in adults. *International Journal of Language and Communication Disorders 44,* 731–747.

Hill, A. J., Theodoros, D. G., Russell, T. G., Ward, E. C., & Wootton, R. (2009). The effects of aphasia severity upon the ability to assess language disorders via telerehabilitation. *Aphasiology, 23,* 627–642.

Hjelm, N. M. (2006). Benefits and drawbacks of telemedicine. In R. Wootton, J. Craig, & V. Patterson (Eds.), *Introduction to Telemedicine* (2nd ed., pp. 135–150). London, UK: Royal Society of Medicine Press.

Kent, R. D., Weismer, G., Kent, J. F., Vorperian, H. K., & Duffy, J. R. (1999). Acoustic studies of dysarthric speech: Methods, progress, and potential. *Journal of Communication Disorders, 32,* 141–186.

Kleim, J. A., & Jones, T. A. (2008). Principles of experience-dependent neuroplasticity: Implications for rehabilitation after brain damage. *Journal of Speech, Language, and Hearing Research, 51,* S225–S239.

Kreiman, J., Gerratt, B. R., Kempster, G. B., Erman, A., & Berke, G. S. (1993). Perceptual evaluation of voice quality: Review, tutorial, and a framework for future research. *Journal of Speech and Hearing Research, 36,* 21–40.

Krupinski, E., Dimmick, S., Grigsby, J., Mogel, G., Puskin, D., Speedie, S., . . . Yellowlee, P. (2006). Research recommendations for the American Telemedicine Association. *Telemedicine & e-Health, 12,* 579–589.

Kully, D. (2000). Telehealth in speech pathology: Applications to the treatment of stuttering. *Journal of Telemedicine and Telecare,* 6(Suppl. 2), 39–41.

Lewis, C., Packman, A., Onslow, M., Simpson, J. M., & Jones, M. (2008). A phase II trial of telehealth delivery of the Lidcombe Program of Early Stuttering Intervention. *American Journal of Speech-Language Pathology, 17,* 139–149.

Loane, M. A, Bloomer, S. E, Corbett, R., Eedy, D. J., Evans, C., Hicks, N., . . . & Wootton, R. (2001). A randomized controlled trial assessing the health economics of real-time teledermatology compared with conventional care: Urban versus rural perspective. *Journal of Telemedicine and Telecare, 7,* 108–118.

Ludlow, C. L., Hoit, J., Kent, R., Ramig, L. O., Shrivastav, R., Strand, E., . . . Sapienza, C. (2008). Translating principles of neural plasticity into research on speech motor control recovery and rehabilitation. *Journal of Speech, Language, and Hearing Research, 51,* S240–S258.

Mashima, P. A., & Doarn, C. R. (2008). Overview of telehealth activities in speech-language pathology. *Telemedicine and e-Health, 14,* 1101–1117.

Mashima, P. A., Birkmire-Peters, D. P., Holtel, M. R., & Syms, M. J. (1999). Telehealth applications in speech-language pathology. *Journal of Healthcare Information Management, 13,* 71–78.

Mashima, P. A., Birkmire-Peters, D. P., Syms, M. J., Holtel, M. R., Burgess, L. P. A., & Peters, L. (2003). Telehealth: Voice therapy using telecommunications technology. *American Journal of Speech-Language Pathology, 12,* 432–439.

McCullough, A. (2001). Viability and effectiveness of teletherapy for preschool children with special needs. *International Journal of Language and Communication Disorders, 36*(Suppl. 1), 321–326.

Myers, C. (2005). Telehealth applications in head and neck oncology. *Journal of Speech-Language Pathology and Audiology, 29,* 125–129.

Muennig, P. (2002). *Designing and conducting cost-effectiveness analyses in medicine and health care.* San Francisco, CA: John Wiley.

O'Brian, S., Packman, A., & Onslow, M. (2008). Telehealth delivery of the Camperdown program for adults who stutter: A phase 1 trial. *Journal of Speech, Language, and Hearing Research, 51,* 184–195.

Palsbo, S. E. (2004). Medicaid payment for telerehabilitation. *Archives of Physical Medicine and Rehabilitation, 85,* 1198–1191.

Palsbo, S. E. (2007). Equivalence of functional communication assessment in speech pathology using videoconferencing. *Journal of Telemedicine and Telecare, 13,* 40–43.

Perlman, A. L., & Witthawaskul, W. (2002). Real-time remote telefluroroscopic assessment of patients with dysphagia. *Dysphagia, 17,* 162–167.

Pickering M., McAllister L., Hagler P., Whitehill, T. L., Penn, C., Robertson, S. J., & McCready, V. (1998). External factors influencing the profession in six societies. *American Journal of Speech-Language Pathology, 7,* 5–17.

Ramig, L. O., Countryman, S., Thompson, L. L. and Horii, Y.(1995). Comparison of two forms of intensive speech treatment for Parkinson disease. *Journal of Speech and Hearing Research, 38,* 1232–1251.

Rosen M. J. (1999). Telerehabilitation. *NeuroRehabilitation, 3,* 3–18.

Rosen, M. J. (2004). Telerehabilitation. *Telemedicine Journal and e-Health, 10,* 115–117.

Russell, T. (2004). *Establishing the efficacy of telemedicine as a clinical tool for physiotherapists: From systems design to randomised controlled trial.* Unpublished doctoral thesis. Brisbane, Australia: The University of Queensland.

Savard, L., Borstad, A., Tkachuck, J., Lauderdale, D., & Conroy, B. (2003). Telerehabilitation consultations for clients with neurologic diagnoses: Cases from rural Minnesota and America Samoa. *NeuroRehabilitation, 18,* 93–102.

Schopp, L. H., Hales, J. W., Brown, G. D., & Quetsch, J. L. (2003). A rationale and training agenda for rehabilitation informatics: Roadmap for an emerging discipline. *NeuroRehabilitation, 18,* 159–170.

Sicotte, C., Lehoux, P., Fortier-Blanc, J., & Leblanc, Y. (2003). Feasibility and outcome evaluation of a telemedicine application in speech-language pathology. *Journal of Telemedicine and Telecare, 9,* 253–258.

Stronge, A. J., Rogers, W. A., & Fisk, A. D. (2007). Human factors considerations in implementing telemedicine systems to accommodate older adults. *Journal of Telemedicine and Telecare, 13,* 1–3.

Temkin, A., Ulicny, G. R., & Vesmarovich, S. (1996). Telerehab: A perspective of the way technology is going to change the future of patient treatment. *Rehabilitation Management, 9,* 28–30.

Theodoros, D. G., Constantinescu, G., Russell, T., Ward, E. C., Wilson, S. J., & Wootton, R. (2006). Treating the speech disorder in Parkinson's Disease online. *Journal of Telemedicine and Telecare, 12*(Suppl. 3), 88–91.

Theodoros, D., & Russell, T. (2008). Telerehabilitation: Current perspectives. In Lafiti, R. (Ed.), *Current principles and practices of telemedicine and e-health* (pp. 191–209). Amsterdam, The Netherlands: IOS Publishing.

Theodoros, D., Hill, A., Russell, T., Ward, E., & Wootton, R. (2008). Assessing acquired language disorders in adults via the Internet. *Telemedicine Journal and e-Health, 14,* 552–559.

Torsney, K. (2003). Advantages and disadvantages of telerehabilitation for persons with neurological disabilities. *NeuroRehabilitation, 18,* 183–185.

United Nations Programme on Ageing (2007). Retrieved on January 27, 2010, from http://www.un.org/esa/socdev/ageing/popageing.html

Vestal, L., Smith-Olinde, L., Hick, G., Hutton, T., & Hart, J. (2006). Efficacy of assessment Alzheimer's disease: Comparing in-person examination and telemedicine. *Clinical Interventions in Aging, 1,* 467–471.

Waite, M., Cahill, L., Theodoros, D., Russell, T., & Busuttin, S. (2006). A pilot study of online assessment of childhood speech disorders. *Journal of Telemedicine and Telecare, 12*(Suppl. 3), 92–94.

Waite, M., Theodoros, D. G., Russell, T., & Cahill, L. (2010). Assessing children's literacy via an Internet-based telehealth system. *Telemedicine and e-Health, 16,* 564–575.

Waite, M., Theodoros, D. G., Russell, T., & Cahill, L. (In press. Internet-based telehealth assessment of language using the CELF-4. *Language Speech and Hearing Services in Schools.*

Ward, E. C., Crombie, J., Trickey, M., Hill, A. J., Theodoros, D. G., & Russell, T. (2009). Assessment of communication and swallowing post-laryngectomy: A remote telerehabilitation trial. *Journal of Telemedicine and Telecare, 15,* 232–237.

Ward, L., White, J., Russell, T., Theodoros, D., Kuhl, M., Nelson, K., & Peters, I. (2007). Assessment of communication and swallowing function post laryngectomy: A telerehabilitation trial. *Journal of Telemedicine and Telecare, 13*(Suppl. 3), 88–91.

Wertz, R. T., Dronkers, N. F., Berstein-Ellis, E., Shubitowski, Y., Elman, R., Shenaut, G. K., & Knight, R. T. (1987). Appraisal and diagnosis of neurogenic communication disorders in remote settings. *Clinical Aphasiology, 17,* 117–123.

Wilson, L., Onslow, M., & Lincoln, M. (2004). Telehealth adaptation of the Lidcombe Program of early stuttering intervention: Five case studies. *American Journal of Speech-Language Pathology, 13,* 81–93.

Winters, J. M. (2002). Telerehabilitation research: Emerging opportunities. *Annual Review Biomedical Engineering, 4,* 287–320.

Winters, J. M., & Winters, J. M. (2004). A Tele-homecare model for optimizing rehabilitation outcomes. *Telemedicine Journal and e-Health, 10,* 200–212.

World Health Organization (2001). *International classification of functioning, disability, and health: ICF.* Geneva: World Health Organization.

10

Biodynamics of Speech and Orofacial Movement

STEVEN M. BARLOW, PH.D., MEREDITH POORE, M.A., SHIN YING CHU, M.A.

Introduction

The speech motor control system, including the chest wall (abdomen and ribcage), larynx, velopharynx, tongue, jaw, and lips, represents an anatomically and biomechanically diverse array of connective tissue—muscle subsystems regulated by a phylogenetically elaborated and distributed neural system. The coordinated actions of more than 100 muscles are required to generate the source excitation and to shape dynamically the vocal tract and upper airway for speech production. Across one's life span, considerable neurological, anatomical, and physiological development and remodeling in health and disease can affect speech production (Barlow, Farley, & Andreatta, 1999). Compared to adults, infants have a proportionately smaller mandible, shorter oral cavity, more anterior tongue body, gently sloping oropharyngeal channel, a more closely approximating velum and epiglottis, higher larynx, and circular-

shaped lips (Kent & Voperian, 1995; Smith, Goffman, & Stark, 1995). The integrity of the underlying performance anatomy, including contractile elements, connective tissue, bone, and the neural substrate, is central to a discussion of motor proficiency during speech. At any point in development, damage to select areas of the nervous system caused by neurological disease, maldevelopment, and traumatic injury can affect the selection, sequencing, and activation of articulatory muscles, degrade speech production, and reduce intelligibility (Guenther, Ghosh, & Tourville, 2006).

Speech production and other oromotor behaviors are highly sensitive to pathological processes or disease that can alter neurobiology, leading to a developmental delay or damage to the brain infrastructure's underlying pattern assembly and the execution of complex acoustic targets for speech production. Speech movement transitions are short, typically on the order of tens of milliseconds, with articulatory velocities approaching 20 cm/sec and an average speaking rate of approximately 8 to 12 sounds per second. Acceleration is an important dynamic property of movement as it relates to the initial and terminal phases of speech movements and ensuing changes in movement direction. As the second derivative of movement, acceleration is related temporally to the maxima of the underlying forcing function and correlates with the peak burst in agonist EMG activity. Typical peak accelerations observed during the production of the sentence "Buy Bobby a puppy" for the upper lip, lower lip, and jaw are 1000 mm/s^2, 3500 mm/s^2, and 3000 mm/s^2 respectively (Figure 10–1). A time series histogram analysis of position, velocity, and acceleration indexed at 24-ms intervals are summarized among the upper lip, lower lip and jaw during the production of "Buy Bobby a puppy" at a comfortable rate and loudness level by a normal speaker (Figure 10–2). As a sensorimotor skill, speech is performed with speed and accuracy, improved with practice, highly adaptive in achieving spatiotemporal goals, and relegated to automaticity in the adult speaker. Compared to adults, infants and toddlers speak more slowly, exhibit more spatiotemporally variable movements, and are less proficient at independent control of vocal tract structures (Green, Moore, & Reilly, 2002; Nip, Green, & Marx, 2009). Speech has a very protracted course of development; some aspects of speech motor control are still developing, even through the teenage years (Smith, 2006).

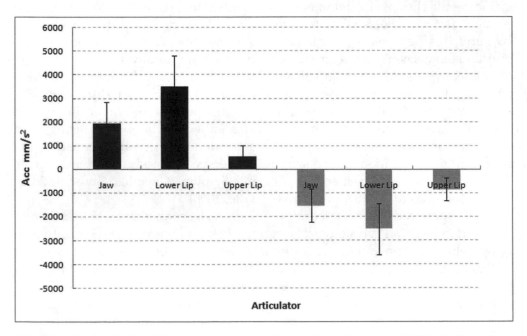

Figure 10–1. Normal adult peak acceleration values (mean and SD) derived from infrared motion capture data sampled during superior and inferior movements of the jaw, lower lip, and upper lip during the production of "Buy Bobby a puppy." (Courtesy of Dr. Jordan Green, University of Nebraska, 2010.)

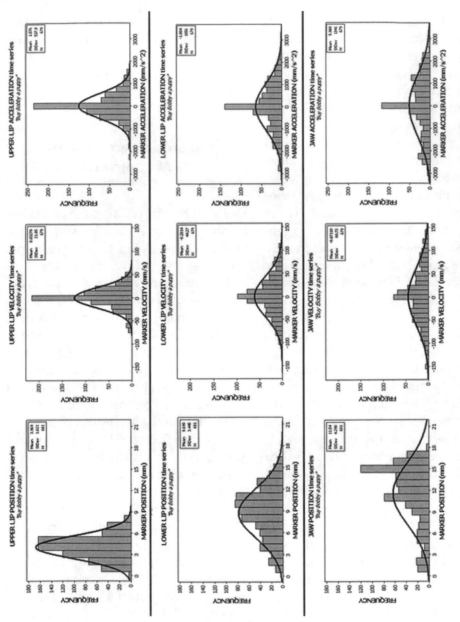

Figure 10–2. Time series histograms of marker trajectories along the Y-dimension (inferior-superior) processed at 24-ms intervals for the upper lip, lower lip, and jaw during production of "Buy Bobby a puppy" in a young normal female adult speaker. (Courtesy of the Communication Neuroscience Laboratories, University of Kansas, 2010.)

Speech performance exhibits the Hebbian principle of motor equivalence, which is defined as the capacity of the motor control system to achieve the same goal or end product with considerable variation among individual components that contribute to the output (Guenther, 1994; Hebb, 1949). In achieving a particular vocal tract goal, the specific contributions of individual speech articulators may vary from one production to another, as long as the desired end-product is achieved. Compensatory vowel articulation, presumably involving the operation of motor equivalence between the lips, tongue, and jaw, is defined as the ability of speakers to generate acceptable vowel qualities in spite of a fixed position of the mandible or other structures. Producing vowels that require a relatively closed jaw position, such as [i] or [u], with a spacer held between the teeth, fixing the jaw into a very open position, confronts a speaker with a new, or at least unfamiliar, task compared to producing the same vowel under normal nonconstrained conditions. Remarkably, speakers are able to produce perceptually adequate vowels that approximate acoustic targets with regard to formant frequency locations on the first trial following the introduction of the bite block (Lindblom, Lubker, & Gay, 1979; Lindblom & Sundberg, 1971). Continued practice with such perturbations leads to improvement in acoustic and perceptual measures of speech (Baum, McFarland, & Diab, 1996; Flege, Fletcher, & Homiedan, 1988; McFarland & Baum, 1995). Bite block manipulations have been used to examine compensatory abilities among speakers with Broca's aphasia and apraxia (Sussman, Marquardt, Hutchinson, & MacNeilage, 1986), nonfluent aphasia

and apraxia (Baum, 1999), and apraxia of speech (Jacks, 2008). Collectively, these studies demonstrate the important role of position sense, somatosensory information, and central brain loci to accurately reset the initial tongue position and shape in reorganizing motor output to achieve the desired acoustic product.

Biomechanics and Movement

The biodynamics of human speech is a fascinating journey of discovery, replete with complex relations among dynamic processes, including motions within and coordination among multiple articulatory systems, and the forces of acceleration inherent to pattern formation and directional change, which is the essence of the rhythms we recognize as human speech. The mechanical properties (e.g., mass, stiffness, viscoelasticity) of bone, cartilage, muscle, tendon, ligament, fat, and skin among articulatory subsystems involved in speech and gesture collectively influence all aspects of movement and must be accounted for in the selection and sequencing of motor program elements. Damage or disease processes affecting peripheral and/or central nervous system function can affect muscle coordination and alter muscle stiffness. Therefore, the biomechanics of orofacial and vocal tract structures should be taken into account when considering the movement patterns and network signaling in the neuromotor control system, in health and disease (Chu & Barlow, 2009; Chu, Barlow, Kieweg, & Lee, 2010; Chu, Barlow, & Lee, 2009; Sanguineti, Laboissière, & Ostry, 1998; Shiller, Laboissière, & Ostry, 2002).

Stiffness as a regulated variable has been hypothesized to play a significant role in movement associated with equilibrium position and end-point accuracy (Feldman & Levin, 2009; Shadmehr, 1993), force recruitment, and velocity scaling among articulators during speech production (Gracco, 1994; Löfqvist & Gracco, 1997; Shaiman & Gracco, 2002). Separate cortical control systems have been hypothesized for movement and stiffness regulation related to reciprocal activation and coactivation of antagonist muscle groups (Humphrey & Reed, 1983). Precise regulation of lip stiffness is essential for the accurate production of fricative sounds, such as /f/ and /v/, (Ito, Gomi, & Honda, 2004) and the duration of lip closure during consonant production (Löfqvist, 2005). Altered stiffness regulation between articulators is another feature of orofacial motor control that could impact facial movements. For example, jaw perturbation experiments revealed that stiffness is up-regulated between the upper lip and jaw in order to maintain the constriction area between lips during the production of a fricative consonants (Gomi, Honda, Ito, & Murano, 2002). Increased jaw stiffness is associated with a decrease in the variability of speech kinematics (Shiller et al., 2002). Stiffness regulation appears to play a central role for speech motor learning and adaptation (Nasir & Ostry, 2006; Tremblay, Houle, & Ostry, 2008).

Measurement of speech-related muscle performance variables, including kinematics and associated dynamics, are central to advancing our understanding of the development and maintenance of speech movements across our life spans, and the response to neurological disease and traumatic injury. Activation of the speech musculature yields a number of measurable outputs including force, displacement, heat, vibration, and electrical activity. Speech kinematic variables typically studied include the amplitude of displacement, velocity, acceleration, phase and relative timing among multiple articulators, reciprocity, spatiotemporal variability, electromyographic-movement relations, and spectral properties of movement and muscle firing patterns (coherence, frequency domain) (Smith, 1992; Steeve & Moore, 2009).

Methods and Studies of Supralaryngeal Speech Kinematics

Radiographic Tracking of Orofacial Movements

The X-ray microbeam is a computer-controlled system that was developed at the Research Institute of Logopedics and Phoniatrics (RILP) at the University of Tokyo in 1968 and later implemented at the University of Wisconsin. Currently, no operating X-ray microbeam system exists in the world. This device was designed to generate a narrow beam of X-rays to localize and track the two-dimensional movements of small gold pellets attached to select structures, including the lips, jaw, tongue, soft palate (Abbs, Nadler, & Fujimura, 1988; Westbury, 1991) and compare to the position of gold pellets attached to skull reference points (bridge of nose, maxillary incisor). The X-ray microbeam system generated an electron beam accelerated by a voltage source of up to 600 kV at a 5 mA current (Fujimura, Kiritani, & Ishida, 1973; Kiritani, Itoh, & Fujimura, 1975). The focal X-ray beam (0.4 mm diameter) was scanned at a high rate across a pellet, producing a recognizable shadow that is registered on a sodium iodide crystal detector. A prediction algorithm based on current and previous positions was used to guide the X-ray beam toward a pellet. At periodic intervals, the location of each pellet (defined as the centroid of its shadow) is assigned rectangular coordinates relative to axes specified by the reference pellets. The sequence of scanning, recognition, prediction, and calculation of location for up to 10 pellets may be completed with an aggregate cycling rate of up to 700 Hz. Each pellet may be assigned its own cycle rate in the range of 40–180 Hz.

The X-ray microbeam system has been used successfully to study the relation between speech rate and velocity profiles of movements of the lower lip and tongue tip during the production of stop consonants in young normal adults (Adams, Weismer, & Kent, 1993). Fast speaking rates yielded symmetrical, single-peaked velocity functions; whereas slow speech produced asymmetrical, multipeaked velocity profiles. Speech produced at fast rates appears to involve unitary movements that may be preprogrammed and executed with little or no dependence on sensorimotor integration; whereas articulatory gestures produced at slow speaking rates may have greater dependence on feedback mechanisms.

X-ray microbeam data also have been combined with cinefluorography to examine the displacement of the tongue body during opening articulatory gestures in deaf and hearing subjects (Tye-Murray, 1991). Speech samples consisted of consonant—vowel—consonant (CVC) syllables embedded within a carrier phrase. Deaf speakers manifested less flexible tongue bodies as a result of compensatory and incorrectly learned principles for constraining tongue movement during speech.

The question of functional regions within the tongue during speech and swallowing was studied by quantifying the strength of coupling among four different tongue locations (Green & Wang, 2003). Tongue-surface movement patterns characterized by calculating the covariance between the vertical displacement time histories of all possible pellet pairs showed that speech and swallowing kinematics are clustered into distinct groups based on their coupling profiles. The study of the coupling relations among tongue regions has the potential to elucidate modes of control for swallowing and speech, as well as advancing our understanding of the differences in the coordinative requirements for these two motor behaviors.

The effects of progressive neuromotor disease on the scaling of orofacial motor control dynamics are evident in a recent study of vowel production. The position and trajectory of markers attached to the jaw, lower lip, tongue blade, and dorsum were sampled using the X-ray microbeam during the production of words (i.e., seed, feed, big, dish, too, shoo, bad, cat, box, and dog), which were embedded into sentences and read at a comfortable rate (Yunusova, Weismer, Westbury, & Lindstrom, 2008). Participants included 19 normal speakers and speakers with dysarthria due to amyotrophic lateral sclerosis (ALS, $n = 8$) or Parkinson disease (PD, $n = 7$). The authors noted that articulator markers do not necessarily move less in speakers with dysarthria due to ALS or PD, as compared to healthy controls but tend to take longer to move the same distances. The tongue manifested disproportionately greater impairments in the scaling of velocity and movement duration, particularly for ALS speakers compared to the healthy controls. The effects of neurologic disease on vowel production often are articulator-, vowel-, and context-specific.

Orofacial Magnetometry

Alternating magnetic field devices, known as magnetometers, represent the predominant technology used to capture movements of the tongue during speech and swallowing (Bartle-Meyer, Goozée, & Murdoch, 2009; Chen, Murdoch, Goozée, & Scott, 2007; Hertrich & Ackermann, 2000; Steele & Van Lieshout, 2004). Part of the magnetometer's appeal in speech physiology research and clinical application is the capability to sample real-time kinematics of intraoral structures without the biohazards associated with cineradiography. One of the earliest versions of a magnetometer sensor for tracking tongue tip movements was described by Sonoda (1974) from Kumamoto University (Japan). A small permanent magnet was fixed on the tongue surface, and two magnetometer units sensitive to horizontal and vertical movements of the tongue were oriented at a right angle to the sagittal plane of the head. With this configuration, the position of the magnet in the mouth could be determined during speech. Hixon (1971) and van der Giet (1977) also used alternating fields and discrete transmitter signals to track

the movement trajectories of the jaw and lips, respectively. These systems did not have a provision for correcting for rotational misalignment between the magnetic field transmitters and the transducers, which could cause undetectable measurement error. Sonoda recognized that magnetometry represented a powerful method for speech physiology research and a promising therapeutic tool for speech correction due to its relative simplicity, safety, economy, and flexibility for signal presentation. For example, real-time visual display of tongue position is an efficient biofeedback tool for correcting articulatory errors due to hearing loss, dysarthria, craniofacial disorders, or second-language acquisition.

By 1980, the development of a multichannel electromagnetic articulometer, based on two transmitter coils and miniature biaxial sensors designed for correction due to rotational misalignment, was well underway at the Massachusetts Institute of Technology (Perkell et al., 1992). It was possible to record movements of multiple midline points on vocal tract structures. Motivated in part by the speech magnetometry work at the MIT laboratory, another development of a two-dimensional electromagnetic articulograph began at the Medical School of the University of Göttingen in 1982. By 1988, Carstens Medizinelektronik (Lenglern, Germany) developed the first commercial articulograph known as the AG100. The AG500 is currently the most completely developed three-dimensional electromagnetic articulograph system and is certified for use as a laboratory apparatus. It does not require the participant to wear a heavy, restraining head mount. This system allows sensor placement at all positions in the oral cavity and in all orientations within a 300-mm spherical measurement area. It features high temporal resolution with either 8 or 12 channels. Each channel is sampled at 100 kHz with 200 Hz demodulated output. A separate channel for sampling the speech acoustic signal is synchronized by the AG500 by the host microprocessor. The principal components of the AG500 include an acrylic case, known as the Ema Cube® (Figure 10–3), small sensor coils that are positioned on and in the subject's mouth, electronic signal conditioning, and a digital interface to a MS Windows-compatible microprocessor. System operation includes a sensor calibration procedure to ensure accurate scaling of displacement among the sensors attached to the tongue, mouth, palate, and mandible. A reference sensor attached to the bridge of the nose provides for head movement correction. Each of the six transmitters fixed on the case produces an alternating magnetic field at different frequencies. The alternating magnetic field induces an alternating current in the sensors and allows the calculation of the distances of each sensor from the six transmitters. The Carstens system provides for motion tracking in

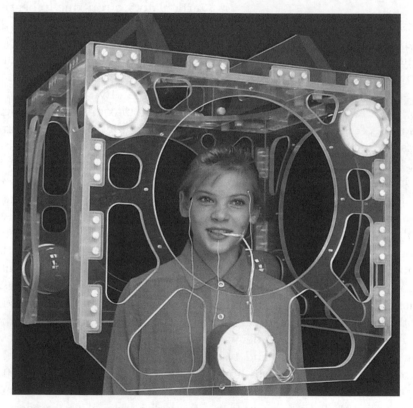

Figure 10–3. Carstens Articulograph AG500 for 3-D recording of facial and intraoral movements. Transduction and subject interface is shown including the EMA Cube and small sensor coils positioned on and in the speaker's mouth. The fixed transmitters are attached to the acrylic case. Reprinted with permission granted by Brigitta Carstens, Carstens Medizinelektronik GmbH, D37120 Lenglern (Germany) (See Color Plate 2).

five degrees of freedom (i.e., three Cartesian and two angular coordinates). An independent laboratory test of the spatial resolution of the AG500 EMA system showed a median error less than 0.5 mm across different types of recordings, with the maximum error ranging between 1 and 2 mm as a function of task and location of the sensors within the recording region of the cube (Yunusova, Green, & Mefferd, 2009).

Optical Tracking of the Face

Studies of lip and jaw coordination during speech, mastication, feeding, and animation in infants, children, and adults have benefited directly from the emergence of sophisticated multichannel video-based movement tracking systems. High-speed video cameras are used to register marker location using either reflective markers (Eagle-4 Digital Real Time® from Motion Analysis Corporation, Santa Rosa, California) or infrared source tracking (Optotrack Certus® from Northern Digital Inc., Ontario, Canada). Reflective markers as small as 2 mm are placed on the face and body (Figure 10–4). The motion of these markers are tracked with submillimeter precision, typically on the order of 0.2 mm or less, using Eagle 4MP digital

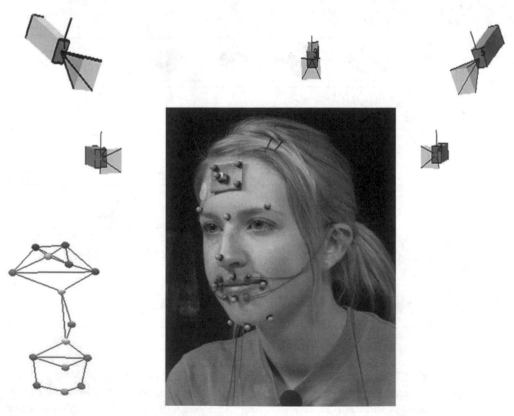

Figure 10–4. A 5-camera (Eagle 4MP, Motion Analysis Corporation) configuration for sampling 4-mm diameter reflective markers on the face simultaneously with two channels of perioral EMG and voice audio. (Courtesy of the Communication Neuroscience Laboratories, University of Kansas, 2010.) (See Color Plate 3)

infrared cameras sampling up to 200 frames per second at full resolution, or up to 10,000 fps at reduced resolution. With advanced data collection software, such as Cortex™ (Motion Analysis Corp.), motion data are synchronized and digitized with other biological signals (audio, electromyographic, force, air pressure, air flow, etc.) along with composite video. Multichannel examples showing motion capture records using a 5-camera system for sampling the upper lip, lower lip, and jaw positions synchronized with voice audio and electromyographic signals for orbicularis oris superior (OOS) and orbicularis oris inferior (OOI) muscles during syllabic production /pa/ and

the sentence "Buy Bobby a puppy" are shown in Figures 10–5 and 10–6. This multichannel capability provides the investigator with flexibility for comprehensive analysis of biobehavioral performance variables.

Many important findings on orofacial movement across one's life span have resulted from optical tracking studies of face motion. For infants, motion capture systems using reflective markers provide a noninvasive and appropriate solution for capturing emerging movements of the face and extremities. For example, at 9 months of age, more than half of infants' recorded orofacial behaviors *do not* include vocalization (Nip et. al., 2009), even though infants at

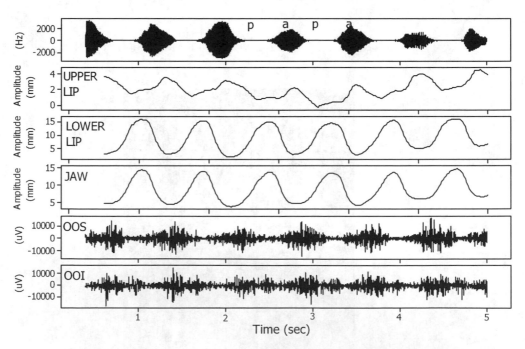

Figure 10–5. Sample record for repetition of the syllable [pa] by a normal adult female (age 26) illustrating synchronized multichannel sampling of orofacial kinematics (inferior-superior trajectories) using Motion Analysis Corporation reflective marker technology with orbicularis oris superior (OOS) and orbicularis oris inferior (OOI) muscle recording sites and voice audio (top channel). (Courtesy of the Communication Neuroscience Laboratories, University of Kansas, 2010.)

this age are well into an important early stage of speech-like vocal behavior, canonical babbling. The number of spontaneous oral movements in fact increases over the first year of life (Green & Wilson, 2006), a type of motor behavior that would not be captured with traditional acoustic measures. Studies of infant orofacial behaviors have revealed numerous differences between infant and adult oral motion. For example, infants are less able to independently move the jaw from lips and upper lip from lower lip (Green et al., 2002; Nip et al., 2009). In general, coordinated jaw movements for speech occur before coordinated lip or tongue movements (Green, Moore, Higashikawa, & Steeve,

2000; Green et al., 2002; Kent, 1999; MacNeilage, Davis, Kinney, & Matyear, 2000), and this is reflected in the acoustic features of their oromotor gestures as well (Nittrouer, 1993). Compared to adults and children, infants' jaw and lip movements are produced at lower velocities over shorter a duration of movement epochs, exhibit decreased coupling among facial regions, with the jaw kinematics approaching maturity sooner than the lip (Green et al., 2002; Green & Wilson, 2006; Nip et al., 2009).

Trotman and colleagues (Trotman & Faraway, 1998; Trotman, Faraway, & Essick, 2000; Trotman, Faraway, Silvester, Greenlee, & Johnston, 1998) found that individual cleft lip patients

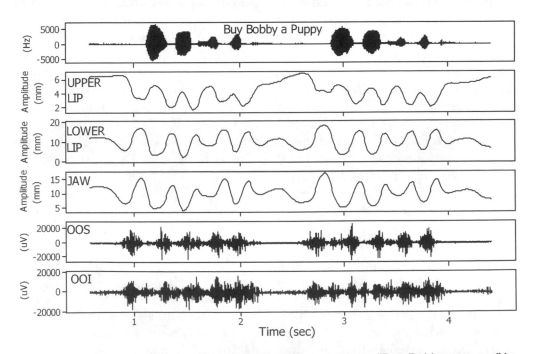

Figure 10–6. Sample record for repetition of the sentence "Buy Bobby a puppy" by a normal adult female (age 26) illustrating synchronized multichannel sampling of orofacial kinematics (inferior-superior trajectories) using Motion Analysis Corporation reflective marker technology with orbicularis oris superior (OOS) and orbicularis oris inferior (OOI) muscle recording sites and voice audio (top channel). (Courtesy of the Communication Neuroscience Laboratories, University of Kansas, 2010.)

exhibited significant asymmetry of facial movements along with changes in the range of displacement during the production of facial gestures. For participants with a cleft lip, force regulation of the circumoral region within the operating range, presumed important for facial and speech animation, is compromised because of impairments in force recruitment, gradation, fractionation, and stability (Trotman, Barlow, & Faraway, 2007). In the presence of a change in upper lip tissue biomechanics due to scarring or neuromotor impairment, the lower lip typically exhibits compensatory motor actions. Thus, assessment of facial kinematics and dynamics should be considered during the course of surgical intervention.

Smith and Zelaznik (2004) used infrared light emitting diode (LED) marker technology to sample and calculate the 3-D motions of the upper lip, lower lip, and jaw markers relative to the head during the production of two sentences in 180 speakers ranging in age from 4 years to 22 years. An acoustic signal sampled at 7.5 KHz was synchronized with the kinematic channels sampled at 250 Hz. An algorithm was developed to provide a quantitative index of spatial and temporal variability (STI) in the trajectory patterns for the facial articulators over repeated productions of a particular utterance. Application of the STI measure to the development of functional synergies among labio-mandibular (Smith & Zelaznik, 2004) and lingua-mandibular systems (Chen et al., 2007) revealed that the time course of development for speech motor coordination is protracted and does not reach adult-like performance until after age 14 years for both males and females, with males lagging on the STI measure.

The STI has been used successfully in limb motor control studies (Atkeson & Hollerbach, 1985; Georgopoulos, Kalaska, & Massey, 1981) and in studies of speech (Cheng et al., 2007; Goffman, Gerken, & Lucchesi, 2007; Smith, Johnson, McGillem, & Goffman, 2000; Smith & Zelaznik, 2004). Recently, this approach has paid dividends to help expand our understanding of ororhythmic pattern formation and development of non-nutritive suck in preterm infants (Poore, Barlow, Wang, Estep, & Lee, 2008; Poore, Zimmerman, Barlow, Wang, & Gu, 2008). In preterm infants, ororhythmic dynamics have been extracted from intraluminal pressure signals sampled during non-nutritive suck. Disease processes and medical interventions associated with prematurity, including respiratory distress syndrome, impose extensive periods of sensory deprivation and motor restriction to the emerging oromotor pattern generating neural circuits, which can degrade significantly the spatiotemporal stability of non-nutritive suck (NNS STI) (Poore, Barlow, et al., 2008). Synthesis and delivery of patterned orocutaneous inputs can enhance significantly ororhythmic pattern formation (Barlow, Finan, Chu, & Lee, 2008) and increase the stability of NNS STI (Poore, Zimmerman, et al., 2008).

Overall, orofacial STI for speech movements tends to decline with age. A brief decline in the spatiotemporal stability of lip and jaw movements for speech, however, is observed at 2 years of age, when language development is at a peak (Green et al., 2002). Children's speech production is more spatiotemporally variable during nonword production tasks but increases in stability with practice. Adult speech motor control, on the other hand, is more spatiotemporally stable regardless of word novelty (Walsh, Smith, & Weber-Fox, 2006). Speech movement variability in adults does increase, however, with increased utterance length and syntactic complexity (Kleinow & Smith, 2006; Maner, Smith, & Grayson, 2000) and while performing visuomotor tracking tasks (Dromey & Bates, 2005).

Tracking Tongue Movements

Motion and conformational change of the tongue hydrostat is very complex and cannot be seen externally with the unaided eye. Early studies in adult speakers relied heavily on radiography (Chiba & Kajiyama, 1958; House, 1967; Kiritani, Itoh, Fujisaki, & Sawashima, 1976; Perkell, 1969; Potter, Kopp, & Green, 1947) and tongue contact devices such as the dynamic palatometer (Fletcher, McCutcheon, & Wolf, 1975; Harley, 1972; Kuzmin, 1962; Kydd & Belt, 1964; Palmer, 1973; Shibata, 1968).

Palatometry (Fletcher, Hasegawa, McCutcheon, & Gilliom, 1980; Fletcher et al., 1975; Johnson, 1969; Michi, Suzuki, Yamashita, & Imai, 1986) involves mapping the place of linguapalatal contact for consonant and vowel articulations. As described by Fletcher (1989), the palatometer employs 96 tiny (0.5 mm) bead electrodes embedded on the oral surface of an acrylic pseudopalate to sense the pattern of tongue contact during speech production. An AC carrier signal at 27.8 KHz is delivered to the palatal electrode array (current limited to 100 μamps) and referenced to the wrist. The system described by Michi et al. (1986) employs a palatal reference electrode and uses considerably less current at just 8 microamperes. Tongue conductance on any electrode in the array is registered as a sensor location in a palatometric display on a video monitor. According to Fletcher, each vowel in English is associated with a unique stationary lingua-palatal contact map. For example, during the stable contact portion of /i/, the tongue is in contact with sensors extending from the cuspid-bicuspid region of the palate to the posterior border of the alveolar ridge. During the /æ/, the contact is against the most posterior-lateral sensors. Diphthongs are characterized by movements between two stable monophthong positions. The glosssometer (optical diode tracking) and palatometer (lingua-palatal contact) have been used in training or retraining vowel space and consonant production in hearing-impaired (Fletcher, 1989; Fletcher, Dagenais, & Critz-Crosby, 1991) and cleft palate patients (Michi et al., 1986).

Many improvements to the EPG have been instantiated through the integration of digital electronics and advanced signal processing (Hardcastle, Gibbon, & Jones, 1991). The Reading EPG3 system, an innovative computer-based tool for assessing and treating speech motor difficulties, enables the speaker to see the placement of his or her tongue during speech and to attempt to correct any lingual palatal errors. The EPG3 records the location and timing of tongue contacts with the hard palate during continuous speech and provides real-time visual feedback of tongue to palate movement. The Reading EPG 3 system consists of an artificial acrylic palate consisting of 62 touch-sensitive electrodes to record tongue-to-palate contacts. The 1.4-mm diameter Ag electrodes are arranged into eight rows and eight columns according to predetermined anatomical landmarks. The first four rows proximal to the incisors constitute the anterior zone, and the last four rows make up the posterior zone. The spacing between the electrodes in the anterior rows is half that of the posterior rows. The artificial acrylic palate is bounded by the central incisors anteriorly (Hardcastle, Jones, Knight, Trudgeon, & Calder, 1989), the side teeth laterally (Gibbon & Nicolaidis, 1999), and the junction between the hard and soft palate posteriorly (Figure 10–7). The anatomical and proportional arrangement of electrodes in the Reading EPG3 system allows comparison across participants with respect to specific rows and electrode positions, even in the presence of different palate shapes and sizes (Hardcastle et al., 1989). Multiplexed tongue contact pattern and acoustic data typically are sampled at 100Hz and 10kHz, respectively (Gibbon & Nicolaidis, 1999). The Reading EPG3 system also is available as an MS Window's XP application, WinEPG.

The development of a prototype 5-channel, pressure-sensing EPG system based on Hall Effect transistor technology has followed (Murdoch, Goozée, Veidt, Scott, & Meyers, 2004). These units are compact, offer high sensitiv-

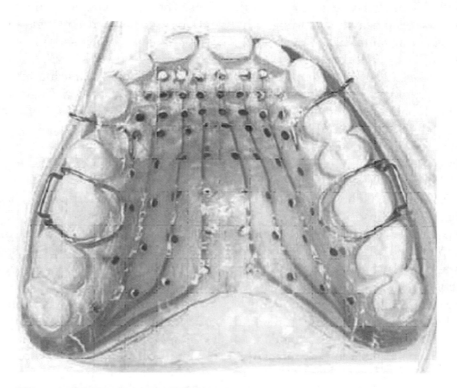

Figure 10–7. Reading EPG3 artificial palate. Permission granted from publisher (Cengage Learning) via Copyright.com for Figure 1, which appeared in Kuruvilla, Murdoch, & Goozée (2008).

ity, and are inexpensive. The pressure-sensing palate was capable of recording dynamic tongue-to-palate pressures during syllable repetition, with minimal disruption to speech detected perceptually. With only five sensors, problems were encountered in optimally positioning the sensors to defect the consonant lingual pressures. The pressure-sensing palate represents a novel enhancement to the EPG. Comprehensive analysis of tongue-to-palate contacts, including pressure measures, is expected to enable more specific and effective therapeutic techniques to be developed for a variety of speech disorders.

The EPG also has found application to address speech motor control and intelligibility problems experienced by many children and young people with Down's syndrome (DS) (Cleland, Timmins, Wood, Hardcastle, & Wishart, 2009; Wood, Wishart, Hardcastle, Cleland, & Timmins, 2009) . These studies have shown that visual supplementation of auditory feedback afforded by EPG offers potential therapeutic benefits for children with intellectual disabilities, many of whom show relative strengths in visual versus auditory and simultaneous versus sequential processing. EPG also provides therapists with an objective measure of articulatory ability and represents a positive approach for improving articulatory patterns in children with DS.

Dysarthria with severe articulatory impairment is a common sequelae following severe traumatic brain injury (TBI). Therapeutic application of EPG as a biofeedback instrument was delivered weekly over a period of 2.5 months in three adolescents who had severe TBI (Morgan, Liegeois, & Occomore, 2007). Perceptual improvements for

phoneme precision and length were correlated with increased precision of spatial EPG measures during phoneme production. The authors concluded that EPG treatment may be effective for improving speech at the isolated phoneme, word, or sentence level of articulation and provide a new intervention to effect speech changes in participants with severe TBI and persistent dysarthria. An analysis of temporal and spatial parameters of lingual-palatal contact patterns during target consonant production in sentence- and syllable-repetition tasks at a habitual rate and loudness level was completed in 11 dysarthric individuals post-severe TBI and 10 age- and sex-matched healthy control speakers (Kuruvilla, Murdoch, & Goozée, 2008). The post-TBI dysarthric speakers manifest prolonged duration of the transitional phases of consonant production, which were attributed to articulatory slowness. The impaired accuracy of lingua-palatal contacts using EPG confirmed spatial programming deficits among the post-TBI speakers.

EPG has been used to study the temporal aspects of speech articulation in individuals with PD at sentence, word, and segment level (McAuliffe, Ward, & Murdoch, 2006). Participants were required to read aloud the phrase "I saw a ____ today" with the EPG palate *in-situ*. Target words included the consonants /l/, /s/ and /t/ in initial position in both the /i/ and /a/ vowel environments. The percept of impaired speech rate for PD speakers was at odds with EPG results of segment durations, which were measured to be generally consistent with age-matched controls, except for the significantly increased duration of the release phase for /la/.

The disparity in articulatory timing measures likely is due to the fact that EPG provides time indexes correlated to tongue-palate contacts, and thus, does not measure the dynamics of the tongue's trajectory towards and away from the hard palate.

Technological advances also have been made in optics, magnetometry, X-ray microbeam, functional magnetic resonance imaging (MRI), and ultrasound for tracking the tongue during speech and swallowing. Ultrasound provides real-time images of the tongue surface in a digital video format during speech and swallowing (Gick, 2002; Peng, Jost-Brinkmann, Miethke, & Lin, 2000; Shawker, Sonies, Stone, & Baum, 1983; Stone, Epstein, & Iskarous, 2004; Stone & Lundberg, 1996; Watkin, 1999). The sounds waves then are reflected back and used to create images of the position and motion of internal structures of the vocal tract, such as the tongue or lateral pharyngeal walls. Classic ultrasound techniques could image only one plane at a time, but 3D technologies now exist at scan rates up to 24 Hz (Epstein & Stone, 2005; Stone, 2005). Images are combined with estimates of the hard palate boundary using ultrasound during the production of command swallows to establish a reference within headspace for coregistration among subjects and calculation of select phonetic measures. Limitations of ultrasound include difficulty imaging the tip and lateral margins of the tongue and also that the images themselves lack a reference structure, which makes it difficult to correct the images for head or neck motion (Stone, 2005). This limitation can be addressed, however, with combination technologies such as the Haskins Optically Corrected Ultra-sound System (HOCUS). The HOCUS combines data from the ultrasound transceiver with optical motion tracking data to correct ultrasound images of the tongue for motion of adjacent supportive musculoskeletal structures (Whalen et al., 2005).

Ultrasound shows that cross-sectional tongue shape is related directly to the position of the tongue, and the lateral and sagittal shape of the tongue (Stone, Shawker, Talbot, & Rich, 1988). In general, midsagittal grooving is evident for all vowel types, with posterior grooves being deeper than anterior grooves. In the /p/ context, posterior grooving is greater than in the /s/ context. Grooving for vowels in the /p/ context demonstrated a continuum, whereas in the anterior /s/ context, two groups of vowels were identified (high group/shallower grooves and back group with deeper grooves). In the anterior /s/ context, tongue shape for /i/ and /u/ was convex. Ultrasound technology is particularly well suited to digitally capture and visualize the complex 3-D surface shapes associated with the lingual groove.

Considerable progress has been made on high-speed 3-D reconstruction of tongue ultrasonic images (Lundberg & Stone, 1999; Stone, Epstein, & Iskarous, 2004; Stone, Epstein, & Sutton, 2003; Sze, Iny, Stone, & Levine, 1999; Watkin & Rubin, 1989; Yang & Stone, 2002) and tagged cineradiographic and MRI images (Dick, Ozturk, Douglas, McVeigh, & Stone, 2000; Stone, Dick, Davis, Douglas, & Ozturk, 2000). Recent work using ultrasound has focused on defining predictable mathematical relations between midsagittal tongue contour shapes and five cross-sectional (coronal) contours (Stone et al., 2003). This prediction was based on earlier work, which found that 3-D tongue surfaces are composed of a concatenation of coronal slices, a subset of which accurately represents the 3-D tongue surface (Stone & Lundberg, 1996). These relations are shown in Figure 10–8. When compared among four tongue-shape phonemic categories (i.e., front raising /i/, back raising /ŋ/, continuous groov- ing /æ/, and two-point displacement /l/), it was found that transitional values exist when exceeded that predict tongue arching versus midsagittal tongue grooving. Even better predictions were noted for the three anterior coronal slices in which strong correlations exist between midline displacement and groove depth to arch height. Stone et al. (2004) concluded that knowledge

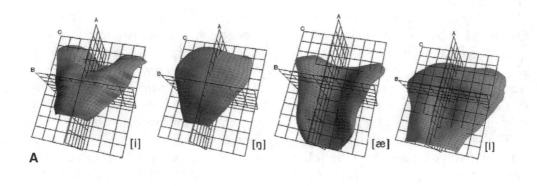

A

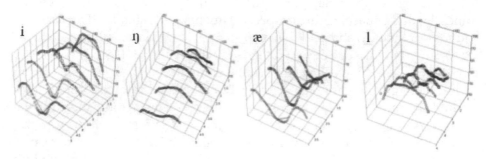

B

Figure 10–8. **(A)** Representative three-dimensional tongue surface shapes for the four shape-based categories, including front-raising /i/, back-raising /ŋ/, continuous groove /æ/, and two-point displacement /l/. Tongue tip shown on the lower left. **(B)** Coronal slices and derived slopes for representation phonemes from each of the four shape-based categories, including front-raising /i/, back-raising /ŋ/, continuous groove /æ/, and two-point displacement /l/. Tongue tip shown on the upper left. Reprinted with permission from Taylor & Francis Group LLC—BOOKS and Dr. Maureen Stone, from Stone, M., Epstein, M. A., Kambhamettu, C., and Li, M. (2006). Predicting 3D tongue shapes from midsagittal contours. In J. Harrington, and M. Tabain, (Eds.), *Speech production: Models, phonetic processes, and techniques* (pp. 315–330). Routledge Publishing, Inc.

of both category and midsagittal displacement provides good prediction of coronal tongue shape.

Tracking Velar Movements

Kinematic studies of the invisible valves of speech, including the velopharynx, is challenging technically due to small size and relative inaccessibility. Acceptable sampling methods in humans usually reflect a concession between the invasiveness of the instrument and the quality of the acquired signals. New technologies that rely on imaging, acoustics, and/or fluid mechanics have come to the forefront. These procedures are described in the following sections.

The velopharynx (VP) is a complex muscular valve consisting of the velum and lateral and posterior pharyngeal walls and is situated strategically to channel acoustic and aerodynamic energy through the oral and nasal cavities. The size of the velar port determines the oral or nasal nature of speech sounds. Methods to study VP kinematics roughly fall into one of two categories: direct and indirect. Direct methods include imaging techniques such as cineradiography or videoflouroscopy, video nasendoscopy, electromechanical, optomechanical transduction of velar displacement, and magnetic resonance imaging (MRI). With the exception of MRI, many of these technologies share a common limitation in resolving movement within a single plane. In most radiographic studies, discrete points are tracked on a frame-by-frame basis, which is useful in resolving velocity and displacement profiles. However, because the radiographic methods are limited to one plane or slice through the velo-

pharynx, one is never certain whether closure has occurred. Velar apertures may exist at locations opposite the lateral pharyngeal walls on one or both sides. The patterns of VP closure are highly variable both within and across adult speakers (Siegel-Sadewitz, & Shprintzen, 1986; Finkelstein, Talmi, Nachmani, Hauben, & Zohar 1992).

From a biodynamical perspective, the velar muscular-connective tissue complex can be modeled as a predominantly viscoelastic system, with considerable intersubject variation in anatomy and kinematic output (Moon & Kuehn, 2004; Kuehn & Perry, 2009). Our knowledge of velar dynamics is limited due in part to its relative inaccessibility compared to the large number of studies on lip, tongue, and jaw kinematics during speech. Cineradiographic tracking of midsagittal velar fleshpoints (100 frames/sec = 10 ms dwell time per frame) relative to the tongue tip and tongue dorsum in two young adults (Kuehn, 1976a) has shown velar movements to be smaller (Displacement$_{Velum}$ = 0.86 * Displacement$_{TongueTip}$) and slower (Velocity$_{Velum}$ = 0.685 * Velocity$_{TongueTip}$) compared to the tongue tip during normal speech rate conditions. Based on these scale factors, this translates to mean velar and tongue tip displacements of 7.25 and 8.4 mm, respectively, with mean velar and tongue tip velocities approximately 7.95 and 11.6 cm/sec, respectively.

It is well known from radiography (Moll, 1962; Moll & Daniloff, 1971), nasoendoscopy (Bell-Berti & Hirose, 1975), direct observation (Bloomer, 1953; Calnan, 1953), photodetection (Dalston, 1989; Keefe & Dalston, 1989; Moon & Lagu, 1987), and acoustic analysis (House & Fairbanks, 1953) that complete velopharyngeal closure is not always achieved during vowel production. Pioneering work aimed at characterizing normal patterns of VP closure using cineflourographic techniques revealed that high vowels exhibit greater VP closure than low vowels, regardless of consonant context (Moll, 1962). Complete closure of the VP is not always present during production of the low vowels or attained on vowels adjacent to a nasal consonant (assimilation). Speech rate (Dwyer, Robb, O'Beirne, & Gilbert, 2009) and age (Thom, Hoit, Hixon, & Smith, 2006) are other factors that significantly can influence the degree of VP closure.

Flexible fiberoptic nasoendoscopy is a powerful imaging tool that helps to resolve some of the uncertainty regarding the dynamics of the velopharyngeal port. Advanced camera, fiberoptics, and digital recording technology provide high-resolution color images of the velopharynx in real-time during speech production. Image recognition software routines assist the investigator in accurate identification of tissue boundaries and kinematic properties of the velopharynx, including computation of portal area and boundary velocity, displacement, and calibration schemes for scaling distance. This information will be invaluable for studies of velopharyngeal motor control in patients with sensorimotor speech disorders. Magnetic resonance imaging (MRI) also can be used to produce images of the velopharynx but is used primarily in research rather than clinical settings due to the high cost. One advantage of MRI is the quality of 3-D images reconstructed, which can be useful for imaging the velopharynx pre- and postsurgery (Perry & Kuehn, 2009), for example. Velopharyn-

geal MRI measurements can be made at rest, during sustained production of consonants or vowels (Tian & Redett, 2009).

Aerodynamic measures of velopharyngeal port function offer some unique perspectives on the fluid dynamics of this valve during speech in adults and children. Current aerodynamic protocols and instrumentation provide reasonably accurate estimates of the subglottal driving air pressures (P_s) and air flows acting on the velopharynx during speech in fluid mechanics terms without the biohazards associated with radiation or the invasiveness of a fiberoptic bundle inserted into the nasal cavity. Area functions (Warren, 1988; Warren & Dubois, 1964), resistance (impedance) estimates (Smitheran & Hixon, 1981), and temporal pattern studies (Samlan & Barlow, 1999; Warren, Dalston, Trier, & Holder, 1985; Zajac & Hackett, 2002) have been used effectively to characterize the activity of the velopharynx during speech.

Numerous reports have described some of the temporal relations between pressure-flow variables during nasalplosive blends to stress the velopharyngeal mechanism and reveal the coarticulatory dynamics between velopharynx and other upper airway structures in normal and cleft palate speakers (Dalston, Warren, & Smith, 1990; Samlan & Barlow, 1999; Warren et al., 1985). For example, studies of VP aerodynamics in repaired cleft palate adults and normal controls revealed that the magnitude of mean intraoral air pressures tend to be slightly less than control speakers (Dalston et al., 1990). Articulatory timing errors were evident as the nasal airflow pulse overlapped into the rising phase and peak of the pressure pulse associated with /p/ in the word "hamper."

A decrease in respiratory effort may represent a compensatory strategy used by patients with repaired cleft palates to achieve adequate velopharyngeal closure and minimize shunting (air leak) through the velopharyngeal port. This conclusion was based on careful study of the temporal relations between the airflow and pressure curves associated with production of the nasal-plosive blend.

Competing Hypotheses on the Neural Infrastructure for Orofacial Movements: Early Ororhythmicity Versus Speech

The development of orofacial movements for speech has been suggested by some to occur quasi-independently from phonatory and respiratory control mechanism with mature speech production ultimately resulting from the integration sensorimotor control from these constituent systems (MacNeilage, 1998; Meier, McGarvin, Zakia, & Willerman, 1997). These authors posit that early nonspeech behaviors provide the building blocks for the coordinative mechanisms underlying the production of early speech behaviors (MacNeilage, 1998; Meier et al., 1997; Thelen, 1991). Challenging this view are physiological studies of mandibular motor control based on the measurement of movement patterns and associated EMG, which were reported to demonstrate the existence of parallel, distinct *coordinative infrastructures* to support early alimentary behaviors, babble, and speech (Green, Moore, Ruark, Rodda, Morvée, & VanWitzenburg, 1997; Moore & Ruark, 1996; Steeve, Moore, Green, Reilly, &

McMurtrey, 2008). Each motor behavior develops along a protracted timeline (Green et al., 1997; Steeve et al., 2008). Based on longitudinal study consisting of 11 sessions of a single infant from 9 to 22 months of age, these authors concluded that the coordinative mechanisms that support suck and mastication do not support the development of early speech production. The question remains as to whether a motor stereotypy, such as jaw, lip, tongue oscillation, relies on a coordinative infrastructure that can be exploited later on for early types of babble productions or whether motor control for jaw oscillation is distinct and develops in parallel with other mandibular behaviors (Steeve & Moore, 2009).

It is not surprising that orofacial kinematics and muscle activation patterns differ between non-nutritive suck, nutritive suck, mastication, babble, and mature speech. In this regard, the studies referenced previously have done an admirable job mapping the topography of orofacial kinematics by age and task complexity. However, one major issue left unresolved from these descriptive studies of orofacial movement in tackling the potential links between early oromotor activity (suck, mastication, lick), canonical babbling, and speech concerns the reference to a coordinative infrastructure. In the writings of Steeve and Moore (2009), use of the term "coordinative infrastructure" refers to a neuroanatomical circuit or network. It is well established that a relatively simple central pattern generator (CPG) can produce a wide range of motor patterns depending on developmental stage (incorporation of inhibitory interneurons to an existing circuit), central neuromodulation (transmitter type and molar concentration, sensory modulation (mechanoreceptor firing rate), changes in body plan, and task dynamics (motor rate, motor intensity, direction, chew soft versus hard foods, etc.) (Barlow & Estep, 2006; Barlow, Lund, Estep, & Kolta, 2010; Grillner, 2003; Grillner, Markram, De Schutter, Silberberg, & LeBeau, 2005; Lund, 1991; Lund & Kolta, 2006; Pearson, 2000). Not all CPGs for motor control are confined to the internuncial central gray of the brainstem or spinal cord but are often components of distributed networks with *Grillnerian* microcircuits localized in cerebral, cerebellar, brainstem, and spinal cord loci capable of dynamic assembly and fractionation as a function of task demands (Grillner et al., 2005; Barlow, et al., 2010). This presents challenges concerning the identification of orofacial coordinative infrastructure for early nonspeech versus later appearing speech-vocalization behaviors.

A recent functional neuroimaging study specifically addressed the issue of shared neural resources during speech and suck and demonstrated highly significant overlap in the blood-oxygen level dependent (BOLD) activated networks during the production of these two oromotor behaviors (Estep, 2009; Estep, Barlow, Auer, Kieweg, & Savage, 2009). This fMRI study utilized a randomized block design with sparse volume acquisition within the context of an audiovisual motor stimulus paradigm to record neural correlates of suck and unvoiced syllabic speech performed at two rates (1 and 3 Hz) by a group of healthy adults. A functionally defined region of interest (ROI) analysis with separate spatial masks created for cerebral and subtentorial (brainstem/cerebellum) provided (1) descriptive analysis

of individual clusters and (2) quantitative analysis of the extent of activation differences between conditions. Both factors (task and rate [1 Hz or 3 Hz]) were shown significantly to affect BOLD signal changes at the cortical, subcortical, and brainstem levels. This study is the first to show that an unvoiced syllable and nonspeech (suck) ororhythmic behaviors are encoded by functionally overlapping brain areas (Estep et al., 2009). The minimal *shared* network or *infrastructure* essential to encode two-rate specific (1 Hz and 3 Hz) oromotor (suck and unvoiced [da]) tasks includes cortical (bilateral precentral gyri, insula, cingulate), subcortical (bilateral basal ganglia, left cerebellum, and thalamus), and brainstem (right dorsal pons, left medulla, and pontomedullary regions) correlates. These results further support the notion of a distributed network of brain areas participating in the ongoing production of the speech task being generated by a subset of areas that also participate in the nonspeech behavior of suck in the adult. These findings are in agreement with other functional neuroimaging studies that describe a basic speech production network activated by producing simple syllable movement sequences to extend beyond the central sulcus to include medial premotor areas, frontal operculum, anterior insula, anterior thalamus, and cerebellum.

Functional Neural Systems for Speech Motor Control

The encoding of force and movement by the brain is central to models of movement and highly relevant to our understanding of the biodynamics of speech. The relation between force control and neural firing patterns in primate motor cortex is correlated strongly with the rate and direction of force change (Evarts, 1968; Georgopolous, Ashe, Smyrnis, & Taira, 1992; Hepp-Reymond, Kirkpatrick-Tanner, Gabernet, Qi, & Weber, 1999; Hepp-Reymond, Wyss, & Anner, 1978; Humphrey, Schmidt, & Thompson, 1970; Moran & Schwartz, 1999; Smith, Hepp-Reymond, & Wyss, 1975) and preferred-torque directions (Herter et al., 2007; Kurtzer, Herter, & Scott, 2006). Primary motor cortex also has been shown to encode functional muscle synergies (Holdefer & Miller, 2002). The cortical mechanisms involved in the regulation of muscle dynamics during the early phases of force recruitment (Cheney & Fetz, 1980; Evarts, Fromm, Kroller, & Jennings, 1983; Fromm & Evarts, 1977; Sanes & Evarts, 1983) may be especially important for orofacial muscles that are characterized by small motor units, which produce finely graded forces for speech (Barlow & Bradford, 1992; Barlow, Bradford, & Andreatta, 1999; Estep & Barlow, 2007). The complex articulatory force dynamics evident among facial muscles during speech is similar in many ways to the precise movements and forces generated by hand and fingers during manipulation. During speech production, the muscles of the perioral system exhibit a streaming repertoire of phasic adjustments in force from resting tonic activation to approximately 10% of the maximum voluntary contraction level (Barlow & Muller, 1991; Muller, Milenkovic, & MacLeod, 1985).

Mounting evidence also suggests that the sensorimotor cortex may participate in the modulation of the reflexive compensatory motor responses in lip muscles during speech (Ito & Gomi, 2007; Ito, Kimura, & Gomi, 2005). The orofacial apparatus appears to utilize mechanosensory information differentially for the early versus later phases of lip force output (Estep & Barlow, 2007), similar to the forelimb (Cheney & Fetz, 1980; Fromm & Evarts, 1977). During speech articulation, longer latency reflex actions presumably involving primary motor cortex correct for the effects of external movement disturbances (Ito, Kimura, & Gomi, 2005). Mechanical inputs delivered to a dynamically contracting lip muscle produce a compound evoked perioral response characterized by phases of excitation and suppression that are absent during static force conditions (Andreatta, Barlow, & Finan, 1994). Under these conditions, compensatory lip movements demonstrate a well-calibrated readjustment (Gracco & Abbs, 1985).

Velocity is one kinematic variable that has been explored in some detail and appears to have a definable neural network. Positron emission tomography (PET) mapping of regional cerebral blood flow (rCBF) has demonstrated a velocity subcircuit that includes the bilateral sensorimotor cortex, basal ganglia (putamen and globus pallidus), and the ipsilateral cerebellum (Turner, Desmurget, Grethe, Crutcher, & Grafton, 2003; Turner, Grafton, Votaw, DeLong, & Hoffman, 1998). Increases in velocity are associated with parallel increases in BG activation. The BG motor circuit may be involved preferentially in controlling or monitoring the scale and/or dynamics of arm movements and also may control articulatory movements at lower frequencies. A dysfunctional BG circuit (i.e., Parkinson's disease, PD) may result in hypophonia (lowered speech volume) and bradykinesia (Barlow & Hammer, 2009). Functional brain imaging of patients with PD during velocity control tasks reveals a significant disruption to the BG circuitry, which may account partially for the pathophysiology of bradykinesia (Turner, Grafton, McIntosh, DeLong, & Hoffman, 2003). Unilateral lesions of the globus pallidus internal (GPi) and globus pallidus external (GPe) result in slowness of movement and abnormal cocontraction of agonist and antagonist muscles and often impair movements of the orofacial, laryngeal, and chest wall systems for speech production.

A positive relation also exists between increases in speech rate and cerebellar activation (Estep et al., 2009), suggesting this brain structure plays a significant role in sequencing syllable streams (Ackermann, 2008; Riecker et al., 2005) and regulation of the velocity of articulatory movements within the frame of time-critical adjustments (Wildgruber, Ackermann, & Grodd, 2001). Motor speech symptoms resulting from cerebellar pathology may reflect a distorted process of articulatory planning and coordination. Cerebellar posterior lobe syndrome often is associated with speech that is perceived as having an "intoxicated-like" ataxic quality (Barlow, Finan, Andreatta, & Boliek, 2008).

Movements associated with intelligible speech are associated with a certain degree of control for articulatory displacement, velocity, and syllable rate. Changes in speech rate are correlated with rescaling of timing, muscle recruitment patterns, and orofacial muscle stiffness (Ostry & Munhall, 1985). Due to inherent biomechanical limitations, orofacial articulators (and presumably other muscle-tissue systems of the vocal tract and chest wall) reorganize their coordination patterns in order to achieve adequate system output for increased speech rates. In most cases, speakers reduce their articulators' displacements and increase velocity to speak more quickly, indicating that in addition to timing reorganization for faster speech, muscle commands are reorganized to increase articulatory effort (Smith & Kleinow, 2000). In some instances, the accurate positioning of one structure (i.e., the lower lip) may be dependent upon another structure (i.e., the mandible). Kinematic studies of speech typically involve recording from multiple structures in an attempt to understand the trading relations between structures, patterns of organization, and reorganization during development, external perturbation, or following brain injury or neurological disease.

During infancy, spontaneous oral movements precede speech. These oral motor movements are accompanied and influenced by other bodily motions, in particular motion of the hands. Sensorimotor events of the hand and mouth specifically affect one another during feeding behaviors such as sucking, linguistic behaviors such as vocalization and canonical syllable production, and motor behaviors such as reaching (e.g., Bernardis, Bello, Pettenati, Stefanini, & Gentilucci, 2008; Butterworth & Hopkins, 1988; Ejiri, 1998; Fogel & Hannan, 1985; Iverson & Fagan, 2004; Locke, Bekken, McMinn-Larson, & Wein, 1995; Pedroso & Rotta, 2004; Thelen, 1981). The effect of both linguistic and nonlinguistic hand and mouth behaviors on one another persists throughout adulthood as well (e.g., Dromey & Shim, 2008; Gentilucci, 2003; Gentilucci, Stefanini,

Roy, & Santunione, 2004; Higginbotham, Isaak, & Domingue, 2008; Kühn & Brass, 2008; Ravizza, 2003) and is reflected in overlapping and influential neural control of the hand and mouth (e.g., Ferrari, Gallese, Rizzolatti, & Fogassi, 2003; Meister et al., 2003; Petrides, Cadoret, & Mackey, 2005; Rizzolatti et al., 1988). This evidence has been used to support a larger theoretical framework for a hand–mouth link in human brain and behavior (e.g., Arbib, 2008; Corballis, 2009; Gentilucci & Volta, 2008; Iverson & Thelen, 1999).

Neural Network Model of Speech Production and Frame/Content Theory

Speech production is a sensorimotor skill and heavily dependent on auditory (Larson, Altman, Liu, & Hain, 2008), somatosensory (Estep & Barlow, 2007; Gracco &Abbs, 1985; Hammer & Barlow, 2010; Ito et al., 2005; Ito & Gomi, 2007), and visual feedback (Auer, 2009; Bernstein, Auer, Wagner, & Ponton, 2008) for its development and maintenance. The search for the neural network(s) that produce speech movements and the wide range of related gestural and ingestive motor behaviors is moving ahead at a rapid pace and includes a combination of functional and anatomical studies. Meta-analyses of this database of information has led to the creation of computational models and simulations of speech and vocalization systems pertinent to test notions about early development, maintenance in the mature speech motor control system, and response to injury or progressive neuromotor disease as it relates to var-

ious forms of dysarthria. These mechanisms also are crucial to invoke mechanisms of plasticity following a sudden insult to the brain (ischemia-reperfusion or hemorrhage) or during the course of a progressive neuromotor disease (i.e., PD). Directions Into Velocities of Articulators (DIVA) is a neural network model of speech motor skill acquisition and speech production developed by Frank Guenther and colleagues (Guenther, 2006; Guenther et al., 2006). In computer simulations, the model includes both feedback and feedforward subsystems and learns to control the movements of a computer-simulated vocal tract in order to produce speech sounds. The DIVA model also generates simulated fMRI activations associated with small populations of synchronously firing neurons from the model's cell activities during computer simulation. The model's neural mappings are tuned during a babbling phase in which auditory feedback from self-generated speech sounds is used to learn the relationship between motor actions and their acoustic and somatosensory consequences. Initial attempts rely heavily on auditory feedback. This leads to the formation and strengthening of feedforward representations of speech sounds and their combinations. After learning, the model can produce arbitrary combinations of speech sounds, even in the presence of constraints on the articulators such as mandibular block. The DIVA model has evolved over the past 15 years and provides unified explanations for a number of long-studied speech production phenomena including motor equivalence, contextual variability, speaking rate effects, anticipatory coarticulation, and carryover coarticulation (Guenther,

Hampson, & Johnson, 1998; Guenther, 1995). The DIVA model posits the existence of a speech sound map (SSM) module in the left ventral premotor cortex and/or posterior inferior frontal gyrus pars opercularis that contains cell groups coding for well-learned speech sounds. The model is schematized in Figure 10–9. Each block in the diagram corresponds to a hypothesized set of neurons in the human speech system. With changes in body plan (i.e., growth of the speech articulators), the auditory feedback control system continues to

provide corrective tuning of the feedback controller over the life span. Consistent with research in other laboratories, it is clear that somatosensory information is central to achieving the precision requirements of speech movements, including consonant and vowel position targets. The neural control of stiffness appears to be a key factor to consider for the somatosensory precision involved in speech production.

The DIVA model has been extended (Bohland, Bullock, & Guenther, 2009) to include paired structure and content

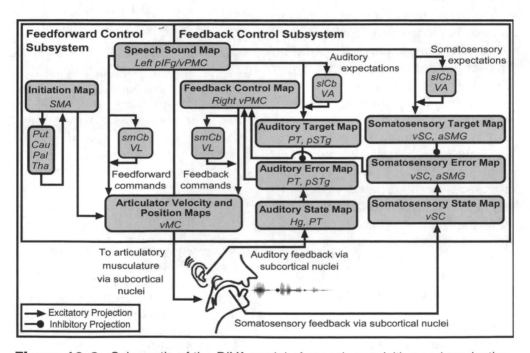

Figure 10–9. Schematic of the DIVA model of speech acquisition and production. Abbreviations: aSMg = anterior supramarginal gyrus; Cau = caudate; Pal = pallidum; Hg = Heschl's gyrus; pIFg = posterior inferior frontal gyrus; pSTg = posterior superior temporal gyrus; PT = planum temporale; Put = Putamen; sICB = superior lateral cerebellum; smCB = superior medial cerebellum; SMA = supplementary motor area; Tha = thalamus; VA = ventral anterior nucleus of the cerebellum; VL = ventral lateral nucleus of the thalamus; vMC = ventral motor cortex; vPMC = ventral premotor cortex; vSC = ventral somatosensory cortex. Reproduced with permission (Golfinopoulos, E., Tourville, J. A., Guenther, F. H. (2009). The integration of large-scale neural network modeling and functional brain imaging in speech motor control. *NeuroImage.*)

subsystems consistent with MacNeilage's frame/content theory of evolution of speech production (MacNeilage, 1998) to assess hypotheses specific to phonological and phonetic processes. This new version is termed *gradient order DIVA* (GODIVA) and provides parallel representations of a future speech plan and mechanisms for interfacing phonological planning representations with learned sensorimotor programs which enable multisyllabic speech plans. The GODIVA's components are hypothesized to be localized to the left inferior frontal sulcus, medial premotor cortex, basal ganglia, and thalamus.

The brain imaging and neurocomputational literature is proliferating rapidly concerning studies of speech production and sensorimotor control of the upper airway. The production of simple vowels and simple oral movements result in similar activation patterns among cortical and subcortical motor systems, with new focus on cerebellar and brainstem loci. More complex polysyllabic utterances are associated with additional activation of the bilateral cerebellum, presumably reflecting increased demands on speech motor control and additional activation of the bilateral temporal cortices thought to subserve phonological processing.

Acknowledgment. This work was supported in part by NIH R01 DC003311, NIH P30 HD02528, NIH P30 DC005803, and The Sutherland Foundation.

References

Abbs, J. H., Nadler, R. D., & Fujimura, O. (1988). X-ray microbeams track the shape of speech. *SOMA, 2,* 29–34.

Ackermann, H. (2008). Cerebellar contributions to speech production and speech perception: Psycholinguistic and neurobiological perspectives. *Trends in Neurosciences, 31*(6), 265–272.

Adams, S. G, Weismer, G., & Kent, R. D. (1993). Speaking rate and speech movement velocity profiles. *Journal of Speech and Hearing Research, 36,* 41–54.

Andreatta, R. D., Barlow, S. M., & Finan, D. S. (1994). Modulation of the mechanically evoked perioral reflex during active force dynamics in young adults. *Brain Research, 646,* 175–179.

Arbib, M. A. (2008). From grasp to language: Embodied concepts and the challenge of abstraction. *Journal of Physiology, 102,* 4–20.

Atkeson, C. G., & Hollerbach, J. M. (1985). Kinematic features of unrestrained vertical arm movements. *Journal of Neuroscience, 5*(9), 2318–2330.

Auer, E. T., Jr. (2009). Spoken word recognition by eye. *Scandinavian Journal of Psychology, 50*(5), 419–425.

Barlow, S. M., & Bradford, P. T. (1992). Measurement and implications of orofacial muscle performance in speech disorders. *Journal of Human Muscle Performance, 1,* 1–31.

Barlow, S. M., Bradford, P. T., & Andreatta, R. D. (1999). Orofacial force physiology. In S. M. Barlow (Ed.), *Handbook of clinical speech physiology* (pp. 303–346). San Diego, CA: Singular.

Barlow, S. M., & Estep, M. (2006). Central pattern generation and the motor infrastructure for suck, respiration, and speech. *Journal of Communication Disorders, 39,* 366–380.

Barlow, S. M., Farley, G. R., & Andreatta, R. D. (1999). Neural systems in speech physiology. In S. M. Barlow (Ed.), *Handbook of clinical speech physiology* (pp. 101–164). San Diego, CA: Singular.

Barlow, S. M., Finan, D. S., Andreatta, R. D., & Boliek, C. (2008). Kinematic measurement of speech and early orofacial movements. In M. McNeil (Ed.), *Clinical management of sensorimotor speech disor-*

ders (pp. 80–99). New York. NY: Thieme Medical.

Barlow, S. M., Finan, D. S., Chu, S., & Lee, J. (2008). Patterns for the premature brain: Synthetic orocutaneous stimulation entrains preterm infants with feeding difficulties to suck. *Journal Perinatology, 28,* 541–548.

Barlow, S. M., & Hammer, M. (2009). Pallidotomy and deep brain stimulation in Parkinson's disease: Effects on speech and voice. In M. McNeil (Ed.), *Clinical management of sensorimotor speech disorders* (pp. 362–364). New York, NY: Thieme Medical.

Barlow, S. M., Lund, J. P., Estep, M., & Kolta, A. (2010). Central pattern generators for orofacial movements and speech. In S. M. Brudzynski (Ed.), *Handbook of mammalian vocalization. An integrative neuroscience approach,* (pp. 351–370). Oxford, UK: Academic Press.

Barlow, S. M., & Muller, E. M. (1991). The relation between interangle span and in vivo resultant force in the perioral musculature. *Journal of Speech and Hearing Research, 34,* 252–259.

Bartle-Meyer, C. J., Goozeé, J. V., & Murdoch, B. E. (2009). Kinematic investigation of lingual movement in words of increasing length in acquired apraxia of speech. *Clinical Linguistics & Phonetics, 23*(2), 93–121.

Baum, S. R. (1999). Compensation for jaw fixation by aphasic patients under conditions of increased articulatory demands: A follow-up study. *Aphasiology, 13,* 513–527.

Baum, S. R., McFarland, D. H., & Diab, M. (1996). Compensation to articulatory perturbation: Perceptual data. *The Journal of the Acoustical Society of America, 99,* 3791–3794.

Bell-Berti, F., & Hirose, H. (1975). Palatal activity in voicing distinctions: A simultaneous fiberoptic and electromyographic study. *Journal of Phonetics, 3,* 69–74.

Bernardis, P., Bello, A., Pettenati, P., Stefanini, S., & Gentilucci, M. (2008). Manual actions affect vocalizations in infants. *Experimental Brain Research, 184,* 599–603.

Bernstein, L. E., Auer, E. T., Jr., Wagner, M., & Ponton, C. W. (2008). Spatio-temporal dynamics of audiovisual speech processing. *Neuroimage, 39*(1), 423–35.

Bloomer, H. (1953). Observations on palatopharyngeal movements in speech and deglutition. *Journal of Speech and Hearing Disorders, 19,* 230–246.

Bohland, J. W., Bullock, D., & Guenther, F. H. (2010). Neural representations and mechanisms for the performance of simple speech sequences. *Journal of Cognitive Neuroscience, 22*(7), 1504–1529.

Butterworth, G., & Hopkins, B. (1988). Hand-mouth coordination in the newborn baby. *British Journal of Developmental Psychology, 6,* 303–314.

Calnan, J. S. (1953). Movements of the soft palate. *British Journal of Plastic Surgery, 5,* 286–296.

Chen, H. Y., Murdoch, B. E., Goozée, J. V., & Scott, D. (2007). Physiologic development of tongue–jaw coordination from childhood to adulthood. *Journal of Speech, Language, and Hearing Research, 50,* 352–360.

Cheney, P. D., & Fetz, E. E. (1980). Functional classes of primate corticomotoneuronal cells and their relation to active force. *Journal of Neurophysiology, 44,* 773–791.

Cheng, H. Y., Murdoch, B. E., & Goozée, J. V. (2007). Temporal features of articulation from childhood to adolescence: An electropalatographic investigation. *Clinical Linguistics & Phonetics, 21*(6), 481–499.

Chiba, T., & Kajiyama, M. (1958). *The vowel, its nature and structure.* Tokyo: Chiyoda Press.

Chu, S., & Barlow, S. M. (2009). Orofacial biomechanics and speech motor control. *Perspectives in Speech Science and Orofacial Disorders—SID 5, 19*(1), 37–43.

Chu, S.-Y., Barlow, S. M., Kieweg, D., & Lee, J. (2010). OroSTIFF: Face-referenced measurement of perioral stiffness in health and disease. *Journal Biomechanics, 43,* 1476–1482.

Chu, S., Barlow, S. M., & Lee, J. (2009). Non-participatory stiffness in the male perioral complex. *Journal of Speech, Language, and Hearing Research, 52*(5), 1353–1359.

Cleland, J., Timmins, C., Wood, S. E., Hardcastle, W. J., & Wishart, J. G. (2009). Electropalatographic therapy for children and young people with Down's syndrome. *Clinical Linguistics & Phonetics, 23*(12), 926–939.

Corballis, M. C. (2010). Mirror neurons and the evolution of language. *Brain and Language, 112*(1), 25–35.

Dalston, R. M. (1989). Using simultaneous photodetection and nasometry to monitor velopharyngeal behavior during speech. *Journal of Speech and Hearing Research, 32,* 195–202.

Dalston, R. M., Warren, D. W., & Smith, L. R. (1990). The aerodynamic characteristics of speech produced by normal speakers and cleft palate speakers with adequate velopharyngeal function. *Cleft Palate Journal, 27*(4), 393–399.

Dick, D., Ozturk, C., Douglas, A., McVeigh, E., & Stone, M. (2000, April). *Three-Dimensional Tracking of Tongue Motion using Tagged MRI.* Poster session presented at the meeting of the International Society for Magnetic Resonance in Medicine, Denver, CO.

Dromey, C., & Bates, E. (2005). Speech interactions with linguistic, cognitive, and visuomotor tasks. *Journal of Speech, Language, and Hearing Research, 48*(2), 295–305.

Dromey, C., & Shim, E. (2008). The effects of divided attention on speech motor, verbal fluency, and manual task performance. *Journal of Speech, Language, and Hearing Research, 51,* 1171–1182.

Dwyer, C. H., Robb, M. P., O'Beirne, G. A., & Gilbert, H. R. (2009). The influence of speaking rate on nasality in the speech of hearing impaired individuals. *Journal of Speech, Language, and Hearing Research, 52,* 1321–1333.

Ejiri, K. (1998) Relationship between rhythmic behavior and canonical babbling in infant vocal development. *Phonetica, 55,* 226–237.

Epstein, M. A., & Stone, M. (2005). The tongue stops here: Ultrasound imaging of the palate. *Journal of the Acoustical Society of America, 118*(4), 2128–2131.

Estep, M. (2009). *Cortical and subcortical correlates of ororhythmic behaviors.* Unpublished doctoral dissertation, University of Kansas, Lawrence.

Estep, M., & Barlow S. M. (2007). Modulation of the trigeminofacial pathway during speech. *Brain Research, 1171,* 67–74.

Estep, M. E., Barlow, S. M., Auer, E. T., Kieweg, D., & Savage, C. R. (2009). November). *Task and Rate Specific Functional Correlates of Human Ororhythmic Behaviors.* Poster session presented at the annual meeting of the Society for Neuroscience, Chicago, IL.

Evarts, E. V. (1968). Relation of pyramidal tract activity to force exerted during voluntary movement. *Journal of Neurophysiology, 31,* 14–27.

Evarts, E. V., Fromm, C., Kroller, J., & Jennings, V. A. (1983). Motor cortex control of finely graded forces. *Journal of Neurophysiology, 49,* 1199–1215.

Feldman, A. G., & Levin, M. F. (2009). The equilibrium-point hypothesis- past, present, and future. In D. Sternad, (Ed.), *Progress in motor control* (pp. 699–726). New York, NY: Springer Science.

Ferrari, P. F., Gallese, V., Rizzolatti, G., & Fogassi, L. (2003). Mirror neurons responding to the observation of ingestive and communicative mouth actions in the monkey ventral premotor cortex. *European Journal of Neuroscience, 17,* 1703–1714.

Finkelstein, Y., Talmi, Y. P., Nachmani, A., Hauben, D. J., & Zohar, Y. (1992). On the variability of velopharyngeal valve anatomy and function: A combined perioral and nasendoscopic study. *Plastic and Reconstructive Surgery, 89*(4), 631–639.

Flege, J. E., Fletcher, S. G., & Homiedan, A. (1988). Compensating for a bite block in /s/ and /t/ production: Palatographic, acoustic, and perceptual data. *The Jour-*

nal of the Acoustical Society of America, 83, 212–228.

Fletcher, S. G. (1989). Palatometric specification of stop, affricate, and sibilant sounds. *Journal of Speech and Hearing Research, 32,* 736–748.

Fletcher, S. G., Dagenais, P. A., & Critz-Crosby, P. (1991). Teaching vowels to profoundly hearing-impaired speakers using glossometry. *Journal of Speech and Hearing Research, 34,* 943–956.

Fletcher, S. G., Hasegawa, A., McCutcheon, M. J., & Gilliom, J. (1980). Use of linguapalatal contact patterns to modify articulation in a deaf adult. In D. L. McPherson (Ed.), *Advances in prosthetic devices for the deaf: A technical workshop.* Rochester, NY: National Technical Institute for the Deaf.

Fletcher, S. G., McCutcheon, M. J., & Wolf, M. B. (1975). Dynamic palatometry. *Journal of Speech and Hearing Research, 18,* 812–819.

Fogel, A., & Hannan, T. E. (1985). Manual actions of nine- to fifteen-week-old human infants during face-to-face interaction with their mothers. *Child Development, 56,* 1271–1279.

Fromm, C., & Evarts, E. V. (1977). Relation of motor cortex neurons to precisely controlled and ballistic movements. *Neuroscience Letters, 5,* 259–265.

Fujimura, O., Kiritani, S., & Ishida, H. (1973). Computer controlled radiography for observation of articulatory and other human organs. *Computers in Biology and Medicine, 3,* 371–384.

Gentilucci, M. (2003). Grasp observation influences speech production. *European Journal of Neuroscience, 17,* 179–184.

Gentilucci, M., Stefanini, S., Roy, A. C., & Santunione, P. (2004). Action observation and speech production: Study on children and adults. *Neuropsychologia, 42,* 1554–1567.

Gentilucci, M., & Volta, R. D. (2008). Spoken language and arm gestures are controlled by the same motor control system. *Quarterly Journal of Experimental Psychology, 61*(6), 944–957.

Georgopoulos, A. P., Ashe, J., Smyrnis, N., & Taira, M. (1992). The motor cortex and the coding of force. *Science, 256,* 1692–1695.

Georgopoulos, A. P., Kalaska, J. F., & Massey, J. T. (1981). Spatial trajectories and reaction times of aimed movements: Effects of practice, uncertainty, and change in target location. *Journal of Neurophysiology, 46*(4), 725–743.

Gibbon, F., & Nicolaidis, K. (1999). Palatography. In W. J. Hardcastle, & N. Hewlett (Eds), *Coarticulation in speech production: Theory, data and techniques* (pp. 229–245). Cambridge, UK: Cambridge University Press.

Gick B. (2002). The use of ultrasound for linguistic phonetic fieldwork. *Journal of the International Phonetics Association, 32,* 113–122.

Goffman, L., Gerken, L., & Lucchesi, J. (2007). Relations between segmental and motor variability in prosodically complex nonword sequences. *Journal of Speech, Language, and Hearing Research, 50*(2), 444–458.

Golfinopoulos, E., Tourville, J. A., and Guenther, F. H. (2010). The integration of large-scale neural network modeling and functional brain imaging in speech motor control. *NeuroImage, 52*(3), 862–874.

Gomi, H., Honda, M., Ito, T., & Murano, E. Z. (2002). Compensatory articulation during bilabial fricative production by regulating muscle stiffness. *Journal of Phonetics, 30,* 261–279.

Gracco, V. L. (1994). Some organizational characteristics of speech movement control. *Journal of Speech, Language, and Hearing Research, 37,* 4–27.

Gracco, V. L., & Abbs, J. H. (1985). Dynamic control of the perioral system during speech: kinematic analyses of autogenic and nonautogenic sensorimotor processes. *Journal of Neurophysiology, 54,* 418–432.

Green, J. R., Moore, C. A., Higashikawa, M., & Steeve, R. W. (2000). The physiologic development of speech motor control: Lip and jaw coordination. *Journal of*

Speech, Language, and Hearing Research, 43, 239–255.

Green, J. R., Moore, C. A., & Reilly, K. J. (2002). The sequential development of jaw and lip control for speech. *Journal of Speech, Language, and Hearing Research, 45*, 66–79.

Green, J. R., Moore, C. A., Ruark, J. L., Rodda, P. R., Morvée, W. T., & VanWitzenburg, M. J. (1997). Development of chewing in children from 12 to 48 months: Longitudinal study of EMG patterns. *Journal of Neurophysiology, 77*, 2704–2727.

Green, J. R., & Wang, Y. (2003). Tongue-surface movement patterns during speech and swallowing. *Journal of Acoustical Society of America, 113*, 2820–2833.

Green, J. R., & Wilson, E. M. (2006). Spontaneous facial motility in infancy: A 3D kinematic analysis. *Developmental Psychobiology, 48*(1), 16–28.

Grillner, S. (2003). The motor infrastructure: From ion channels to neuronal networks. *Nature Reviews Neuroscience, 4*, 573–586.

Grillner, S., Markram, H., De Schutter, E., Silberberg, G., & LeBeau, F.E.N. (2005). Microcircuits in action—from CPGs to neocortex. *Trends in Neurosciences, 28*(10), 525–533.

Guenther, F. H. (1994). A neural network model of speech acquisition and motor equivalent speech production. *Biological Cybernetics, 72*, 43–53.

Guenther, F. H. (1995). Speech sound acquisition, coarticulation, and rate effects in a neural network model of speech production. *Psychological Review, 102*, 594–621.

Guenther, F. H. (2006). Cortical interactions underlying the production of speech sounds. *Journal of Communication Disorders, 39*(5), 350–365.

Guenther, F. H., Ghosh, S. S., & Tourville, J. A. (2006). Neural modeling and imaging of the cortical interactions underlying syllable production. *Brain and Language, 96*, 280–301.

Guenther, F. H., Hampson, M., & Johnson, D. (1998). A theoretical investigation of reference frames for the planning of speech movements. *Psychological Review, 105*, 611–633.

Hammer, M. J., & Barlow, S. M. (2010). Laryngeal somatosensory deficits in Parkinson's disease: Implications for speech respiratory and phonatory control. *Experimental Brain Research, 201*(3), 401–409.

Hammer, M. J., Barlow, S. M., Lyons, K. E., & Pahwa, R. (2010). Subthalamic nucleus deep brain stimulation changes speech respiratory and laryngeal control in Parkinson's disease.*Journal of Neurology.* PMID: 20708741

Hardcastle, W. J., Gibbon, F. E., & Jones, W. (1991). Visual display of tongue-palate contact: Electropalatography in the assessment and remediation of speech disorders. *The British Journal of Disorders of Communication, 26*(1), 41–74.

Hardcastle, W., Jones, W., Knight, C., Trudgeon, A., & Calder, G. (1989). New developments in electropalatography state-of-the-art report. *Clinical Linguistics & Phonetics, 3*, 1–38.

Harley, W. T. (1972). Dynamic palatography—A study of linguapalatal contacts during the production of selected consonant sounds. *Journal of Prosthodontic Dentistry, 27*, 364–376.

Hebb, D. O. (1949). *The organization of behavior: A neuropsychological theory.* New York, NY: Wiley.

Hepp-Reymond, M. C., Kirkpatrick-Tanner, M., Gabernet, L., Qi, H. X., & Weber, B. (1999). Context-dependent force coding in motor and premotor cortical areas. *Experimental Brain Research, 128*, 123–133.

Hepp-Reymond, M. C., Wyss, U. R., & Anner, R. (1978). Neuronal coding of static force in the primate motor cortex. *Journal of Physiology (Paris), 74*, 287–291.

Herter, T. M., Kurtzer, I., Cabel, D. W., Haunts, K. A., & Scott, S. H. (2007). Characterization of torque-related activity in primary motor cortex during a multijoint postural task. *Journal of Neurophysiology, 97*(4), 2887–2899.

Hertrich, I., & Ackermann, H. (2000). Lip-jaw and tongue-jaw coordination during rate-controlled syllable repetitions. *The Journal of the Acoustical Society of America, 107,* 2236–2247.

Higginbotham, D. R., Isaak, M. I., & Domingue, J. N. (2008). The exaptation of manual dexterity for articulate speech: an electromyogram investigation. *Experimental Brain Research, 186,* 603–609.

Hixon, T. J. (1971). An electromagnetic method for transducing jaw movements during speech. *Journal of the Acoustical Society of America, 49,* 603–606.

Holdefer, R. N., & Miller, L. E. (2002). Primary motor cortical neurons encode functional muscle synergies. *Experimental Brain Research, 146,* 233–243.

House, R. A. (1967). *A study of tongue body motion during selected speech sounds.* Unpublished doctoral dissertation, University of Michigan, Ann Arbor.

House, A. S., & Fairbanks, G. (1953). The influence of consonant environment upon the secondary acoustical characteristics of vowels. *Journal of the Acoustical Society of America, 25,* 105–113.

Humphrey, D. R., & Reed, D. J. (1983). Separate cortical systems for control of joint movement and joint stiffness: reciprocal activation and coactivation of antagonist muscles. In J. E. Desmedt (Ed.), *Motor control mechanisms in health and disease* (pp. 347–372). New York, NY: Raven Press.

Humphrey, D. R., Schmidt, E. M., & Thompson, W. D. (1970). Predicting measures of motor performance from multiple cortical spike trains. *Science, 179,* 758–762.

Ito, T., & Gomi, H. (2007). Cutaneous mechanoreceptors contribute to the generation of a cortical reflex in speech. *NeuroReport, 18(9),* 907–910.

Ito, T., Gomi, H., & Honda, M. (2004). Dynamical simulation of speech cooperative articulation by muscle linkages. *Biological Cybernetics, 91,* 275–282.

Ito, T., Kimura, T., & Gomi, H. (2005). The motor cortex is involved in reflexive compensatory adjustment of speech articulation. *NeuroReport, 16,* 1791–1794.

Iverson, J. M., & Fagan, M. K. (2004). Infant vocal-motor coordination: Precursor to the gesture-speech system? *Child Development, 74(4),* 1053–1066.

Iverson, J. M., & Thelen, E. (1999). Hand, mouth, and brain. *Journal of Consciousness Studies, 6(11–12),* 19–40.

Jacks, A. (2008). Bite block vowel production in apraxia of speech. *Journal of Speech, Language, and Hearing Research, 51,* 898–913.

Johnson, K. (1969). Mapping the movements of the human tongue. *The Atom, 6,* 12–16.

Keefe, M. J., & Dalston, R. M. (1989). An analysis of velopharyngeal timing in normal adult speakers using a microcomputer based photodetector system. *Journal of Speech and Hearing Research, 32,* 39–48.

Kent, R. D. (1999). Motor control: Neurophysiology and functional development. In A. Caruso & E. Strand (Eds.), *Clinical management of motor speech disorders in children.* New York, NY: Thieme Medical.

Kent, R. D., & Voperian, H. K. (1995). Development of the craniofacial-oral-laryngeal anatomy: A review. *Journal of Medical Speech-Language Pathology, 3(3),* 145–190.

Kiritani, S., Itoh, K., & Fujimura, O. (1975). Tongue-pellet tracking by a computer-controlled X-ray microbeam system. *Journal of the Acoustical Society of America, 57(6),* 1516–1520.

Kiritani, S., Itoh, K., Fujisaki, H., & Sawashima, M. (1976). Tongue pellet movement for the Japanese CV syllables— Observations using the X-ray microbeam system. *Annual Bulletin of the Research Institute of Logopedics and Phoniatrics (Univ of Tokyo), 10,* 19–27.

Kleinow, J., & Smith, A. (2006). Potential interactions among linguistic, autonomic, and motor factors in speech. *Developmental Psychobiology, 48(4),* 275–287.

Kuehn, D. P. (1976a). A cineradiographic investigation of velar movement variables in two normals. *Cleft Palate Journal, 13,* 88–103.

Kuehn, D. P. (1976b). A cineradiographic study of VC and CV articulatory velocities. *Journal of Phonetics, 4,* 303–320.

Kuehn, D. P., & Perry, J. L. (2009). Anatomy and physiology of the velopharynx. In J. L. Losee & R. E. Kirschner (Eds.), *Comprehensive cleft care.* New York, NY: McGraw-Hill Medical.

Kühn, S., & Brass, M. (2008). Testing the connection of the mirror system and speech: How articulation affects imitation in a simple response task. *Neuropsychologia, 46*(5), 1513–1521.

Kurtzer, I., Herter, T. M., & Scott, S. H. (2006). Nonuniform distribution of reach-related and torque-related activity in upper arm muscles and neurons of primary motor cortex. *Journal of Neurophysiology, 96,* 3220–3230.

Kuruvilla, M. S., Murdoch, B. E., & Goozée, J. V. (2008). Electropalatographic (EPG) assessment of tongue-to-palate contacts in dysarthric speakers following TBI. *Clinical Linguistics & Phonetics, 22*(9), 703–725.

Kuzmin, Y. I. (1962). Mobile palatography as a tool for acoustic study of speech sounds. *Report of Fourth International Congress on Acoustics,* Copenhagen, G35.

Kydd, W., & Belt, D. A. (1964). Continuous palatography. *Journal of Speech and Hearing Disorders, 29,* 489–492.

Larson, C. R., Altman, K. W., Liu, H., & Hain, T. C. (2008). Interactions between auditory and somatosensory feedback for voice F0 control. *Experimental Brain Research, 187*(4), 613–21.

Lindblom, B., Lubker, J., & Gay, T. (1979). Formant frequencies of some fixed-mandible vowels and a model of speech motor programming by predictive simulation. *Journal of Phonetics, 7,* 147–161.

Lindblom, B. E. F., & Sundberg, J. (1971). *Neurophysiological representation of speech sounds.* Paper presented at the 15th World Congress of Logopedics and Phoniatrics, Buenos Aires, Argentina.

Locke, J. L., Bekken, K. E., & McMinn-Larson, L., Wein, D. (1995). Emergent control of manual and vocal-motor activity in relation to the development of speech. *Brain and Language, 51,* 498–508.

Löfqvist, A. (2005). Lip kinematics in long and short stop and fricative consonants. *Journal of the Acoustical Society of America, 117,* 858–878.

Löfqvist, A., & Gracco, V. L. (1997). Lip and jaw kinematics in bilabial stop consonant production. *Journal of Speech, Language, and Hearing Research, 40,* 877–893.

Lund, J. P. (1991). Mastication and its control by the brain stem. *Critical Reviews of Oral Biology and Medicine, 2*(1), 33–64.

Lund, J. P., & Kolta, A. (2006). Generation of the central masticatory pattern and its modification by sensory feedback. *Dysphagia, 21*(3), 167–174.

Lundberg, A. & Stone, M. (1999). Three-dimensional tongue surface reconstruction: Practical considerations for ultrasound data. *Journal of the Acoustical Society of America, 106,* 2858–2867.

MacNeilage, P. F. (1998). The frame/content theory of evolution of speech production. *Behavioral and Brain Sciences, 21,* 499–546.

MacNeilage, P. F., Davis, B. L., Kinney, A., & Matyear, C. L. (2000). The motor core of speech: A comparison of serial organization patterns in infants and languages. *Child Development, 71,* 153–163.

Maner, K. J., Smith, A., & Grayson, L. (2000). Influences of utterance length and complexity on speech motor performance in children and adults. *Journal of Speech, Language, and Hearing Research, 43,* 560–573.

McAuliffe, M. J., Ward, E. C., & Murdoch, B. E. (2006). Speech production in Parkinson's disease: II. Acoustic and electropalatographic investigation of sentence, word and segment durations. *Clinical Linguistics & Phonetics, 20*(1), 19–33.

McFarland, D. H., & Baum, S. R. (1995). Incomplete compensation to articulatory perturbation. *The Journal of the Acoustical Society of America, 97,* 1865–1873.

Meier, R. P., McGarvin, L., Zakia, R. A. E., & Willerman, R. (1997). Silent mandibular oscillations in vocal babbling. *Phonetica, 54,* 153–171.

Meister, I. G., Boroojerdi, B., Foltys, H., Sparing, R., Huber, W., & Töpper, R. (2003). Motor cortex hand area and speech: Implications for the development of language. *Neuropsychologia, 41*(4), 401–406.

Michi, K.-I., Suzuki, N., Yamashita, Y., & Imai, S. (1986). Visual training and correction of articulation disorders by use of dynamic palatography: Serial observation in a case of cleft palate. *Journal of Speech and Hearing Disorders, 51,* 226–238.

Moll, K. L. (1962). Velopharyngeal closure on vowels. *Journal of Speech and Hearing Research, 5,* 30–37.

Moll, K. L., & Daniloff, R. G. (1971). Investigation of the timing of velar movements during speech. *Journal of the Acoustical Society of America, 50,* 673–684.

Moon, J., & Kuehn, D. (2004). Anatomy and physiology of normal and abnormal velopharyngeal function for speech. In K. Bzoch (Ed.), *Communicative disorders related to cleft lip and palate* (5th ed.). Austin, TX: Pro-Ed.

Moon, J. B., & Lagu, R. K. (1987). Development of a second-generation phototransducer for the assessment of velopharyngeal activity. *Cleft Palate Journal, 24*(3), 240–243.

Moore, C. A., & Ruark, J. L. (1996). Does speech emerge from earlier appearing motor behaviors? *Journal of Speech and Hearing Research, 39,* 1034–1047.

Moran, D. W., & Schwartz, A. B. (1999). Motor cortical representation of speed and direction during reaching. *Journal of Neurophysiology, 82,* 2676–2692.

Morgan, A. T., Liegeois, F., & Occomore, L. (2007). Electropalatography treatment for articulation impairment in children with dysarthria post-traumatic brain injury. *Brain Injury, 21*(11), 1183–1193.

Muller, E. M., Milenkovic, P. H., & MacLeod, G. E. (1985). Perioral tissue mechanics during speech production. In C. DeLisi & J. Eisenfeld (Eds.), *Proceedings of the Second IMAC International Symposium on Biomedical Systems Modeling* (pp. 363–371). Amsterdam, Netherlands: North-Holland Publishers.

Murdoch, B. E., Goozée, J. V., Veidt, M., Scott, D. H., & Meyers, I. A. (2004). Introducing the pressure-sensing palatograph—The next frontier in electropalatography. *Clinical Linguistics & Phonetics, 18*(6–8), 433–445.

Nasir, S. M., & Ostry, D. J. (2006). Somatosensory precision in speech production. *Current Biology, 16,* 1918–1923.

Nip, I. S. B., Green, J. R., & Marx, D. B. (2009). Early speech motor development: Cognitive and linguistic considerations. *Journal of Communication Disorders, 42,* 286–298.

Nittrouer, S. (1993). The emergence of mature gestural patterns is not uniform: Evidence from an acoustic study. *Journal of Speech and Hearing Research, 36*(5), 959–972.

Ostry, D. J., & Munhall, K. G. (1985). Control of rate and duration of speech movements. *Journal of the Acoustical Society of America, 77*(2), 640–648.

Palmer, J. M. (1973). Dynamic palatography—General implications of locus and sequencing patterns. *Phonetica, 28,* 76–85.

Pearson, K. G. (2000). Neural adaptation in the generation of rhythmic behavior. *Annual Review Physiology, 62,* 723–753.

Pedroso, F. S., & Rotta, N. T. (2004). Babkin reflex and other motor responses to appendicular compression stimulus of the newborn. *Journal of Child Neurology, 19*(8), 592–596.

Peng, C. L., Jost-Brinkmann, P. G., Miethke, R. R., & Lin, C. T. (2000). Ultrasonographic measurement of tongue movement during swallowing. *Journal of Ultrasound Medicine, 19,* 15–20.

Perkell, J. S. (1969). Physiology of Speech Production: Results and Implications of a Quantitative Cineradiographic Analysis. *Research Monograph No. 53.* Cambridge, MA: MIT Press.

Perkell, J. S., Cohen, M. H., Svirsky, M. A., Matthies, M. L., Garabieta, I., & Jackson, M. T. T. (1992). Electromagnetic midsagittal articulometer systems for transducing speech articulatory movements. *Journal of the Acoustical Society of America, 92*, 3078–3096.

Perry, J. L., & Kuehn, D. P. (2009). Magnetic resonance imaging and computer reconstruction of the velopharyngeal mechanism. *Journal of Craniofacial Surgery, 20*, 1739–1749.

Petrides, M., Cadoret, G., & Mackey, S. (2005). Orofacial somatomotor responses in the macaque monkey homologue of Broca's area. *Nature, 435*(7046), 1235–1238.

Poore, M., Barlow, S. M., Wang, J., Estep, M.E., & Lee, J. (2008). Respiratory treatment history predicts suck pattern stability in preterm infants. *Journal of Neonatal Nursing, 14*, 185–192.

Poore, M., Zimmerman, E., Barlow, S. M., Wang, J., & Gu, F. (2008). NTrainer therapy increases suck spatiotemporal stability in preterm infants. *Acta Paediatrica, 97*(7), 920–927.

Potter, R. K., Kopp, G. A, & Green, H. C. (1947). *Visible speech*. New York, NY: Van Nostrand.

Ravizza, S. (2003). Movement and lexical access: Do noniconic gestures aid in retrieval? *Psychonomic Bulletin & Review, 10*(3), 610–615.

Riecker, A., Mathiak, K., Wildgruber, D., Erb, M., Hertrich, I., Grodd, W., & Ackermann, H. (2005). fMRI reveal two distinct cerebral networks subserving speech motor control. *Neurology, 64*, 700–706.

Rizzolatti, G., Camarda, R., Fogassi, L., Gentilucci, M., Luppino, G., & Matelli, M. (1988). Functional organization of inferior area 6 in the macaque monkey. II. Area F5 and the control of distal movements. *Experimental Brain Research, 71*, 491–507.

Samlan, R., & Barlow, S. M. (1999). The effects of transition rate and vowel height on velopharyngeal airway resistance. In S. M. Barlow (Ed.), *Handbook of clinical speech physiology* (pp. 247–264). San Diego, CA: Singular.

Sanes, J., & Evarts, E. V. (1983). Regulatory role of proprioceptive input in motor control of phasic or maintained voluntary contractions in man. In J. Desmedt (Ed.), *Motor control mechanisms in health and disease* (pp. 47–59). New York, NY: Raven Press.

Sanguineti, V., Laboissière, R. G., & Ostry, D. J. (1998). A dynamic biomechanical model for neural control of speech production. *Journal of Acoustical Society America, 103*, 1615–1627.

Shadmehr, R. (1993). Control of equilibrium position and stiffness through postural modules. *Journal of Motor Behavior, 25*, 228–241.

Shaiman, S., & Gracco, V. L. (2002). Task-specific sensorimotor interactions in speech production. *Experimental Brain Research, 146*, 411–418.

Shawker, T. H., Sonies, B., Stone, M., & Baum, B. J. (1983). Real-time ultrasound visualization of tongue movement during swallowing. *Journal of Clinical Ultrasound, 11*, 485–490.

Shibata, S. (1968). A study of dynamic palatography. *Annual Bulletin of the Research Institute of Logopedics and Phoniatrics (Univ of Tokyo), 2*, 28–36.

Shiller, D. M., Laboissière, R. G., & Ostry, D. J. (2002). Relationship between jaw stiffness and kinematic variability in speech. *Journal of Neurophysiology, 88*, 2329–2340.

Siegel-Sadewitz, V. L., Shprintzen, R. J. (1986). Changes in velopharyngeal valving with age. *International Journal of Pediatric Otorhinolaryngology, 11*(2), 171–182.

Smith, A. (1992). The control of orofacial movements in speech. *Critical Reviews in Oral Biology Medicine, 3*(3), 233–267.

Smith, A. (2006). Speech motor development: Integrating muscles, movements, and linguistic units. *Journal of Communication Disorders, 39*(5), 331–349.

Smith, A., & Kleinow, J. (2000). Kinematic correlates of speaking rate changes in stuttering and normally fluent adults.

Journal of Speech, Language, and Hearing Research, 43(2), 521–536.

Smith, A., Goffman, L., & Stark, R. E. (1995). Speech motor development. *Seminars in Speech and Language, 16*(2), 87–98.

Smith, A. M., Hepp-Reymond, M.-C., & Wyss, U. R. (1975). Relation of activity in precentral cortical neurons to force and rate of force change during isometric contractions of finger muscles. *Experimental Brain Research, 23,* 315–332.

Smith, A., Johnson, M., McGillem, C., & Goffman, L. (2000). On the assessment of stability and patterning of speech movements. *Journal Speech, Language, Hearing Research, 43,* 277–286.

Smith, A., & Zelaznik, H. N. (2004). Development of functional synergies for speech motor coordination in childhood and adolescence. *Developmental Psychobiology, 45*(1), 22–33.

Smitheran, J., & Hixon, T. J. (1981). Clinical method for estimating laryngeal airway resistance during vowel production. *Journal of Speech and Hearing Disorders, 46,* 138–146.

Sonoda, Y. (1974). Observation of tongue movements employing magnetometer sensor. *IEEE Transactions on Magnets, 10*(3), 954–957.

Steele, C. M., & Van Lieshout, P. H. H. M. (2004). The use of electromagnetic midsagittal articulography in the study of swallowing. *Journal of Speech, Language, and Hearing Research, 47,* 342–352.

Steeve, R. W., & Moore, C. A. (2009). Mandibular motor control during the early development of speech and nonspeech behaviors. *Journal of Speech, Language, and Hearing Research, 51*(6), 1530–1554.

Steeve, R. W., Moore, C. A., Green, J. R., Reilly, K., & McMurtrey, J. (2008). Babbling, chewing, and sucking: Oromandibular coordination at 9 months. *Journal of Speech, Language, and Hearing Research, 51*(6), 1390–1404.

Stone, M. (2005). A guide to analyzing tongue motion from ultrasound images. *Clinical Linguistics & Phonetics, 19*(6/7), 455–501.

Stone, M., Dick, D., Davis, E., Douglas, A., & Ozturk, C. (2000, May). *Modeling the Internal Tongue Using Principal Strains.* Paper presented at the Proceedings of the Fifth Speech Production Seminar, Kloster-Seeon, Germany.

Stone, M., Epstein, M. A., & Iskarous, K. (2004). Functional segments in tongue movement. *Clinical Linguistics & Phonetics, 18,* 507–522.

Stone, M., Epstein, M. A., Kambhamettu, C., & Li, M. (2006). Predicting 3D tongue shapes from midsagittal contours. In J. Harrington, and M. Tabain, (Eds.), *Speech production: Models, phonetic processes, and techniques* (pp. 315–330). Sussex, UK: Psychology Press.

Stone, M., Epstein, M. A., & Sutton, M. W. (2003, December) *Predicting 3D tongue shapes from midsagittal contours.* Poster presented at the Proceedings of the 6th International Seminar on Speech Production, Sydney, Australia.

Stone, M., & Lundberg, A. (1996). Three-dimensional tongue surface shapes of English consonants and vowels. *Journal of the Acoustical Society of America, 99*(6), 3728–3737.

Stone, M., Shawker, T., Talbot, L., & Rich, A. (1988). Cross-sectional tongue shape during the production of vowels. *Journal of the Acoustic Society of America, 83*(4), 1586–1596.

Sussman, H., Marquardt, T., Hutchinson, J., & MacNeilage, P. (1986). Compensatory articulation in Broca's aphasia. *Brain and Language, 27,* 56–74.

Sze, C.-F., Iny, D., Stone, M., & Levine, W. (1999). Reconstructing three-dimensional tongue motion from ultrasound images. *Proceedings of the Conference of the International Federation for Automatic Control, Beijing, China, 1,* 97–102.

Thelen, E. (1981). Kicking, rocking, and waving: Contextual analysis of rhythmical stereotypies in normal human infants. *Animal Behavior, 29,* 3–11.

Thelen, E. (1991). Motor aspects of emergent speech: A dynamic approach. In N.

A. Krasnegor, D. M. Rumbaugh, R. L. Schiefelbusch, & M. Studdert-Kennedy (Eds.), *Biological and behavioral determinants of language development* (pp. 339–362). Hillsdale, NJ: Erlbaum.

Thom, S. A., Hoit, J. D., Hixon, T. J., & Smith, A. E. (2006). Velopharyngeal function during vocalization in infants. *Cleft Palate Craniofacial Journal, 43*(5), 539–546.

Tian, W, & Redett, R. J. (2009). New velopharyngeal measurements at rest and during speech: implications and applications. *Journal of Craniofacial Surgery, 20*(2), 532–539.

Titze, I. R. (1990). Interpretation of the electroglottographic signal. *Journal of Voice, 4*, 1–9.

Tremblay, S., Houle, G., & Ostry, D. J. (2008). Specificity of speech motor learning. *Journal of Neuroscience, 28*, 2426–2434.

Trotman, C-A., Barlow, S. M., & Faraway J. J. (2007). Functional outcomes of cleft lip surgery. Part 3. Measurement of lip forces. *Cleft Palate–Craniofacial Journal, 44*(6), 617–623.

Trotman, C.-A., & Faraway, J. J. (1998). Sensitivity of a method for the analysis of facial motility: II. Interlandmark separation. *Cleft Palate–Craniofacial Journal, 35*, 142–153.

Trotman, C.-A., Faraway, J. J., & Essick, G. K. (2000). Three-dimensional nasolabial displacement during movement in repaired cleft lip and palate patients. *Plastic Reconstructive Surgery, 105*, 1273–1283.

Trotman, C.-A., Faraway, J. J., Silvester, K. T., Greenlee, G. M., & Johnston, L. E. (1998). Sensitivity of a method for the analysis of facial motility: I. Vector of displacement. *Cleft Palate–Craniofacial Journal, 35*, 132–141.

Turner, R. S., Desmurget, M., Grethe, J., Crutcher, M. D., & Grafton, S. T. (2003). Motor subcircuits mediating the control of movement extent and speed. *Journal of Neurophysiology, 90*(6), 3958–3966.

Turner, R. S,, Grafton, S. T., McIntosh, A. R., DeLong, M. R., & Hoffman, J. M. (2003). The functional anatomy of parkinsonian bradykinesia. *NeuroImage, 19*(1), 163–179.

Turner, R. S., Grafton, S. T., Votaw, J. R., & DeLong, M. R. (1998). Motor subcircuits mediating the control of movement velocity: A PET study. *Journal of Neurophysiology, 80*, 2162–2176.

Tye-Murray, N. (1991). The establishment of open articulatory postures by deaf and hearing talkers. *Journal of Speech and Hearing Research, 34*, 453–459.

van der Giet, G. (1977). Computer-controlled method for measuring articulatory activities. *Journal of the Acoustical Society of America, 61*(4), 1072–1076.

Walsh, B., Smith, A., & Weber-Fox, C. (2006). Short-term plasticity in children's speech motor systems. *Developmental Psychobiology, 48*(8), 660–674.

Warren, D. W. (1988). Aerodynamics of speech. In N. J. Lass (Ed.), *Handbook of speech-language pathology and audiology*. Toronto, B.C.: Decker.

Warren, D. W., Dalston, R. M., Trier, W. C., & Holder, M. B. (1985). A pressure-flow technique for quantifying temporal patterns of palatopharyngeal closure. *Cleft Palate Journal, 22*, 11–19.

Warren, D. W., & DuBois, A. (1964). A pressure-flow technique for measuring velopharyngeal orifice area during continuous speech. *Cleft Palate Journal, 1*, 52–71.

Watkin, K. L. (1999). Ultrasound and swallowing. *Folia Phoniatrica Logopedics, 51*, 183–198.

Watkin, K. L., & Rubin, J. M. (1989). Pseudo-three-dimensional reconstruction of ultrasonic images of the tongue. *Journal of the Acoustical Society of America, 85*(1), 496–499.

Westbury, J. R. (1991). The significance and measurement of head position during speech production experiments using the x-ray microbeam system. *Journal of the Acoustical Society of America, 89*(4), 1782–1791.

Whalen, D. H., Iskarous, K., Tiede, M. K., Ostry, D. J., Lehnert-LeHouillier, H.,

Vatikiotis-Bateson, E., & Hailey, D. S. (2005). The Haskins optically corrected ultrasound system (HOCUS). *Journal of Speech, Language, and Hearing Research, 48*(3), 543–553.

Wildgruber, D., Ackermann, H., & Grodd, W. (2001). Differential contributions of motor cortex, basal ganglia, and cerebellum to speech motor control: Effects of syllable repetition rate evaluated by fMRI. *NeuroImage, 13*, 101–109.

Wood, S., Wishart, J., Hardcastle, W., Cleland, J., & Timmins, C., (2009). The use of electropalatography (EPG) in the assessment and treatment of motor speech disorders in children with Down's syndrome: Evidence from two case studies. *Developmental Neurorehabilitation, 12*(2), 66–75.

Yang, C., & Stone, M. (2002). Dynamic programming method for temporal registration of three-dimensional tongue surface motion from multiple utterances. *Speech Communication, 38,* 199–207.

Yunusova, Y., Green, J. R., & Mefferd, A. (2009). Accuracy assessment for AG500, electromagnetic articulograph. *Journal of Speech, Language, and Hearing Research, 52*, 547–555.

Yunusova, Y., Weismer, G., Westbury, J. R., & Lindstrom, M. J. (2008). Articulatory movements during vowels in speakers with dysarthria and healthy controls. *Journal of Speech, Language, and Hearing Research, 51*, 596–611.

Zajac, D. J., & Hackett, A. M. (2002). Temporal characteristics of aerodynamic segments in the speech of children and adults. *Cleft Palate–Craniofacial Journal, 39*(4), 432–438.

11

Assessment of Rhythm

LAURENCE WHITE, PH.D., JULIE M. LISS, PH.D., AND VOLKER DELLWO, PH.D.

Introduction

A motor speech disorder (MSD) can be characterized, in part, by the impact of the specific neurological defect on the flow of speech, resulting in a percept of disturbed speech rhythm. Darley, Aronson, and Brown (1969a) applied terms such as *excess and equal stress, reduced stress, short rushes of speech,* and *prolonged segments,* among others, to characterize the perceptual experience of rhythmic disturbance. Darley et al. (1969a) asserted a causal relationship between the nature of the neuropathophysiology and the resulting speech-deficit pattern, such that similar rhythmic abnormalities are expected within a given neurological disease and severity level (Darley, Aronson, & Brown, 1969a, 1969b; Kent & Kim, 2003). Thus, accurate quantification and classification of the rhythmic disorder may assist in differential diagnosis of the underlying pathology, as well as guiding clinicians in their recommendation(s) for appropriate speech therapeutic intervention.

A prerequisite for the assessment of rhythmic disruption in motor speech disorder is a clear definition of what we mean by the term "speech rhythm." It was once believed that there is a coordination of metrical units in time, with stressed syllables in languages like English occurring at regular intervals, but evidence for such isochrony is lacking (e.g., Dauer, 1983). Speech production may nevertheless be considered "contrastively" rhythmical, based on the prominence distinction between stressed and unstressed syllables, at least in the languages of the world that maintain such a distinction. There are multiple cues to lexical stress, and languages differ in their use of variation in duration, fundamental frequency, amplitude, spectral tilt, and vowel quality. However, as we review in this chapter, recent research on typology of contrastive rhythm has focused on duration and, specifically, on how the degree of durational contrast between stressed and unstressed syllables varies between languages. As terms such as *excess and equal stress* demonstrate, MSDs may also be marked by variation from normal patterns of temporal stress contrast, and so it is reasonable to expect that quantification methods appropriate to cross-linguistic studies of contrastive rhythm may also have some utility in the assessment of MSDs.

In the following section, we introduce a variety of metrics that have been applied to the quantification of cross-linguistic differences in contrastive rhythm in nondisordered speech. We then consider the nature and origin of the manifest disturbances of rhythm and timing that arise in MSDs and review studies that have applied contrastive rhythm metrics specifically to examine rhythm in MSDs. As the majority of published work has applied metrics of speech rhythm to English, this is necessarily the focus of our discussion. We conclude with some practical guidelines for researchers and clinicians wishing to use contrastive rhythm metrics for the diagnosis and assessment of MSDs.

Metrics of Contrastive Speech Rhythm

Multiple factors contribute to cross-linguistic variation in contrastive rhythm (Dauer, 1983). In high temporal stress contrast languages (e.g., English), un-stressed vowels have reduced articulation and are much shorter than stressed vowels, whereas unstressed vowels in low temporal stress contrast languages (e.g., Spanish) are minimally reduced and not greatly shorter than stressed vowels.[1] These languages also differ in terms of syllable onset and coda phonotactics, with Spanish having a predominant pattern of open (consonant-vowel, CV) syllables and no relationship between syllable weight and stress placement, whereas English has a much greater range of permissible syllable types, with the heaviest syllables (those with complex codas, for example) tending to attract stress.

A number of duration-based rhythm metrics have been devised to quantify these cross-linguistic differences in temporal stress contrast. The first step in deriving scores for such metrics is a segmentation of the speech string into vocalic and consonantal intervals (see Practical Details of Rhythm Metric Calculation later in this chapter). The simplest metrics of durational variation in such intervals were proposed by Ramus, Nespor, and Mehler (1999): %V, the proportion of the utterance that is vocalic, and ΔC and ΔV, the standard deviation of consonantal (C) and vocalic (V) interval durations, respectively (Table 11–1 summarizes definitions of all metrics discussed here). A cross-linguistic comparison of these acoustic parameters revealed that languages of different putative rhythmic classes (in the terms employed by Ramus et al., 1999: "stress-timed," "syllable-timed,

---

[1]We prefer the terms "high/low temporal stress contrast" rather than the traditional "stress-timed" and "syllable-timed," as the latter imply a coordination of metrical units in time for which there is little empirical support.

Table 11–1. Definitions of Acoustic Interval-based Rhythm Metrics

Measures	Description
ΔV	Standard deviation of vocalic interval duration (Ramus, et al., 1999).
ΔC	Standard deviation of consonantal interval duration (Ramus et al., 1999).
%V	Percentage of utterance duration composed of vocalic intervals (Ramus et al., 1999).
VarcoV	Standard deviation of vocalic interval duration divided by mean vocalic duration and multiplied by 100 (White & Mattys, 2007a).
VarcoC	Standard deviation of consonantal interval duration divided by mean consonantal duration and multiplied by 100 (Dellwo, 2006).
VarcoVC	Standard deviation of vocalic + consonantal interval duration divided by mean vocalic + consonantal interval duration and multiplied by 100 (Liss et al., 2009).
Normalized pairwise variability index (nPVI)	Overall mean of the differences between successive pairs of intervals divided by their sum and multiplied by 100 (Low, Grabe, & Nolan, 2000). $$nPVI = 100 \times \left(\sum_{k=1}^{m-1} \left| (d_k - d_{k+1}) / ((d_k + d_{k+1})/2) \right| \right) / (m-1)$$ (Where m is the number of intervals and d is the duration of the kth interval.)
nPVI-V	Normalized pairwise variability index for vocalic intervals
nPVI-VC	Normalized pairwise variability index for vocalic + consonantal intervals
Raw pairwise variability index (rPVI)	Overall mean of the differences between successive pairs of intervals (Grabe & Low, 2002). $$rPVI = \left(\sum_{k=1}^{m-1} \left| d_k - d_{k+1} \right| \right) / (m-1)$$ (Where m is the number of intervals and d is the duration of the kth interval.)
rPVI-C	Raw pairwise variability index for consonantal intervals.

Note. Metric scores generally are calculated separately for each utterance of each speaker, based on interval durations measured in milliseconds.

and "mora-timed") are best separated by %V and ΔC. Thus, for example, Spanish has low ΔC because of its relative scarcity of onset or coda consonant clusters, making consonant intervals less variable than in languages like English. English has low %V, both because unstressed vowels are greatly shortened in English and because of its relative preponderance of consonant clusters (as also influences ΔC scores).

Comparison between groups of speakers with different articulation rates is problematic with ΔV and ΔC, however, as scores for both metrics show an inverse relationship with rate (Barry, Andreeva, Russo, Dimitrova, & Kostadinova, 2003; Dellwo & Wagner, 2003; White & Mattys, 2007a). This is unsurprising: when articulation rate is higher, mean interval durations are lower, and other things being equal, standard deviation tends to be lower as well. Ramus (2002) suggested a straightforward normalization procedure, implemented by Dellwo (2006) and White and Mattys (2007a): VarcoV and VarcoC are the coefficients of variability of V and C interval duration standard deviations, respectively (standard deviation of interval durations divided by the mean; see Table 11–1). White and Mattys (2007a, 2007b) showed that these normalized metrics are robust to variation in articulation rate. For %V, rate normalization is not required as scores do not show any systematic relation to rate (White & Mattys, 2007a, 2007b; Dellwo, in press).

A somewhat different approach to assessing variation in vocalic and consonantal interval durations was proposed by Francis Nolan and implemented initially by Low, Grabe, and Nolan (2000).

The Pairwise Variability Index (PVI) was intended to address the fact that standard deviation metrics take no account of the sequential pattern of durational variation within an utterance, presumably a crucial aspect of the perceptual experience of speech rhythm. The PVI is derived from durational differences between successive pairs of intervals, with these pairwise differences averaged over the utterance. This method would find a difference between, for example, a sequence of three long and three short vowels (schematically, VVVvvv) and an alternating sequence of long and short vowels (VvVvVv), which would not be picked up by standard deviation-based metrics.

The mathematical formulae for vocalic and consonantal PVI (nPVI-V and rPVI-C, respectively) are given in Table 11–1. As with standard deviation metrics, it was recognized as important to control for articulation rate variation in the vocalic PVI (hence nPVI-V, indicating "normalized"), in this case by dividing the difference between successive vowel durations by their sum. Rate normalization was not considered appropriate for consonantal interval PVI (rPVI-C, indicating "raw"), as differences between languages in intrinsic mean consonant interval duration could work in the direction of reducing variation between successive intervals; that is, high stress contrast languages would have both a larger numerator for consonantal interval variation, due to their greater differences between successive intervals, and a larger denominator, due to their longer mean consonantal interval durations (based on intrinsic—and therefore, linguistically significant

—factors rather than simply arising due to idiosyncratic variation in segment-by-segment articulation).[2] This issue of rate with regard to consonant intervals is further confounded because cross-linguistic differences in syllables-per-second articulation rate are strongly affected by consonant complexity. At the same rate of segment production, there will be more Spanish-typical CV syllables per second than English-typical CVC syllables. Dellwo (in press) argues that—exactly because of this relationship between rate and C interval durations—rate normalization is necessary to establish whether C variation is intrinsic or due to performance factors.

The metrics introduced previously (ΔV, ΔC, VarcoV, VarcoC, nPVI-V, rPVI-C, %V) have been the most widely utilized thus far. White & Mattys (2007a, 2007b) evaluated their relative efficacy and found that VarcoV and %V were the most discriminative—when there were pre-existing reasons for expecting differences—between various European languages, between first and second language speakers, and between accents of English. As discussed, scores for the nonrate normalized metrics (ΔV, ΔC, rPVI-C) were strongly inversely correlated with articulation rate, and the rate-normalized consonantal metric (VarcoC) showed no discrimination between language groups. Scores for

the two rate-normalized metrics of vocalic interval duration were highly correlated, with VarcoV being slightly more discriminative than nPVI-V. Presumably, this correlation arises because the languages studied did not strongly deviate from a fairly regular alternation of stressed and unstressed syllables.

Scores for the optimal combination of metrics found by White and Mattys (2007a, 2007b) are shown in Figure 11–1 for a range of European languages. The pattern illustrated is typical of many studies exploiting rhythm metrics, which tend to show a gradient variation in rhythm scores between high and low temporal stress contrast languages, with English and Spanish the most extreme examples of these respective types studied thus far. Also evident from Figure 11–1 is the strong inverse correlation between %V and VarcoV. This is partly because increased unstressed vowel shortening will tend to make VarcoV higher and %V lower, and partly because unstressed vowel shortening and high consonant cluster complexity tend to co-occur in the languages examined here.

There are languages in which variation in vowel and consonant duration is not correlated: Polish, for example, has high C complexity but low V variation (Ramus et al., 1999). Indeed, one rationale for the separation of vocalic

---

[2]A numerical example from the data of White & Mattys (2007a) makes this clear. Mean vowel durations are almost identical for Spanish (76 ms) versus English (76 ms), but mean consonantal durations are very different for Spanish (87 ms) versus English (125 ms). Thus, in the normalization, the higher mean, deriving from intrinsic not performance factors, overcompensates and reduces the real difference in interval duration variation. This is indeed what was found by White & Mattys (2007a): the rate-normalized VarcoC did not show any differences between the languages Dutch/English versus French/Spanish (the logic regarding the scaling of both numerator and denominator applies similarly to VarcoC and rPVI-C).

	VarcoV	SE VarcoV	%V	SE %V
ABN	64.99633	1.463427	41.258	1.195757
Bristol	56.93267	2.201255	40.946	0.545523
Fr Fr	49.98	0.876285	44.83033	0.809055
Ib Sp	40.95467	2.015844	47.935	0.797958
Paduan	50.25495	0.50226	46.73851	1.124807
Orkney	52.58433	1.950845	40.45033	1.042776
Shetland	58.72767	1.158839	38.796	0.616218
Sicilian	47.33242	1.791554	45.71559	1.212553
SSBE	64.47933	1.657666	37.96367	0.529927
Valleys	52.66233	1.821142	41.71033	0.713291

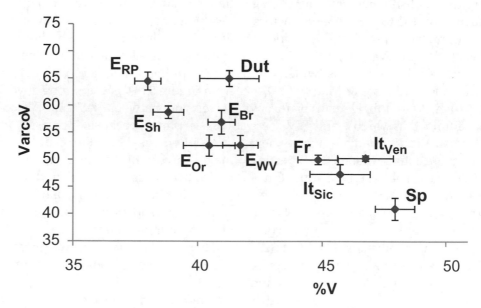

Figure 11–1. VarcoV and %V scores for the nondisordered speech of a range of languages. Key: Dut = Standard Dutch; Fr = Standard French; Sp = Castilian Spanish. It$_{Sic}$ = Sicilian Italian; It$_{Ven}$ = Venetan Italian; E$_{RP}$ = Standard Southern British English; E$_{Sh}$ = Shetland English; E$_{Or}$ = Orkney English; E$_{Br}$ = Bristolian English; E$_{WV}$ = Welsh Valleys English. *Sources:* White and Mattys (2007a, 2007b); White, Payne, and Mattys (2009).

and intervocalic intervals in cross-linguistic studies is this possibility of independent variation in unstressed vowel shortening and consonant clustering.

In the clinical context, variation within rather than between languages is the focus, and so the logic for considering vocalic and consonantal intervals separately does not apply. Thus, for the assessment of MSDs, a number of composite (V + C) metrics have also been proposed, including Varco-VC and nPVI-VC (Liss et al., 2009; see Table 11–1 for definitions); these results are discussed in the following sections. (Taking a phonological rather than acoustic approach to interval definition, Ackerman and Hertrich, 1994, propose the durational scanning index, which utilizes whole syllable durations.)

Rhythm metrics are influenced by within-language variation between sentences and speakers (Dellwo, in press; Wiget et al., 2010). Focusing on the three most reliable metrics (%V, VarcoV, nPVI-V), Wiget et al. (2010) found intersentence variation particularly marked for nPVI-V, an unsurprising finding given the local rather than global nature of its derivation. Rhythm scores also show significant variation between speakers of a common variety (Dellwo & Koreman, 2008, for standard German; Wiget et al., 2010, for standard southern British English). Indeed, %V has been shown to have a high degree of speaker dependence, showing within-speaker consistency even under extreme rate variation (Dellwo & Koreman, 2008). Among the other metrics considered by Wiget et al., those of consonantal interval variation (ΔC, VarcoC, rPVI-C) were particularly subject to interspeaker and intersentence variability. Even for the most reliable metrics (%V, VarcoV, nPVI-V), variation was sufficient to strongly argue against using single, or very few, speakers as representative of a particular population.

Between studies, intralanguage variation in rhythm scores may potentially arise as a result of researchers applying different criteria to identify boundaries between vowels and consonants. Wiget et al. found, however, that reliability between independent measurers working to a common protocol was high for %V, VarcoV, and nPVI-V.

In conclusion, three metrics are particularly discriminative between language groups expected to differ rhythmically: %V, VarcoV, nPVI-V, with scores for VarcoV and nPVI-V tending to be highly correlated. Consonant interval metrics are problematic: scores for nonnormalized metrics are strongly affected by articulation rate, but normalization— necessary and effective for vocalic intervals—tends for consonants to eliminate genuine cross-linguistic differences. Within a language group, rhythm scores vary at least moderately between speakers, with greater speaker-based variation for consonantal metrics. Scores for all metrics vary substantially between sentences.

Assessment of Rhythmic Disturbance in Motor Speech Disorders

The selection of metrics and their experimental utilization for assessment of rhythmic disturbance in MSDs may be determined by considerations somewhat different to those that apply in the case of cross-linguistic studies. Between-language variation in contrastive rhythm, as indexed by rhythm metrics, is assumed to be based on stable differences in phonological properties, such as consonant phonotactics and vowel reduction; however, rhythmic variation in MSDs, where it exists, derives rather from idiosyncratic articulatory implementation of these phonological properties. In addition, the quantification of contrastive rhythm in MSDs may be undertaken for a variety of different purposes: for differential diagnosis of the underlying neuropathology; for quantification of the severity of this pathology; for assessment of the impact of the MSD on communicative function; for the identification of goals for therapeutic action.

As discussed previously, certain metrics—%V, nPVI-V, VarcoV—are particularly sensitive to cross-linguistic differences in temporal stress contrast, while others are not robust for this purpose, being, for example, strongly affected by articulation rate. However, disturbances of perceived rhythm in MSDs have multiple underlying causes, and, thus, metrics may be differentially suitable according to the nature of the disorder. With regard to rate: most MSDs, as discussed in the following section, are characterized both by reduction in articulation rate (with the rate of production of segments themselves being slowed) and by a reduction in speech rate (with multiple pauses between and, according to the severity of the deficit, within words). Thus, measures of rate will serve to distinguish most MSDs of reasonable severity from nondisordered speech. However, the optimum method appears to be a combination of rate and specific contrastive rhythm metrics, according, as reviewed in the following section, to the nature of the disorder.

Rhythmic Disturbance in Specific MSDs

The nature of rhythmic abnormalities in MSDs varies according to the loca-

tion and extent of neurological impairment. Central and/or peripheral lesions that cause hyper- or hypotonicity and muscular weakness may constrain the global rate at which one produces speech, thereby affecting breath groups (Tjaden & Turner, 2000; Turner & Weismer, 1993; Weismer, Jeng, Laures, Kent, & Kent, 2001). Damage to the cerebellar circuits responsible for regulating the force, timing, rhythm, direction, speed, and overall coordination of speech (and other) movements may also produce articulatory speed abnormalities, as well as disruptions in the durational relationships among stressed and unstressed syllables and phrase-level timing abnormalities (Ackermann & Hertrich, 1994; Casper, Raphael, Harris, & Geibel, 2007; Hartelius, Runmarker, Andersen, & Nord, 2000; Kent et al., 2000; Kent, Netsell, & Abbs, 1979; LeDorze, Ryalls, Brassard, Boulanger, & Ratte, 1998; Ziegler & Wessel, 1996). Basal ganglia circuitry impairment interferes with appropriate motor program scaling, suppression of adventitious movement, and smooth movement execution (Hallet & Khoshbin, 1980). This can result in a variety of rate abnormalities associated with reduced articulatory excursions or inadequate suppression of involuntary movement (Caliguiri, 1989; Hertrich & Ackermann 1994; McAuliffe, Ward, & Murdoch, 2006; Spencer & Slocomb, 2007; Weismer, 1984). It is well documented that rhythmic disturbances are a hallmark of apraxia of speech from cortical damage or mal-development that affects speech motor programming (Kent & Rosenbek, 1983; Strand & McNeil, 1996; Shriberg, Campbell, et al., 2003; Shriberg, Green, Campbell, McSweeney, & Scheer, 2003). Finally, it is of note that rate reduction in any MSD may be, in part, compensatory to facilitate reaching articulatory-acoustic goals or to reduce the amount of effort required to achieve them (e.g., Turner & Weismer, 1993).

The majority of investigations that have studied rhythm abnormalities in MSDs have done so within the context of the Mayo Classification System (Darley et al., 1969a, 1969b) and the associated presumptions about speech patterns and underlying neuropathologies. Perhaps the most studied are the rhythm abnormalities associated with ataxic and hypokinetic dysarthria and the mixed dysarthria associated with amyotrophic lateral sclerosis (ALS). Particularly with regard to ataxic and hypokinetic dysarthrias, rhythm analysis has been used as a window to underlying central timing abnormalities or aberrant motor programs (see, for example, Ackermann & Hertrich, 1994; Casper et al., 2007; Hartelius et al., 2000; LeDorze, Ryalls, Brassard, Boulanger, & Ratte, 1998; Spencer & Slocomb, 2007). The following descriptions of motor speech disorders summarize this literature for speakers with a moderately severe level of involvement within each diagnostic classification. It is acknowledged that the clinical presentations for mild or severe patients may be both qualitatively and quantitatively different (see Weismer, 2008).

Flaccid Dysarthria

Because central control of motor program scaling and specification is not directly affected by peripheral lesions, speech rate and rhythm are relatively preserved in the flaccid dysarthrias. Abnormalities of stress-based timing relationships among syllables in flaccid dysarthria have not specifically been reported. It is conceivable, however, for rate and timing abnormalities to occur in the context of multiple and bilateral cranial nerve involvement (Darley et al., 1969b). For example, excessive air wastage associated with vocal fold paralysis and velopharyngeal dysfunction may result in shortened breath groups. Slowed speech may occur in the context of lingual, labial, facial, and velopharyngeal flaccid paralysis when sufficiently severe.

Spastic Dysarthria

A mild perceptible and transient speech disturbance may occur with a unilateral upper motor neuron lesion (unilateral upper motor neuron dysarthria; Duffy, 1995). However, bilateral lesions of the fiber tracts that course from the motor cortex to their synapse in the brainstem can have severe effects on speech rhythm. Spastic dysarthria is associated with slow and labored articulation rate. As the timing aspects of motor programs should be relatively preserved, it has been suggested that the rate decrements arise from the hypertonicity and muscle weakness (Darley et al., 1969b; Weismer, Yunusova & Westbury, 2003; Yunusova, Weismer, Westbury, & Lindstrom, 2008). Nonetheless, rhythm abnormalities also may be present in spastic dysarthria—perhaps as a consequence of the hypertonus—and include syllable segregation (that is, speaking each syllable or word as a distinct unit in time); prolonged phonemes; and a tendency toward excess and even stress. Because it has been demonstrated that individuals with spastic dysarthria can manipulate duration to signal stress, at least some of the profile can be explained by compensatory slowing and increased effort to overcome the weakness and hyperreflexia associated with the spastic paralysis (Patel, 2002; Patel & Campellone, 2009).

Mixed Flaccid-Spastic Dysarthria

The rate and rhythmic disturbance associated with the mixed dysarthria of amyotrophic lateral sclerosis (ALS) has been studied extensively (e.g., Kent, Kent, Rosenbek, & Weismer, 1992; Tjaden & Turner, 2000; Turner & Weismer, 1993). The mixed flaccid-spastic dysarthria of ALS is the result of both lower and upper motor neuron degeneration (see Tomik & Guiloff, 2008, for a review). Speech is slow and prolonged, and breath groups are small due to deficits in respiratory support, the valving defects associated with glottal stenosis (strained-strangled vocal quality), and impaired velopharyngeal function. Movement velocities of articulators, especially the tongue, are slow (Weismer et al., 2003; Yunusova et al., 2008). Liss et al. (2009) reported that speakers with ALS were discriminated from those with other types of dysarthria by metrics (such as VarcoV, nPVI-V, and %V) that captured the prolongation of vowels and the lack of temporal distinction between vowels produced in stressed versus unstressed syllables. In fact, ALS speech had the most elongated, syllable-by-syllable production, with the most regular ("scanning") rhythm of the four dysarthria groups studied. Given the high incidence of pausing, measures of speech rate as well as articulation rate are also likely to be distinctive.

Hypokinetic Dysarthria

Ideopathic Parkinson's disease (PD) and parkinsonian syndromes are associated with hypokinetic dysarthria. Although speech may be slow, it is the relatively normal or supra-normal articulation rate that distinguishes many speakers with hypokinetic dysarthria from other subtypes. Rhythm abnormalities result from inappropriate silences (inability to initiate movement), disfluencies, and short rushes of speech. As articulator movements in PD are shown to be slow, it is believed that the reduced excursions of the articulators secondary to basal ganglia dysfunction give rise to the perceptual experience of rushed speech in the context of normal or supra-normal rates (e.g., Caliguiri, 1989; Weismer, 1984; Yusunova et al., 2008). Converging evidence shows that the underlying temporal structure of the speech motor program is relatively preserved in hypokinetic dysarthria. For example, Liss et al. (2009) showed that metrics of consonantal and combined intervals were similar to values obtained from healthy speakers. This is consistent with observations of other motor systems in basal ganglia disease, which show the motor program for a task is essentially intact, but that it is implemented in a scaled-down spatial domain (Berardelli, Dick, Rothwell, Day, & Marsden, 1986; Hallett & Khoshbin, 1980). Normalized vowel intervals metrics nPVI-V and VarcoV did show some reduction in contrast compared with nondisordered speech, although less than that for other dysarthrias.

Hyperkinetic Dysarthria

The seemingly random bursts of vocalization and intrusive and extraneous orofacial movements result in variable breakdown of the forward flow of speech in hyperkinetic dysarthria of the choreic (quick) type (Hartelius, Carlstedt, Ytterberg, Lillvik, & Laakso, 2003). This variable breakdown manifests as increased interutterance variation in utterance duration (speech rate) and voice onset time (Hertrich & Ackermann, 2000), as well as voice stoppages and inappropriate silences. Liss et al. (2009) reported that metrics capturing the high variability of consonantal segment durations were important for distinguishing speakers with choreic hyperkinetic dysarthria from those with other types of dysarthria: VarcoC and VarcoVC scores are supra-normal (scores for other dysarthrias are lowered). Discrimination from other dysarthrias is better with longer stretches of speech, given the random nature of the intrusive orofacial movements that affect articulation.

Like chorea, dystonic hyperkinetic dysarthria presumably arises from the failure of the basal ganglia to provide sufficient physiological inhibition to the thalamus and brainstem. This manifests in the orofacial region with involuntary and repetitive contractions of the tongue, lip, jaw, and pharyngeal musculature, that can cause uncontrolled mouth opening or closing, jaw deviation, facial grimace, and tongue protrusion (see Lee, Gollamudi, Ozelius, Kim, & Jeon, 2007, for a review). Although rhythm abnormalities have not been the explicit target of research in this relatively rare condition, Darley et al. (1969a, 1969b) characterized dystonic dysarthria as being slow with rhythmic abnormalities tending toward either prosodic excess (excess and equal) or prosodic insufficiency (reductions).

Ataxic Dysarthria

The relatively large body of literature that has reported on rate and rhythm in ataxic dysarthria attributes patterns to the unpredictably abnormal timing, force, range and direction of articulatory movement. Interestingly, speakers

with ataxic dysarthria do not exhibit a homogeneous pattern of rhythmic disturbance despite the presumed common involvement of cerebellar circuitry. Darley et al. (1969b) described three perceptual subsets of ataxic dysarthria, the first predominated by irregular articulatory breakdown (Articulatory); the second predominated by slow rate, excess and equal stress, and prolonged phonemes and intervals (Prosodic Excess); and the third with phonatory disturbance and reduced prosodic variation (Phonatory-Prosodic). These subclasses likely account for the variety of findings regarding rhythm abnormalities in ataxic dysarthria. Whereas some speakers exhibit slow speech with high degrees of excess and equal stress and a strong tendency toward syllabic isochrony (scanning speech), other speakers exhibit high degrees of irregularity both in interutterance articulation rate and defects in phrase-level timing patterns (see, for example, Ackermann & Hertrich, 1994; Hartelius et al., 2000). Liss et al. (2009) found that a combination of VarcoC (near-normal values) and various other metrics (including nPVI-V, %V) served best to discriminate ataxic from other dysarthrias. Vocalic intervals, as indexed by nPVI-V and VarcoV, were more regular than nondisordered speech (see also Henrich, Lowit, Schalling, & Mennen, 2006), but less excess and equal than in ALS speech.

Apraxia of Speech

Because apraxia of speech (AOS) is thought to be a fundamental disturbance of motor programming, it follows that rhythmic abnormalities in the flow of speech are a hallmark of the disorder. AOS is characterized by slowed speaking rate, prolongation of transitions, intersyllable pauses, initiation difficulties, and inappropriate silences (Kent & Rosenbek, 1983). Articulatory groping for targets, false starts, and error revisions further disturb speech rhythm, and all of these features vary with utterance length and linguistic complexity (Strand & McNeil, 1996).

Childhood Apraxia of Speech

Like AOS in adults, children who present with a developmental form of AOS (cAOS) exhibit prolonged and disrupted coarticulatory transitions between sounds and syllables, and inappropriate duration relations for the marking of lexical or phrasal stress (Shriberg, Campbell, et al., 2003; Shriberg, Green, et al, 2003; Velleman & Shriberg, 1999). Also like the adult form, evidence suggests that the abnormal rhythm is the result of a central timing deficit rather than attributable to phonological or linguistic factors (Shriberg, Campbell, et al., 2003). Shriberg and his colleagues have evaluated the patterns of reduced temporal distinctiveness as a diagnostic marker for cAOS using a ratio of the coefficients of variation of pause and interpause (i.e., speech event) durations.

Guidelines for Researchers and Clinicians

In the final section, we present a practical guide for the use of metrics of con

trastive rhythm, suggest factors that may influence the choice of metrics and the design of studies in the clinical context, and consider the potential impact of future developments.

Practical Details of Rhythm Metric Calculation

In order to derive scores for duration-based acoustic metrics of contrastive rhythm such as those detailed in Table 11–1, it is necessary to divide the speech string into vocalic and intervocalic intervals. Identification of the boundaries between vowels and consonants in speech is typically carried out through visual inspection of the waveform and spectrogram in a speech analysis program such as Praat (Boersma & Weenink, 2006). Standard phonetic criteria are used to identify segmental boundaries in speech (see, for example, Peterson & Lehiste, 1960; Turk, Nakai, & Sugahara, 2006).

Figure 11–2 provides an example of a vocalic-consonantal segmentation, showing that the phonological constituency of speech segments is generally ignored, with successive consonants (or vowels) being included within the same interval, even when they are heterosyllabic.[3] Likewise, the division between vowels and consonants is made on purely acoustic criteria: syllabic consonants or underlying vowels that are wholly devoiced in their realization are included in the adjacent consonantal intervals (Grabe & Low,

---

[3]Ramus, Nespor, and Mehler (1999) motivate this step with reference to infant acquisition of the native-language-appropriate rhythmic typological category, reasoning that the neonate has no knowledge of language-specific syllable structure but may be able distinguish vowels from consonants (or, more specifically, sonority peaks from troughs).

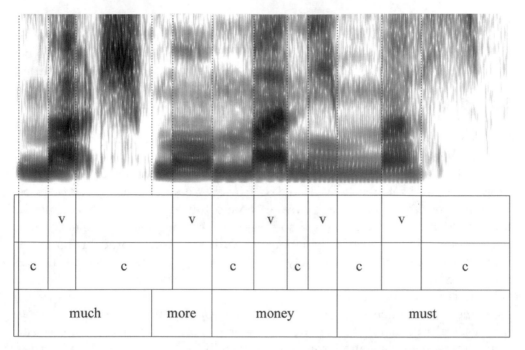

Figure 11–2. Example segmentation of a speech string into vocalic (*v*) and conso-nantal (*c*) intervals. The third label tier shows the orthographic transcription. The com-bination of heterosyllabic intervals is illustrated in the second "*c*" interval, which includes the coda consonant of *much* and the onset consonant of *more*.

2002). Minor variations exist between researchers in what counts as vocalic and what as consonantal: Ramus et al. (1999), for example, classified approxi-mants preceding a vowel as consonan-tal and following a vowel as vocalic; other researchers, such as White and Mattys (2007a, 2007b), have used speech samples that eliminate approximants for ease of measurement. It is unlikely, however, that such variations have a major influence on the overall statistical picture: Liss et al. (2009), for example, found little differences in patterns of scores for approximant-controlled and uncontrolled read speech samples.

By convention, hesitation or bound-ary pauses are excluded and vowel-vowel or consonant-consonant inter-vals are summed across the boundary (Grabe & Low, 2002). Further specific details of a typical segmentation proce-dure for the purposes of rhythm metric calculation are given in White and Mattys (2007a).

After an utterance has been seg-mented, through the placement of boundary labels, into a string of vocalic and consonantal intervals, the durations of both sets of intervals are calculated for each utterance. If using Praat, various scripts are available for the automated extraction of interval durations, one of which can be downloaded from http://language.psy.bris.ac.uk/contrastive _rhythm_metrics. These vowel and con-sonantal interval durations are the raw materials for the derivation of rhythm metric scores; a spreadsheet for the cal-culation of scores for various rhythm metrics discussed in this paper is also available from http://language.psy.bris.ac.uk/contrastive_rhythm_metrics.

Selection of Rhythm Metrics

With regard to the selection of metrics: as Liss et al. (2009) found, no single metric optimally discriminates between all MSDs discussed previously. Most dysarthrias, other than hypokinetic dysarthria, are distinguished from nondisordered speech by reduced articulation rate, but from each other by a variety of metrics, as summarized in Table 11–2. As stated previously, the purpose of the assessment will influence the selection of metrics. If the primary goal is to determine the speaker's deviation from nondisordered speaking patterns, articulation rate must be included, together with rate-normalized metrics that include vocalic interval duration (some of VarcoV, nPVI-V, VarcoVC, %V, the first two being highly correlated). All dysarthrias, except for the hypokinetic type, show substantial lowering of articulation rate relative to normal, and all are characterized by relative leveling of vowel interval durational variation (particularly ataxic and flaccid-spastic dysarthria). However, if the primary goal is diagnostic and, thus, distinction between metrics is required, the most useful metric varies according to the disorder. Thus, ataxic dysarthria is typically characterized as having "excess and equal" rhythm, but scores for metrics of vocalic interval variation are higher (nearer-normal) scores than for flaccid-spastic dysarthria. In fact, ataxic dysarthria is distinguished from other dysarthrias in part by its relatively normal VarcoC scores.

Table 11–2. Typical Temporal and Rhythmic Characteristics of Specific MSDs and Rhythm Metrics Shown To Be Useful in Distinguishing Each Disorder from the Others

Motor Speech Disorder	Articulation Rate	Rhythmic Features	Relevant Objective Metrics
Flaccid dysarthria	Generally normal	Speech rhythm is generally preserved	
Spastic dysarthria	Slow, labored	Tendency toward syllabic segregation and isochrony, excess and equal stress	VarcoV, nPVI-V, VarcoVC, nPVI-VC
Hypokinetic dysarthria	Normal to supra-normal, less often slowed	Rhythm marked by episodic short rushes of speech; relative preservation of the temporal relationships between adjacent syllables; inappropriate silences	nPVI-V, VarcoV (somewhat lower than normal, but higher than other dysarthrias)

Table 11–2. *continued*

Motor Speech Disorder	Articulation Rate	Rhythmic Features	Relevant Objective Metrics
Hyperkinetic dysarthria (Choreic type)	Variable rate, slowed	Irregular articulatory breakdown, inappropriate silences, prolonged phonemes, voice stoppages, irregular durations, involuntary bursts	VarcoC, VarcoVC (supra-normal scores; other dysarthrias have lowered VarcoVC)
(Dystonic Type)	Slowed	Silences, short phrases, prolonged phonemes	
Ataxic dysarthria	Normal to slowed; rate variations	Subclasses of predominant rhythmic patterns: (1) "scanning" with the perception of equal and even syllable rate; (2) irregular articulatory breakdown; prolonged phonemes, prolonged intervals	VarcoC (similar to normal), combined with other metrics. nPVI-V, VarcoV lowered, but less than ALS.
Mixed dysarthria, Flaccid-Spastic (ALS)	Slow, labored	Tendency toward syllabic segregation, short breath groups, frequent pauses, excess and equal stress	VarcoV, nPVI-V lower than other dysarthrias; %V higher.
Apraxia of Speech (acquired)	Slow, labored	Prolongation of transitions, intersyllable pauses, initiation difficulties and inappropriate silences; articulatory groping for targets, false starts, and error revisions	
Childhood Apraxia of Speech	Variations in rate	Both sound prolongations and prolonged pauses between sounds, syllables, or words thereby segregating them for the percept of staccato rhythm; excessive equal stress, with all or most syllables receiving stress	VarcoVC. Pause/speech event coefficient of variation ratio (see Shriberg, Green et al., 2003).

Future Directions in Rhythmic Assessment

All metrics presented in Table 11–1 are based on raw interval durations. However, Dellwo (in press) argued that the calculation of standard deviation and coefficient of variation metrics on absolute interval durations may be problematic, since the underlying distributions of C and V intervals durations are highly positively skewed and show a large amount of positive kurtosis. To normalize the data, interval durations may be logarithmically transformed (each interval duration expressed as a logarithm to the base e). Calculated on logarithmically transformed data, ΔC was found not to correlate with speech rate even for speech data that are extremely variable in rate (Dellwo, in press).

Hand-labeling of speech data is time-consuming and subject to the vagaries of subjective interpretation, although Wiget et al. (2010) found that trained phoneticians operating independently but according to an agreed protocol showed substantial agreement on scores. However, an automated approach based on forced alignment showed no more variation in scores from the human measurers than they did from each other. In this technique, an automatic speech recognition program determined segment boundaries based an orthographic transcription of the utterances. The reliability of forced alignment techniques for the measurement of disordered speech rhythm has not yet been assessed.

Automated methods may also be possible based on different units of measurement. Dellwo, Fourcin, and Abberton (2007) found that deriving rhythm scores based on voiced and voiceless interval durations, rather than vocalic and consonantal interval durations, also provided evidence for cross-linguistic "rhythm class" differences. This method has the advantage that the units under observation are relatively easy to obtain using standard pitch detection algorithms. It remains to be demonstrated whether these units are valuable for the assessment of disordered speech.

As discussed previously, there are many alternative methods of quantifying rhythm variation to those based simply on interval durations. Given that the occurrence of multiple pauses characterizes different disorders to varying degrees, one direction likely to be profitable is an integration of estimates of pause frequency and duration with standard interval durations. The speech-silence coefficient of variation ratio of Shriberg, Green, et al. (2003) for the characterization of childhood apraxia of speech is one such approach. Shriberg, Campbell, et al. (2003) widened their data sources by including nondurational measurements: their lexical stress ratio was based on a weighted sum of durational, frequency, and amplitude measures. Liss, LeGendre, and Lotto (in press) found that automatically extracted envelope modulation spectra allowed discrimination between dysarthrias comparable to that obtained from using rhythm metrics.

Finally, as discussed at the outset, speech is only rhythmical in the contrastive sense, that is, based on the prominence distinction between stressed and unstressed syllables. Indeed, the temporal organization of speech derives primarily not from metrical structure —the division of the speech string into prominence-delimited groups— but from the arrangement of speech into linguistically meaningful units. This prosodic structure is generally taken to reflect the syntactic organization of speech, while not actually being isomorphic with syntactic structure (e.g., Nespor & Vogel, 1986; Selkirk, 1996). In English, the primary timing consequences of prosodic structure are the increased durations of segments associated with the edges and heads of prosodically defined domains: word-final lengthening (e.g., Oller, 1973); phrase-final lengthening (e.g., Wightman, Shattuck-Hufnagel, Ostendorf, & Price, 1992); stressed syllable lengthening (e.g., Klatt, 1976); accentual lengthening (i.e., the increased duration of segments in word that carry phrasal stress/pitch accent; e.g., Turk & White, 1999). Discussion of the consequences of MSDs for prosodic speech timing and the assessment of these patterns is beyond the scope of this review; however, van Santen, Tucker, Prud'hommeaux, and Black (2009) propose methods for the automated assessment of a range of prosodic features, including boundary phenomena as well as stress contrast.

Recommendations

1. The most appropriate metric for distinguishing between disorders varies according to the comparison being made, and so any one metric should not be relied on for all cases. Some combination of rate-normalized vocalic and composite interval-based metrics (VarcoV, nPVI-V, Varco-VC, nPVI-VC) together with articulation rate (or speech rate, or both) is likely to be most effective in providing a general gauge of the severity of the disorder.

2. Rhythm scores are affected by the nature of the spoken materials. Measurements should be based on a range of sentences, read or spontaneous, and care taken when comparing scores derived from different materials. PVI -based metrics are particularly sensitive to the nature of individual utterances.

3. When comparison between disordered speakers has to be made on the basis of distinct corpora of utterances for each speaker, calculation of a baseline difference between the sentences themselves, derived from nondisordered speech, would facilitate interpretation of the observed patterns for disordered speech.

4. Rhythm metrics seem particularly well suited to longitudinal studies of individual speakers, to track the deterioration in a speaker's prosody or the efficacy of ameliorative speech therapy. A comparable set of sentence materials should be used at each stage wherever possible.

5. Where multiple measurers are used, they should all work to a clearly agreed protocol. Automated segmentation methods, based on forced alignment of an orthographic or phonetic transcription, have been shown to be as reliable as using multiple measurers, at least for nondisordered speech.

References

Ackerman, H., & Hertrich, I. (1994). Speech rate and rhythm in cerebellar dysarthria: An acoustic analysis of syllabic timing. *Folia Phoniatrica et Logopaedica, 46,* 70–78.

Barry, W. J., Andreeva, B., Russo, M., Dimitrova, S., & Kostadinova, T. (2003). Do rhythm measures tell us anything about language type? *Proceedings of the 15th International Congress of Phonetics Sciences, Barcelona* (pp. 2693–2696).

Berardelli, A., Dick, J. P. R., Rothwell, J. C., Day, B. L., & Marsden, C. D. (1986). Scaling of the size of the first agonist EMG burst during rapid wrist movements in patients with Parkinson's disease. *Journal of Neurology, Neurosurgery, and Psychiatry, 49,* 1273–1279.

Boersma, P., & Weenink, D. (2006). Praat: Doing phonetics by computer (version 4.3.04) [computer program]. Retrieved March 21, 2006, from http://www.praat .org/

Caliguiri, M. (1989). The influence of speaking rate on articulatory hypokinesia in parkinsonian dysarthria. *Brain and Language, 36,* 493–502.

Casper, M. A., Raphael, L. J., Harris, K. S., & Geibel, J. M. (2007). Speech prosody in cerebellar ataxia. *International Journal of Language and Communication Disorders, 42,* 407–426.

Darley, F. L., Aronson, A. E., & Brown, J. R. (1969a). Differential diagnostic patterns of dysarthria. *Journal of Speech and Hearing Research, 12,* 246–269.

Darley, F. L., Aronson, A. E., & Brown, J. R. (1969b). Clusters of deviant speech dimensions in the dysarthrias. *Journal of Speech and Hearing Research, 12,* 462–496.

Dauer, R. M. (1983). Stress-timing and syllable-timing reanalyzed. *Journal of Phonetics, 11,* 51–62.

Dellwo, V. (in press). Influences of speech rate on the acoustic correlates of speech rhythm: An experimental phonetic study based on acoustic and perceptual evidence. PhD Thesis, University of Bonn. eBibilothek, University of Bonn (http:// hss.ulb.uni-bonn.de/diss_online/).

Dellwo, V. (2006) Rhythm and speech rate: A variation coefficient for deltaC. In P. Karnowski & I. Szigeti (Eds.), *Language and language-processing* (pp. 231–241). Frankfurt am Main, Germany: Peter Lang.

Dellwo, V., Fourcin, F. & Abberton, E. (2007). Rhythmical classification of languages based on voice parameters. *Proceedings of the 16th International Congress of Phonetic Sciences, Saarbrücken* (pp. 1129–1132).

Dellwo, V., & Koreman, J. (2008). How speaker idiosyncratic is measurable speech rhythm? *Proceedings of the Annual Meeting of the International Association of Forensic Phonetics and Acoustics* (http:// www.iafpa.net/IAFPA2008-abstracts .pdf).

Dellwo, V., & Wagner, P. (2003). Relations between language rhythm and speech rate. *Proceedings of the 15th International Congress of Phonetics Sciences, Barcelona* (pp. 471–474).

Duffy, J. R. (1995). *Motor speech disorders: Substrates, differential diagnosis, and management.* St. Louis, MO: Mosby-Year Book.

Grabe, E., & Low, E. L. (2002). Durational variability in speech and the rhythm class hypothesis. In N. Warner & C. Gussenhoven (Eds.), *Papers in laboratory phonology 7* (pp. 515–546). Berlin, Germany: Mouton de Gruyter.

Hallett, M., & Khoshbin, S. (1980). A physiological mechanism of bradykinesia. *Brain, 103,* 301–314.

Hartelius, L., Carlstedt, A., Ytterberg, M., Lillvik, M., & Laakso, K. (2003). Speech disorders in mild and moderate Huntington disease: Results of dysarthria assessments of 19 individuals. *Journal of Medical Speech-Language Pathology, 11,* 1–14.

Hartelius, L., Runmarker, B., Andersen, O., & Nord, L. (2000). Temporal speech characteristics of individuals with multiple sclerosis and ataxic dysarthria: 'Scanning speech' revisited. *Folia Phoniatrica et Logopaedica, 52,* 228–238.

Henrich, J., Lowit, A., Schalling, E., & Mennen, I. (2006). Rhythmic disturbance in ataxic dysarthria: A comparison of different measures and speech tasks. *Journal of Medical Speech-Language Pathology, 14,* 291–296.

Hertrich, I., & Ackermann, H. (1994). Acoustic analysis of speech timing in Huntington's disease. *Brain and Language, 47,* 182–196.

Kent, R. D., Kent, J. F., Duffy, J. R., Thomas, J. E., Weismer, G., & Stuntebeck, S. (2000). Ataxic dysathria. *Journal of Speech, Language and Hearing Research, 43,* 1275–1289.

Kent, J. F., Kent, R. D., Rosenbek, J. C., & Weismer, G. (1992). Quantitative description of the dysarthria in women with amyotrophic lateral sclerosis. *Journal of Speech and Hearing Research, 35,* 723–733.

Kent, R. D., & Kim, Y. J. (2003). Toward an acoustic typology of motor speech disorders. *Clinical Linguistics & Phonetics, 17,* 427–445.

Kent, R. D., Netsell, R., & Abbs, J. H. (1979). Acoustic characteristics of dysarthria associated with cerebellar disease. *Journal of Speech and Hearing Research, 22,* 627–648.

Kent, R. D., & Rosenbek, J. C. (1983). Acoustic patterns of apraxia of speech. *Journal of Speech and Hearing Research, 26,* 231–249.

Klatt, D. H. (1976). Linguistic uses of segmental duration in English: Acoustic and perceptual evidence. *Journal of the Acoustical Society of America, 59,* 1208–1220.

LeDorze, G., Ryalls, J., Brassard, C., Boulanger, N., & Ratte, D. (1998). A comparison of the prosodic characteristics of the speech of people with Parkinson's disease and Friedreich's ataxia with neurologically normal speakers. *Folia Phoniatrica et Logopaedica, 50,* 1–9.

Lee, J. Y., Gollamudi, S., Ozelius, L. J., Kim J. Y., & Jeon, B. S. (2007). ATP1A3 mutation in the first asian case of rapid-onset dystonia-parkinsonism. *Movement Disorders, 22,* 1808–1809.

Liss, J. M., LeGendre, S., & Lotto, A. (2010). Discriminating dysarthria type from envelope modulation spectra. *Journal of Speech, Language, and Hearing Research, 53,* 1246–1255.

Liss, J. M., White, L., Mattys, S. L., Lansford, K., Lotto, A. J., Spitzer, S. M., & Caviness, J.N. (2009). Quantifying speech rhythm abnormalities in the dysarthrias. *Journal of Speech, Language, and Hearing Research, 52,* 1334–1352.

Low, E. L., Grabe, E., & Nolan, F. (2000). Quantitative characterizations of speech rhythm: "syllable-timing" in Singapore English. *Language and Speech, 43,* 377–401.

McAuliffe, M. J., Ward, E. C., & Murdoch, B. E. (2006). Speech production in Parkinson's disease: II. Acoustic and electropalatographic investigation of sentence, word and segment durations. *Clinical Linguistics & Phonetics, 20,* 19–33.

Nespor, M., and Vogel, I. (1986). *Prosodic phonology.* Dordrecht, The Netherlands: Foris.

Oller, D. K. (1973). The effect of position in utterance on speech segment duration in English. *Journal of the Acoustical Society of America, 54,* 1235–1247.

Patel, R. (2002). Prosodic control in severe dysarthria: Preserved ability to mark the question-statement contrast. *Journal of Speech, Language and Hearing Research, 45,* 858–870.

Patel, R., & Campellone, P. (2009). Acoustic and perceptual cues to contrastive stress in dysarthria. *Journal of Speech, Language & Hearing Research, 52,* 206–222.

Peterson, G., & Lehiste, I. (1960). Duration of syllable nuclei in English. *Journal of the Acoustical Society of America, 32,* 693–703.

Ramus, F., Nespor, M., & Mehler, J. (1999). Correlates of linguistic rhythm in the speech signal. *Cognition, 73,* 265–292.

Ramus, F. (2002). Acoustic correlates of linguistic rhythm: Perspectives. In B. Bel &

I. Marlien (Eds.), *Proceedings of speech prosody 2002* (pp. 115–120). Aix-en-Provence, France.

Selkirk, E. O. (1996). The prosodic structure of function words. In J. L. Morgan & K. Demuth (Eds.), *Signal to syntax: Bootstrapping from speech to grammar in early acquisition* (pp. 187–213). Mahwah, NJ: Lawrence Erlbaum.

Shriberg, L. D., Campbell, T. F., Karlsson, H. B., Brown, R. L., McSweeny, J. L., & Nadler, C. J. (2003). A diagnostic marker for childhood apraxia of speech: The lexical stress ratio. *Clinical Linguistics & Phonetics, 17*, 549–574.

Shriberg, L. D., Green, J. R., Campbell, T. F., McSweeny, J. L., & Scheer, A. R. (2003). A diagnostic marker for childhood apraxia of speech: The coefficient of variation ratio. *Clinical Linguistics & Phonetics, 17*, 575–595.

Spencer, K. A., & Slocomb, D. L. (2007). The neural basis of ataxic dysarthria. *The Cerebellum, 6*, 58–65.

Strand, E. A., & McNeil, M. R. (1996). Effects of length and linguistic complexity on temporal acoustic measures in apraxia of speech. *Journal of Speech and Hearing Research, 39*, 1018–1033.

Tjaden, K., & Turner, G. (2000). Segmental timing in amyotrophic lateral sclerosis. *Journal of Speech, Language and Hearing Research, 43*, 683–696.

Tomik, B., & Guiloff, R. J. (2008, October). Dysarthria in amyotrophic lateral sclerosis: A review. *Amyotrophic lateral sclerosis: official publication of the World Federation of Neurology Research Group on Motor Neuron Diseases*, 1–12.

Turk, A., Nakai, S., & Sugahara, M. (2006). Acoustic segment durations in prosodic research: A practical guide. In S. Sudhoff, D. Lenertova, R. Meyer, S. Pappert, P. Augurzky, I. Mleinek, N. Richter, & J. Schliesser (Eds.), *Methods in empirical prosody research* (pp. 1–28). Berlin, Germany: De Gruyter.

Turk, A. E., & White, L. (1999). Structural influences on accentual lengthening in English. *Journal of Phonetics, 27*, 171–206.

Turner, G. S., & Weismer, G. (1993). Characteristics of speaking rate in the dysarthria associated with amyotrophic lateral sclerosis. *Journal of Speech and Hearing Research, 36*, 1134–1144.

van Santen, J. P. H., Tucker Prud'hommeaux, E., & Black, L. M. (2009). Automated assessment of prosody production. *Speech Communication, 51*, 1082–1097.

Velleman, S. L., & Shriberg, L. D. (1999). Metrical analysis of the speech of children with suspected developmental apraxia of speech. *Journal of Speech and Hearing Research, 42*, 1444–1460

Weismer, G. (1984). Articulatory characteristics of Parkinsonian dysarthria: Segmental and phrase-level timing, spirantization and glottal-supraglottal coordination. In M. R. McNeil, J. C. Rosenbek, & A. E. Aronson (Eds.), *The dysarthrias: Physiology, acoustics, perception, management* (pp. 101–130). San Diego, CA: College-Hill Press.

Weismer, G. (2008). Speech intelligibility. In M. J. Ball, M. R. Perkins, N. Müller, & S. Howard (Eds.), *The handbook of clinical linguistics* (pp. 568–582). Oxford, UK: Blackwell.

Weismer, G., Jeng, J., Laures, J. S., Kent, R. D., & Kent, J. F. (2001). Acoustic and intelligibility characteristics of sentence production in neurogenic speech disorders. *Folia Phoniatrica et Logopaedica, 53*, 1–18.

Weismer, G., Yunusova, Y., & Westbury, J.R. (2003). Interarticulator coordination in dysarthria: An X-ray microbeam study. *Journal of Speech, Language and Hearing Research, 46*, 1247–1261.

White, L., & Mattys, S. L. (2007a). Calibrating rhythm: First language and second language studies. *Journal of Phonetics, 35*, 501–522.

White, L., & Mattys, S.L. (2007b). Rhythmic typology and variation in first and second languages. In P. Prieto, J. Mascaró, & M.-J. Solé (Eds.), *Segmental and prosodic issues in romance phonology. Current issues in linguistic theory series* (pp. 237–257). Amsterdam, The Netherlands: John Benjamins.

White, L., Payne, E., & Mattys, S. L. (2009). Rhythmic and prosodic contrast in Venetan and Sicilian Italian. In M. Vigario, S. Frota, & M. J. Freitas (Eds.), *Phonetics and phonology: Interactions and interrelations* (pp. 137–158). Amsterdam, The Netherlands: John Benjamins.

Wiget, L., White, L., Schuppler, B., Grenon, I., Rauch, O., & Mattys, S. L. (2010). How stable are acoustic metrics of contrastive speech rhythm? *Journal of the Acoustical Society of America, 127,* 1559–1569.

Wightman, C. W., Shattuck-Hufnagel, S. Ostendorf, M., & Price, P. (1992). Segmental durations in the vicinity of prosodic phrase boundaries. *Journal of the Acoustical Society of America, 91,* 1707–1717.

Yunusova, Y., Weismer, G., Westbury, J. R., & Lindstrom, M. J. (2008). Articulatory movements during vowels in speakers with dysarthria and healthy controls. *Journal of Speech, Language and Hearing Research, 51,* 596–611.

Ziegler, W., & Wessel, K. (1996). Speech timing in ataxic disorders: Sentence production and rapid repetitive articulation. *Neurology, 47,* 208–214.

12

Assessment of Intonation

**ANJA KUSCHMANN, M.A., NICK MILLER, PH.D.,
ANJA LOWIT, PH.D., AND INEKE MENNEN, PH.D.**

Introduction

Disturbances of intonation are a frequent accompaniment to acquired motor speech disorders, be it as a direct consequence of the neurological disorder, as a result of compensatory strategies, or as a side effect of treatment for other speech components.

For instance, in the dysarthrias, the underlying neuromuscular disturbance may lead to altered fundamental frequency and loudness control, with reduced envelopes of variation or sudden excessive deviations to pitch and loudness (e.g., Casper, Raphael, Harris, & Geibel, 2007; Darley, Aronson, & Brown, 1969; Duffy, 2005; Patel, 2003; Skodda, Rinsche, & Schlegel, 2009; Wang, Kent, Duffy, & Thomas, 2005). Apraxia of speech, despite intact underlying primary neuromuscular parameters, also is typified by intonation problems in addition to the typically slowed, dysfluent speech caused by difficulties initiating words and syllables (e.g., Boutsen & Christman, 2002; Kent & Rosenbek, 1983; McNeil, Robin, & Schmidt, 2008; Van Putten & Walker, 2003). In both

types of disorder, the pattern of overall fundamental frequency declination commonly is no longer smooth, but may proceed in a series of discrete part-falls or a succession of separate falls without overall declination. There may be a tendency to equalization of stress and syllabic speech. The speaker also may rely on a restricted repertoire of intonational patterns.

Another speech disorder that has been the focus of research on intonation problems is Foreign Accent Syndrome (FAS). FAS is a relatively rare neurologically based speech disorder that is characterized by changes in prosodic and articulatory patterns leading to a perceived foreign accent in speech. Studies investigating speech in FAS frequently have identified an underlying disturbance in rhythm and intonation as a main factor contributing to the perceived foreign accent (e.g. Blumstein, Alexander, Ryalls, Katz, & Dworetzky, 1987; Blumstein & Kurowski, 2006; Kurowski, Blumstein, & Alexander, 1996).

In any type of motor speech disorder, disturbed intonation has the potential to impact on intelligibility, whether, for example, through impaired signalling of word or phrase boundaries, ambiguity from accent (mis)placement, pragmatic disturbances from mis-signalling of new versus given information, or altered cues to turn initiation or ending. The same disturbances considerably impact on affective intelligibility—the speaker is unable to convey the intended tone of voice, irony, or happiness. Listeners may misapprehend the mood or intention of the speaker, interpreting them as depressed or indifferent, angry or sarcastic when none of these impressions are intended. The resulting breakdown in communication or simply the perception that the voice sounds "strange" may act as a demotivating factor in communication activities and participation.

In all the preceding cases, the identification of the origins and manifestations of the prosodic problems ultimately should help to design effective rehabilitative exercises appropriate for the specific type of disturbance. In this respect, detailed assessment of intonation fulfills an important role in charting current status and change across time associated with disease progression or therapeutic input. Aside from clinical issues, though, focused intonation evaluation can address important questions concerning the nature of the underlying disturbance and, thus, inform the debate on the nature of breakdown in different disorders.

One significant limitation of previous research on disordered intonation in motor speech disorders has been that most descriptive and analytical approaches have been restricted to rather general acoustic-phonetic measures such as fundamental frequency modulation, as expressed by F0 range or standard deviation. Without linking the phonetic

features to the corresponding linguistic functions, little can be said about the impact of the observed deviations on the overall communicative ability of the speakers. This void in research may be one of the reasons why, despite its central role in communication, intonation often still takes a backseat when it comes to assessment and intervention. With "the prosodic transcription of pathological speech samples being far from routine" (Crystal, 2009, p. 257), new approaches for intonation analysis are needed to narrow the gap between theory and practice. One promising approach that has the potential to assess intonation from a linguistic perspective is the autosegmental-metrical (AM) framework of intonation theory (Pierrehumbert, 1980; Pierrehumbert & Beckman, 1988). This chapter reviews the potential of this framework to capture intonational deviances in a range of speech disorders and addresses methodological issues that need to be considered when applying this analysis method.

Capturing Intonation— The AM Approach

The ability to vary pitch in order to structure speech is a highly important aspect of communication, and research has shown that this ability often is affected in a range of speech disorders. However, designing an adequate assessment tool to comprehensively capture the features of disordered intonation has proven difficult. One of the major criticisms has been the fact that most protocols are largely based on perceptual analysis; thus introducing a high degree of subjectivity to the assessment of intonation (see Lowit-Leuschel & Docherty, 2000, for an overview of perceptual assessment protocols and methodological issues associated with them). However, with the advancement of technology, new speech analysis tools are becoming more readily available—for example, Praat (Boersma & Weenink, 2009) and Wavesurfer (Sjölander & Beskow, 2000) to name but a few—triggering the development of new approaches toward intonational analysis based on acoustic evidence. The access to analysis tools along with increasing knowledge of the nature of intonation in normal speech has the potential to open up new avenues for the analysis of disordered intonation. Interestingly, until recently, linguistic approaches have not had any noteworthy impact in the clinical setting (Lowit-Leuschel & Docherty, 2000), in which assessment procedures mostly concentrate on the phonetic level of pitch variation in nonspeech tasks. Given the importance of phonetic parameters in the linguistic use of intonation in speech, bridging the gap between these two aspects appears vital to achieve a comprehensive assessment of a client's abilities. A step in the right direction has been made by Peppé and McCann (2003) who recently introduced the PEPS-C test (Profiling Elements of Prosodic Systems —Children) that examines functional aspects of intonation in children (see Diehl & Paul, 2009, for an extensive review of the PEPS-C).

The potential of using recent theoretical frameworks for intonation analysis to investigate disordered speech has been recognized by Kent and Kim (2003). They particularly underlined the potential of the ToBI system for transcribing intonation patterns of spoken language (Beckman & Ayers Elam, 1997), which is based on the autosegmental-metrical (AM) framework of intonational analysis. The framework —originally developed to analyze the intonation of American English—rapidly was developed further and adapted successfully to many other languages. As a result, the AM approach is now well established within the international research community and can be regarded as one of the predominant approaches for analyzing intonation. Within the AM framework, intonation contours are analyzed in terms of a string of abstract phonological categories—the so-called High (H) or Low (L) tones—which are associated with either accented syllables or phrase boundaries. These underlying phonological representations are mapped to acoustic parameters following language specific rules. Consequently, two levels of intonation—phonological representation and phonetic implementation— are distinguished within the AM framework. It is this feature that renders the AM approach so valuable for the investigation of disordered speech. The structural make-up of the AM framework permits one to determine whether the changes observed in disordered intonation are the result of deficits at the underlying representational level or the result of problems affecting the phonetic implementation of the tonal structure.

Despite its potential to differentiate between phonological and phonetic aspects of intonation, only a few studies so far have applied the AM approach or relevant language versions of ToBI to disordered speech (Arbisi-Kelm, 2006; Green & Tobin, 2009; Lowit, Kuschmann, MacLeod, & Mennen, 2010; Mennen,

Schaeffler, Watt, & Miller, 2008). Mennen et al. (2008), for example, used the AM approach to investigate the intonation of read speech in two individuals with hypokinetic dysarthria and could demonstrate that phonological elements of intonation appeared to be preserved in Parkinson's Disease induced dysarthria. However, differences in distribution and phonetic realization suggest difficulties when implementing the phonological categories. These promising findings strengthen the position of the AM framework as an appropriate tool to investigate clinical data, although further research including more participants, different speech disorders, different text styles and varying intonational functions needs to be conducted to determine the degree to which these results can be generalized.

The AM Framework and the Different Dimensions of Intonation

As indicated, the AM framework's main goal is to characterize intonation contours in terms of a sequence of abstract phonological categories and to map those phonological representations onto a phonetic representation. Apart from describing intonation in relation to phonological and phonetic properties, the AM framework also is deemed suitable to answer more fundamental questions of intonation research, such as whether universal features can be found across intonation systems (Jun, 2005; Ladd, 1996). That is, employing the AM framework to a number of typologically different languages would

allow one to identify common universals versus language-specific characteristics. Ladd (1996) suggested four intonational dimensions (systemic, realizational, phonotactic, and semantic), which together would describe the intonation system of a language, language variety or dialect comprehensively (Ladd, 1996, p. 119). Mennen et al. (2008) adopted these four levels in order to describe the intonation system of individuals with speech disorders:

1. Systemic level: The inventory of intonation patterns (i.e., types of pitch accents and boundary tones)
2. Realizational level: The phonetic realization of these patterns
3. Phonotactic level: The distribution of these patterns (e.g., frequency of occurrence)
4. Semantic level: The use of these patterns to signal linguistic functions (e.g., sentence modality, focus).

The information obtained from these four levels has the potential to provide a comprehensive picture of the disordered intonation system, permitting the identification of underlying levels of impairment and a consideration of appropriate management options. Using this approach also ensures that each level of intonation is given equal importance in contributing to the overall picture rather than limiting the analysis to specific aspects of intonation such as phonetic representation or linguistic function, as has been the case in the past.

Each of the four levels will now be described and discussed in relation to what it can tell us about the intonational difficulties of a range of speakers.

Inventory of Intonation Patterns

As described previously, the AM approach represents intonation contours as a string of discrete phonological events (Ladd, 1996), whereby two main types of events can be distinguished: pitch accents and boundary tones. Pitch accents are local intonational features associated with prominent syllables, whereas boundary tones are linked with the edges of prosodic constituents such as intonation phrases. The association with either syllables or the beginnings and ends of phrases reflects the function of both categories: Pitch accents are used to highlight specific information within an utterance; boundary tones are used to structure utterances.

In autosegmental-metrical phonology, pitch accents are analyzed as sequences or combinations of two types of abstract tonal values, H (High) and L (Low). These two tones also are referred to as primitives and constitute the basic elements of the pitch contour. Simple pitch accents are marked using an H or L, respectively; more complex pitch accents are indicated by a combination of both tones. That is, a falling pitch accent is indicated by HL; a rising pitch accent is signalled by LH. In all types of pitch accents, the tone that is associated with the prominent syllable is assigned an asterisk. As an example, H*L describes a falling pitch accent in which the fundamental frequency peak (i.e., the H tone) is associated with the prominent syllable.

Boundary tones also are described by the primitives H and L. They are marked with an % sign, which is placed before or after the tone to indicate whether they describe initial bound-aries (e.g., %L) or final boundaries (e.g., H%). The inventory of pitch accents and boundary tones is language- and dialect-specific. That is, the type and number of pitch accents and boundary tones can differ considerably across languages or language varieties.

The assessment of this level of intonation can help to determine whether individuals with disordered intonation have the full range of pitch accents and boundary tones used in their language or dialectal variety at their disposal. Based on this information, it could be possible to establish whether the mental representations of the phonological categories are retained or affected. For instance, a speaker who has intonation difficulties, but displays the full range of pitch accents, is likely to have problems at the level of implementation rather than higher order processing deficits. On the other hand, the use of a very limited inventory of pitch accents could indicate impaired mental representations.

Realization of Intonation Patterns

Although the inventory of pitch accents for a given language variety is well-defined at the abstract phonological level, phonetically the pitch accents can be realized in very different ways. Several factors are known to have a role in defining the overall phonetic implementation of intonation contours. A common aspect influencing the shape of a contour involves natural physiological processes such as declination. In healthy speech, fundamental frequency tends to decline over the course of phrases. That is, pitch accents realized toward the end of a phrase are usually lower in fundamental frequency than pitch accents in initial position.

This interaction of local and global features that shape the phonetic realization of phonological categories in healthy speech is not necessarily present in disordered intonation. Depending on the nature of the speech disorder, a lack of breath support, muscle control, or planning difficulties may considerably influence the way the different abstract categories are realized phonetically. For example, due to muscle weakness, a person with Parkinson's Disease (PD) might realize a falling pitch accent (H*L) in a flattened way compared to a healthy speaker (Figure 12–1A and B). Although the pitch range in the two speakers differs considerably, the underlying pattern (i.e., the H*L pitch accent) remains the same in both cases.

A further aspect that can impact considerably on the way intonation patterns are realized in disordered speech is the (involuntary) break-up of intonation phrases into smaller units due to for example, inappropriate pause placement. A healthy speaker can produce between five and eight words in one intonation phrase (Crystal, 1969). Speakers with difficulties such as poor breath support might not be able to achieve this and instead break an utterance up into smaller intonational units, each with their own boundary tones and pitch accents. This may give rise to an impression of over-accentuation, which in this case would be due purely to physiological factors and not higher order phonological planning problems. That is, intonational difficulties can be secondary to changes in the phrasing of utterances.

Distribution of Intonation Patterns

The distributional analysis of elements concerns the position and frequency of pitch accents and boundary tones. Assessing those patterns can provide information on the potential restrictions occurring within the intonation system. These restrictions, alongside information from other levels of intonation, can provide insight into the mechanism underlying the intonation disturbance.

The assessment of the distribution patterns of *pitch accents* is useful to get information as to the prevailing pitch accent used by a speaker. In British English dialects (with some notable exceptions such as Newcastle or Belfast English), the most common pitch accent is the falling accent (Grabe, Post, Nolan, & Farrar, 2000; Willems, 1982). Some patients, however, might show a prevalence of L*H, or H* (Figure 12–2A and B). Such differences in pitch pattern distribution can be indicative of problems in the planning of the pitch movements, as well as difficulties reaching the intended target quickly enough due to physiological weakness, or indeed a compensatory strategy—for example, trading intonational accuracy against articulatory precision or as a way of holding a conversational place.

An analysis of the use and position of *boundary tones* has the potential to provide information regarding the phrasing abilities of speakers and the factors contributing to the way the phrases are realized. In normal speech, pauses and boundary tones often are placed in positions that coincide with syntactic boundaries. Individuals with speech disorders, however, might struggle to

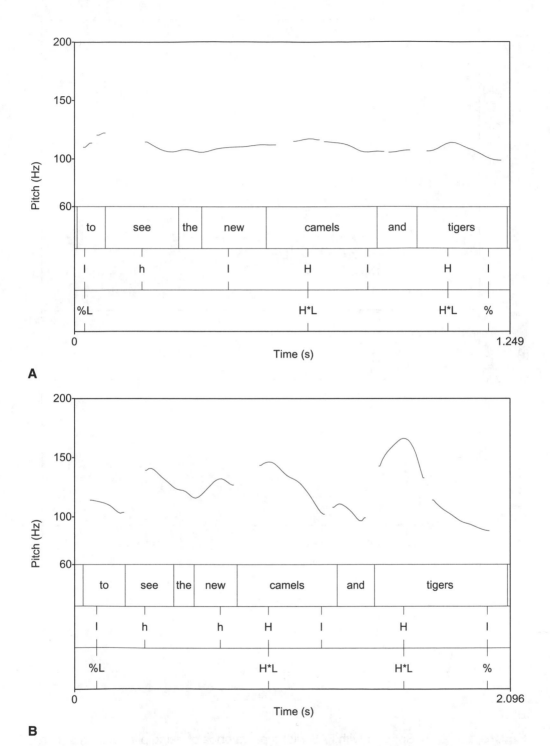

Figure 12–1. A. Example of a flattened contour with H*L pitch accents by a speaker with PD (tier 1: word level; tier 2: phonetic labels; tier 3: phonological labels). **B.** The same phrase produced by a control speaker.

259

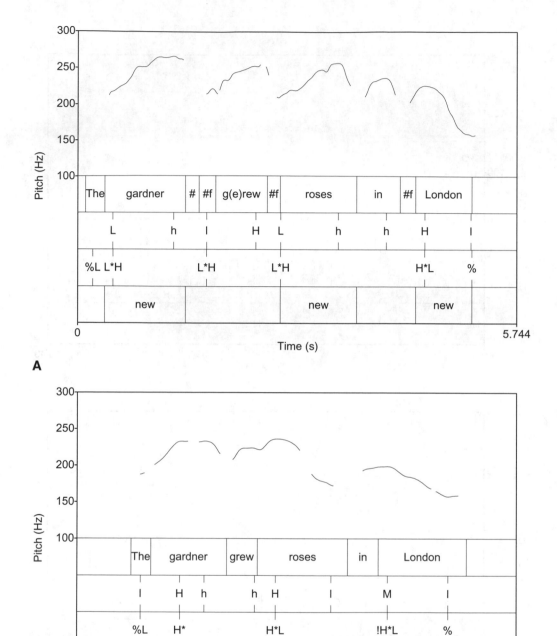

Figure 12–2. A. Speaker with FAS with a prevalence of rising pitch accents (tier 1: word level; tier 2: phonetic labels; tier 3: phonological labels; tier 4: function, marking of givenness; # = pause, #f = filled pause). **B.** The same sentence produced by a control speaker, in which a variety of pitch accents can be observed.

do so. Mennen et al. (2008); Kuschmann, Lowit, Miller, and Mennen (2008); and Heselwood (2007), for example, found that their clients had smaller phrasing units than the control speakers, and often had to take breaths within intonation phrases. That is, pauses often indicated by boundary tones were found at inappropriate places such as in the middle of a verbal phrase and, thus, did not coincide with syntactic boundaries. The inappropriate pausing patterns of the speakers were almost certainly caused by poor breath control (though not exclusively, see Weismer, 1997, for other physiological factors affecting speech breathing) and, therefore, are likely to be found in other populations with disordered speech, too.

Functions of Intonation

The term *intonation* refers to the meaningful pitch variation in speech. In spoken language, intonation serves diverse functions that can be classified according to the type of information they convey: extralinguistic, paralinguistic, or linguistic. The following section provides a brief overview of the diverse functions of intonation, with a main emphasis on the linguistic function and its relation to the remaining dimensions of intonation (for more exhaustive descriptions of intonational functions, see Cruttenden, 1997, and Gussenhoven, 2004).

Extralinguistic intonation provides information on the biological features of a speaker including aspects such as age, sex, and anatomical features; paralinguistic aspects of intonation reflect a speaker's attitude or status or the emotional state of the person. In both instances, the modification of intonation typically is not directly under the speaker's volitional control, reflecting the nonsystematic nature of extra- and paralinguistic aspects. By contrast, linguistic intonation can be controlled purposefully by speakers, and its systematic use is inherent to other linguistic levels such as grammar or pragmatics. The linguistic use of intonation ranges from indicating sentence modality to structuring discourse by means of focus and givenness. Although there is no one-to-one relationship between pitch patterns and linguistic meaning, it is accepted generally that intonation patterns can differentiate between various linguistic and pragmatic meanings. In other words, depending on the linguistic function, the manifestation of intonation—that is, the use of pitch accents and boundary tones—can differ considerably.

A number of linguistic functions can be investigated using the approach proposed here. This includes the aforementioned assessment of sentence modality, but also the pragmatic structuring of discourse. Both linguistic functions are described in greater detail later in this section. In this context, we also will assess how the different functions model the distribution and realisation patterns, and how difficulties in that area may affect a speaker's communicative abilities.

The indication of sentence modality (e.g., question versus statement) is one of the most undisputed linguistic functions of intonation. A common perception is that a rising pitch at the end of an utterance indicates a question, whereas falling pitch would signal a statement (cf., He is \leaving. versus He is /leaving?). However, this dichotomy of rising and falling intonation becomes redundant when sentence modality is signalled grammatically, such as in wh-questions, which can be produced with both rising and falling pitch patterns (cf., Where is he /going? versus What's he \doing?). The ability to vary pitch at the end of phrases is not only important to differentiate between questions and statements but also for turn-taking in dialogue situations. A low pitch at the end of phrases can signal the end of a turn, whereas a high pitch can express the intention to keep the turn. Cases in which the varying of pitch is affected, interpersonal communication might be more difficult as the speaker may struggle to indicate questions and statements, or his intention to keep the turn. At the same time, the interlocutor may experience difficulties in interpreting intentions and react inappropriately (e.g., Patel, 2002; 2003, and Chapter 4 this book).

Another important linguistic function of intonation is the pragmatic organization of information in discourse. Generally, a speaker selects the information units he considers to be important or new(sworthy) and highlights them (Gussenhoven, 2004). This way, the listener's attention is directed to the important information in an utterance. In West-Germanic languages, new information, or the information in focus, usually is marked by a pitch accent, while post-focal materials are de-accented. The salience of new information is signalled using a number of perceptual cues including pitch, loudness, and length, with pitch being the primary cue (Beckman, 1986). However, in dis-

ordered speech, acoustic cues might be traded in order to compensate for parameters over which there is no or only limited control. In other words, a speaker may employ only those parameters s/he can effectively control. In this case, pitch might not necessarily be the most important cue for prominence.

When assessing information structure, it is important to check whether the ability to highlight specific words in an utterance is retained, and if so, which parameters are employed for this. Where modulation of intonation is affected, it is important to find out how this deficit manifests itself in speech. For example, too many or too few words might be highlighted, making it harder for the listener to detect the relevant information. A similar effect can arise from difficulties with de-accentuation.

A detailed assessment of these four levels potentially can aid the identification of factors underlying the intonational disturbance, contribute information for differential diagnosis, and provide the detail necessary for effective treatment planning. For example, a comprehensive inventorial assessment might contribute to the perennial debate of whether the altered intonational use observed in Parkinson's Disease is due to physiological reasons or higher order planning problems (e.g., Penner, Miller, Hertrich, Ackermann, & Schumm, 2001, 2006; Van Lancker Sidtis, Pachana, Cummings, & Sidtis, 2006). Similarly, the analysis may aid the differential diagnosis of apraxia of speech (as a putative breakdown of phonetic encoding of well formed phonological specifications) and phonemic paraphasia (as a possible impairment of phonology, and from the perspective of intonation, of the assignment of prosodic features at a premotoric stage in output, e.g., Baum & Pell, 1999; McNeil et al., 2008; Odell, McNeil, Rosenbek, & Hunter, 1991). Identifying whether speakers with intonation deficits have full access to the range of pitch accents in their language also is crucial for the decision on how to approach the management of the intonational impairment. Where the phonological representations are retained and accessible, it stands to reason to concentrate on the factors affecting the implementation of the categories.

There, thus, exists a clear argument for the application of the AM approach to disordered speech. Anyone endeavouring to adopt this methodology will be aided by the fact that a significant corpus of research results is already available, profiling how healthy speakers signal meaning through intonation at the various levels described. However, what often is not immediately evident from the existing literature are the potential problems that may arise from the approach, particularly when used with participants with motor speech disorders. The following section addresses some of the methodological issues that should be considered when applying the AM approach to this speaker population.

Methodological Issues

Potential Problems

By its very nature, intonational analysis has to rely on the perception of pitch and an acoustic and visual inspection of the fundamental frequency signal. This is, of course, not without its problems particularly in disorders that are neurological in origin. The AM approach

to intonational analysis does not escape these problems. For example, it is difficult to obtain a reliable F0 trace when the voice quality is poor. In some cases, such as PD, the voice of the speaker may be so weak that an F0 trace cannot be computed. More frequently, the F0 contour is distorted, rendering the obtained F0 values unreliable. This may be the case with laryngeal problems, in which a speaker's voice may sound very husky or creaky. At times, these problems may render the acoustic signal so poor that an analysis of pitch is virtually impossible (Figure 12–3). F0 values in speakers with significant tremor in the voice also should be considered with caution, as the tremor may produce a shaky pitch contour that may be difficult to interpret. Some of these cases may be correctable through manual rather than automatic pitch analysis. However, this is time consuming and unrealistic for large data samples. If the voice problem is fluctuating, capturing a large amount of data (e.g., more test items or repetitions thereof) can solve the problem partly as very poor samples can be disregarded from the analysis without affecting the overall power of results too much. If a client presents with a voice problem so significant that no or very few useable pitch traces can be obtained, the current approach will not be suitable.

A further point for consideration in intonational analysis is the fact that intonation patterns may differ substantially depending on the type of elicitation. Differences in intonational inventories (i.e., pitch accents and boundary tones) were observed across text styles (e.g., Grice, Savino, & Refice, 1997), highlighting the relevance of the data elicitation method for the modeling of

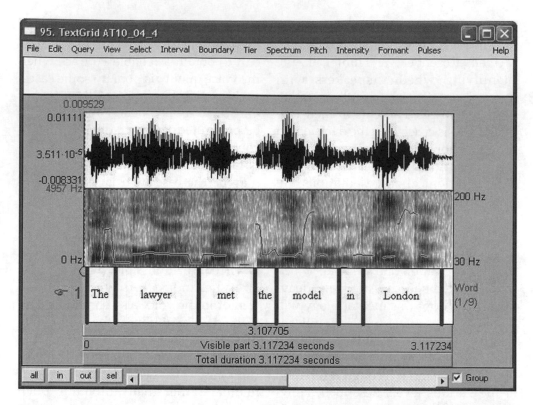

Figure 12–3. Distorted F0 contour due to creaky voice in a speaker with ataxic dysarthria.

intonation. This observation in healthy individuals may be of even more importance for the analysis of disordered intonation as the neurological condition can have an impact on the way different tasks are understood and executed. Reading a text passage, for example, may be easier for certain speakers than producing spontaneous speech, in which the planning component adds to the overall cognitive effort needed to produce speech. This difference in cognitive demand could have an impact on an individual's intonational inventory. Similar to any other type of speech evaluation (cf., intelligibility, rate, etc.), it is, therefore, important to assess speakers across a range of speaking styles to gain a full picture of their abilities.

It also should be kept in mind that some of the differences in relation to the inventory and distribution of categories in healthy as well as disordered speech can further be attributed to normal variation. That is, speakers of a language variety may differ regarding the use of certain categories and the way phonetic cues are exploited to indicate linguistic function.

Minimizing Potential Methodological Problems

Although the previously mentioned problems can complicate the analysis of intonation, they do not preclude the application of the AM approach to disordered speech. Careful construction of elicitation materials can go some way to reducing the potential impact of disordered features on the analysis.

In order to facilitate pitch track analysis, it is important to construct sentences or choose materials that contain as many sonorant elements as possible. That way, the F0 traces are more likely to be correctly computed and not affected by spurious measures such as octave errors or various micro-prosodic effects on the F0 trace due to consonantal perturbations such as bursts of F0 dips (Figure 12–4).

Another aspect to consider when choosing or devising materials is the length of utterances to be elicited. Where breath control problems are evident, longer utterances are likely to be split up in to shorter phrasing units. As discussed previously, this can have an impact on the shape of the intonation contour and the way intonation is used functionally. When designing sentence materials, it may, therefore, be advisable to vary lengths of sentences, combining shorter and longer utterances to evaluate the effect of length on speaker performance.

Alongside choosing the materials wisely, it is furthermore important to keep in mind that one is dealing with individuals who suffer(ed) from a neurological condition. Fatigue is a principal factor likely to have an effect on overall speech performance, giving poorer voice quality or flatter intonation contours.

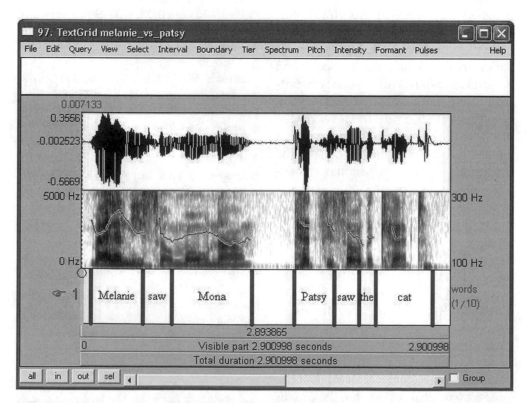

Figure 12–4. Influence of sonorance on the pitch contour display: Melanie saw Mona (*left*) versus Patsy saw the cat (*right*).

Accordingly, the duration of the assessment should be considered carefully in order to obtain optimum data. The length of the assessment procedure, however, will need to be balanced with the amount of data necessary to yield sound statistical results. Depending on the nature of the speech disorder, some utterances might need to be excluded. Collecting the right amount of data but preventing fatigue may not always be easy, and researchers should contemplate whether the advantages of assessing intonation over two sessions may outweigh its disadvantages.

Conclusion

By applying the AM approach to disordered speech, one is able to obtain comprehensive information as to the categorical, realizational, distributional, and functional aspects of intonation patterns. By using this framework, it may be possible to identify the level of disturbance and to explain how the deficit relates to the problems that arise in the functional use of intonational categories. The analysis of intonation patterns using the AM approach has the potential to highlight how different underlying causes can surface and manifest as similar intonation difficulties. It is this ability of the AM approach to differentiate between different underlying causes that makes it so valuable for the investigation of disordered speech. Although there are clear benefits from using such an approach not just in research, but also in clinical management, there is still a long way to go to overcome the practical challenges that the comprehensive transcription of intonation poses in

such settings. However, trying to incorporate and routinely establish "a reasonable prosodic transcription" (Crystal, 2009, p. 257) already would be a step in the right direction.

Acknowledgment. This work was supported by the British Academy, award number SG-44232, and by Ataxia UK. The final author was supported by the ESRC grant RES-000-22-2419.

References

Arbisi-Kelm, T. R. (2006). *An Intonational Analysis of Disfluency Patterns in Stuttering.* Doctoral Dissertation, University of California, Los Angeles.

Baum, S. R. & Pell, M. D. (1999). The neural bases of prosody: Insights from lesion studies and neuroimaging. *Aphasiology, 13*(8), 581–608.

Beckman, M. E. (1986). *Stress and non-stress accent.* Dordrecht, Holland: Foris.

Beckman, M. E., & Ayers Elam, G. (March, 1997). *Guidelines for ToBI labeling* (version 3). The Ohio State University Research Foundation.

Blumstein, S. E., & Kurowski, K. (2006). The foreign accent syndrome: A perspective. *Journal of Neurolinguistics, 19*, 346–355.

Blumstein, S. E., Alexander, M. P., Ryalls, J. H., Katz, W., & Dworetzky, B. (1987). On the nature of the foreign accent syndrome: A case study. *Brain & Language, 31*, 215–244.

Boersma, P., & Weenink, D. (2009). *Praat: Doing phonetics by computer.* Institute of Phonetic Sciences of the University of Amsterdam.

Boutsen, F. R., & Christman, S. S. (2002). Prosody in apraxia of speech. *Seminars in Speech and Language, 23*(4), 245–256.

Casper, M. A., Raphael, L. J., Harris, K. S., & Geibel, J. M. (2007). Speech prosody in cerebellar ataxia. *International Journal of Language and Communication Disorders,* 42(4), 407–426.

Cruttenden, A. (1997). *Intonation.* Cambridge, UK: Cambridge University Press.

Crystal, D. (1969). *Prosodic systems and intonation in English.* Cambridge, UK: Cambridge University Press.

Crystal, D. (2009). Persevering with prosody. *International Journal of Speech-Language Pathology,* 11(4), 257.

Darley, F. L., Aronson, A. E., & Brown, J. R. (1969). Clusters of deviant speech dimensions in the dysarthrias, *Journal of Speech and Hearing Research,* 12, 462–496.

Diehl, J. J., & Paul, R. (2009). The assessment and treatment of prosodic disorders and neurological theories of prosody. *International Journal of Speech-Language Pathology,* 11(4), 287–292.

Duffy, J. (2005). *Motor speech disorders* (2nd ed.). St Louis, MO: Mosby.

Grabe, E., Post, B., Nolan, F., & Farrar, K. (2000). Pitch accent realization in four varieties of British English. *Journal of Phonetics,* 28, 161–195.

Green, H. & Tobin, Y. (2009). Prosodic analysis is difficult . . . but worth it: A study in high functioning autism. *International Journal of Speech-Language Pathology,* 11(4), 308–315.

Grice, M., Savino, M., & Refice, M. (1997). The intonation of questions in Bari Italian: Do speakers replicate their spontaneous speech when reading? *Phonus,* 3, 1–7.

Gussenhoven, C. (2004). *The phonology of tone and intonation.* Cambridge, UK: Cambridge University Press.

Heselwood, B. (2007). Breathing-impaired speech after brain haemorrhage: A case study. *Clinical Linguistics & Phonetics,* 21, 577–604.

Jun, S-A. (2005). *Prosodic typology: The phonology of intonation and phrasing.* Oxford, UK: Oxford University Press.

Kent, R. D., & Rosenbek, J. C. (1983). Acoustic patterns of apraxia of speech. *Journal of Speech and Hearing Research,* 26(2), 231–249.

Kent, R. D., & Kim, Y.-J. (2003). Toward an acoustic typology of motor speech disorders. *Clinical Linguistics & Phonetics,* 17(6), 427–445.

Kurowski, K. M., Blumstein, S. E., & Alexander, M. (1996). The foreign accent syndrome: A reconsideration. *Brain & Language,* 54, 1–25.

Kuschmann, A, Lowit, A., Miller, N., & Mennen, I. (2008). *Intonational realisation of information status in foreign accent syndrome (FAS).* Poster presented at the BAAP colloquium, March/April 2008, Sheffield, UK.

Ladd, D. R. (1996). *Intonational phonology.* Cambridge, UK: Cambridge University Press.

Lowit, A., Kuschmann, A., MacLeod, J. & Mennen, I. (2010). *Rhythm and intonation in ataxic dysarthria.* Paper presented at 15th Biennial Conference on Motor Speech. Savannah, GA.

Lowit-Leuschel, A., & Docherty, G. (2000). Dysprosody. In R. D. Kent and M. J. Ball (Eds.), *The handbook of voice quality measurement* (pp. 59–72). San Diego, CA: Singular.

McNeil, M., Robin, D., & Schmidt, R. (2008). Apraxia of speech. In M. McNeil (Ed.), *Clinical management of sensorimotor speech disorders* (pp. 249–268). New York, NY: Thieme.

Mennen, I., Schaeffler, F., Watt, N., & Miller, N. (2008). An auto-segmental-metrical investigation of intonation in people with Parkinson's Disease. *Asia Pacific Journal of Speech, Language, and Hearing,* 11(4), 205–219.

Odell, K., McNeil, M. R., Rosenbek, J. C., & Hunter, L. (1991). Perceptual characteristics of vowel and prosody production in apraxic, aphasic, and dysarthric speakers. *Journal of Speech and Hearing Research,* 34(1), 67–80.

Patel, R. (2002). Prosodic control in severe dysarthria: Preserved ability to mark the question-statement contrast. *Journal of Speech, Language, and Hearing Research,* 45(5), 858–870.

Patel, R. (2003). Acoustic characteristics of the question-statement contrast in severe dysarthria due to cerebral palsy. *Journal of Speech, Language, and Hearing Research, 46*(6), 1401–1415.

Penner, H., Miller, N., Hertrich, I., Ackermann, H., Schumm, F. (2001). Dysprosody in Parkinson's disease: An investigation of intonation patterns. *Clinical Linguistics and Phonetics, 15*, 551-566.

Penner, H., Miller, N., Hertrich, I., Ackermann, H., & Schumm, F. (2006). Is impaired intonation in speakers suffering from Parkinson's disease caused at a motor or at a planning level? *Journal of the Neurological Sciences, 248*(1–2), 279.

Peppé, S., & McCann, J. (2003). Assessing intonation and prosody in children with atypical language development: The PEPS-C test and the revised version. *Clinical Linguistics & Phonetics, 17*, 345–354.

Pierrehumbert, J. (1980). *The phonology and phonetics of English intonation.* Doctoral dissertation. Cambridge, MA: MIT.

Pierrehumbert, J., B., & Beckman, M. E. (1988). *Japanese tone structure.* Cambridge, MA: MIT.

Sjölander, K., & Beskow, J. (2000). Wavesurfer An open source speech tool. *ICSLP 2000,* (4), 464–467.

Skodda, S., Rinsche, H., & Schlegel, U. (2009). Progression of dysprosody in Parkinson's disease over time-a longitudinal study. *Movement Disorders, 24*(5), 716–722.

Van Lancker Sidtis, D., Pachana, N., Cummings, J. L., & Sidtis, J. J. (2006). Dysprosodic speech following basal ganglia insult: Toward a conceptual framework for the study of the cerebral representation of prosody. *Brain & Language, 97*(2), 135–53.

Van Putten, S. M., & Walker, J. P. (2003). The production of emotional prosody in varying degrees of severity of apraxia of speech. *Journal of Communication Disorders, 36*(1), 77–95.

Wang, Y. T., Kent, R. D., Duffy, J. R., & Thomas, J. E. (2005). Dysarthria in traumatic brain injury: A breath group and intonational analysis. *Folia Phoniatrica et Logopaedica, 57*(2), 59–89.

Weismer, G. (1997). Motor speech disorders. In W. J. Hardcastle and J. Laver (Eds.), *The handbook of phonetic sciences* (pp. 191–219). Cambridge, MA: Blackwell.

Willems, N. (1982). *English intonation form a Dutch point of view.* Dordrecht, Holland: Foris.

13

Variability and Coordination Indices and Their Applicability to Motor Speech Disorders

PETER HOWELL, PH.D., ANDREW ANDERSON, PH.D., AND ANJA LOWIT, PH.D

Introduction

Controlling the articulators to produce fluent, intelligible speech is a complex motor control activity. Articulatory movements have to be executed quickly, as well as being precisely targeted and coordinated. In addition, articulatory maneuvers need to be adaptable to retain phonetic stability in different speaking circumstances, such as different phonetic environments (co-articulation), different speaking rates, or when external influences are imposed (e.g., obstructions in the oral cavity in the form of a bite block, etc.).

The question of how speakers are able to achieve and maintain precise control in the context of internal and external constraints on speech production is a growing area of research inter-est, both in relation to unimpaired speakers, as well as in speakers with a range of disorders (including dysarthria, apraxia, stammering, and cleft palate). Instrumental analysis techniques have served to illuminate some of the processes involved in speech motor control and have been able to point to disturbances in underlying pathology that were not readily apparent in perceptual analyses. In addition, instrumental measurements of speech and motor indicators of control have the potential to identify which speech subsystems need to be addressed in therapy and which technique is most effective in doing so.

Developments in instrumental analysis include advances and refinements in available techniques and in data evaluation procedures. One area of growing interest is speech variability.

Although two productions of the same syllable, word, or utterance may appear identical perceptually, subtle variations across productions are the norm, even in healthy speakers. Disordered speech commonly is considered to be more variable than unimpaired articulation, both at the segmental and suprasegmental level. Initially measures of variability were relatively crude, based upon speech segment duration, or pitch and volume of salient speech features. In the last 15 years more, refined variability indices for analyzing variation over time have started to be used routinely. Using these variability indices, researchers have attempted to quantify what amount of variation is natural (i.e., the amount that occurs in competent adult speakers) in order to capture differences in motor control in response to changes in internal and external task demands, in developing or aging speakers or in people with speech disorders. In addition, techniques currently are being developed further that establish how well a speaker can achieve coordinated movement of the articulators.

For variability and coordination indices to be used in such investigations, both for research and possibly for clinical purposes, they should be easy to obtain procedurally and computationally, have external validity, and be sensitive to features of disorders that are expressed in different deficits. The aim of this chapter is to provide a guide to currently available variability and coordination indices for speaker- and task-variability.

The following sections will focus on (1) terminology; (2) popular speech tasks that have been employed and their associated requirements; (3) the collection of articulatory data; (4) analysis of the articulatory movement data; (5) a description of the statistics available; (6) software resources for estimating variability and coordination; and (7) an illustration of the applicability of these techniques to motor speech disorder.

Terminology

Variability

Variability can be measured on a repetition of a single action. In the present context, this could be a measure from a single articulator. The spatial and temporal dimensions of speech signals can be estimated together to give a joint measure of both dimensions or separately to give variability measures of each dimension. When considered separately, the spatial component represents displacement, that is, the degree of movement excursion whereas the temporal component represents the sequencing of actions (see Smith and Goffman, 2004, for a review of variability).

Coordination

Fluent speech is highly reliant on synchronization across articulators. If a gesture in one articulator is not appropriately timed relative to others, speech may be dysfluent.

Coordination indices give a measure of the relative timing precision of two or more articulators. One technique is described by Smith and Zelaznik (2004) who examined variability in lower lip and upper lip separately and then compared this to lip aperture (the magnitude of lower lip and upper lip displacement summed). An alternative measure described by Howell, Anderson, and Lucero (2010) involves the use of a time-warping procedure to generate independent estimates of relative timing error in different signals to support estimation of coordination. Further details on how coordination is measured are provided below.

Tasks and Associated Requirements

A number of tasks have been used to assess variability and coordination, ranging from highly structured to more naturalistic.

Spontaneous Speech Tasks

Spontaneous speech is a natural activity for most people, and it has the highest external validity (in the sense that there is the least experimentally introduced bias). The downside of high external validity is that there is little control of the exact material the speaker produces. It is thus difficult to ensure that the necessary elements to calculate variability are present in the data (such as several repetitions of a syllable of word in the appropriate context). One measure that can be applied to spontaneous speech is the pairwise variability index (PVI) or related measures (cf., Varco V or C, % V, etc., see Chapter 11, "Assessment of Rhythm," by White, Liss, & Dellwo, this book). However, it should be noted that such indices have been developed primarily to capture rhythmic differences across languages, or more recently between disordered

and healthy speakers, rather than to identify the level of movement variability indicative of motor control function that is the focus of this chapter. Spontaneous speech is, thus, not particularly suitable to assess movement variability in the current sense.

Metronome Speaking

Whilst spontaneous speech tasks index natural rhythmic activity, experimental techniques have employed more structured tasks to account for the type of variability discussed in this chapter. These constrain participants in various ways. In contrast to spontaneous speech tasks, the procedures have high control over what is said, but low external validity. One technique, originally developed for studying isochronous finger tapping, has been modified for use with speech sounds (Wing & Kristofferson, 1973). In the tapping task, subjects start by tapping along with an isochronous metronome click. After responses are entrained to the metronome's rate, the click is switched off and participants continue the response sequence alone. In the speech version of the task, speakers repeat a syllable at an isochronous rhythm.

Exact Phrase Repetition

As its name suggests, in exact phrase repetition, speakers attempt to repeat the same phrase identically. Signals representing direct (Smith & Goffman, 2004) or indirect (Howell, Anderson, Bartrip, & Bailey, 2009) measures of articulation are obtained. The task has lower external validity than spontaneous speech, but in principle analyzes the same articulatory maneuvers and is more natural than isochronous repetition of a single syllable. The data obtained can be examined in a variety of ways to establish how variable speakers are. Techniques that have been used include measurements of the timing of oral opening and closing actions (Gracco & Lofqvist, 1994), Smith's spatiotemporal index (Smith, Goffman, Zelaznik, Ying, & McGillem, 1995) and functional data analysis (Lucero, Munhall, Gracco, & Ramsay, 1997; Ramsay & Silverman, 1997). The latter two are discussed more fully below (Linear and Non-Linear Estimators).

Measures of Articulatory Movement

In taking methodological decisions it is important to consider which parameters can characterize task performance or how a disorder may affect speech control.. For example, one popular extract used in exact phrase repetition is "Buy Bobby a puppy." This is convenient as it involves a lot of lip movement that can be relatively easily measured through kinematic analysis. Also, it has proven success, as it has been shown to be sensitive to various task manipulations and has provided evidence of differences between participant groups (Smith & Goffman, 2004). However, lip movement may not be the best way of assessing every speech disorder. For a start, specialized equipment is necessary to capture the data accurately. The kinematic data capturing procedure can raise ethical issues when used with young children or

clients with disorders. Furthermore, material assessing lip movement would not necessarily be suited to capture all types of speech perturbations. Measures other than lip movement may be required including those suited to registering movement of articulators internal to the vocal tract for some purposes. In this section we consider some readily available direct and indirect measurements that can be applied to articulators, including the lips and tongue. For a more detailed discussion of these techniques, refer to Chapter 10, "Biodynamics of Speech and Orofacial Movement," by Barlow, Poore, & Chu as well as Chapter 3, "Physiological Assessment," by Murdoch in this book.

Direct External Measurements

Lip movement can be measured in various ways. One of the earliest forms was the Abbs' headcage. This apparatus obtains upper lip, lower lip, and jaw movement signals using strain gauge transducers, which measure movement along a superior-inferior plane. The transducers are suspended from a headcage superstructure, which consists of a low-mass tubular aluminum assembly that is adjustable in order to accommodate variations and asymmetries of head size (Barlow, Cole, & Abbs, 1983). The cantilever/strain gauge modules are connected to an integrated circuit socket and the output from each of the strain gauge transducers is passed, after amplification and filtering, to a computer for data processing.

More recent studies use the Optotrack system to track lip movement (see current work by Smith). Markers are placed on the face that the Optotrack apparatus tracks. This is easier to use than the headcage support system (for instance, stability can be a problem with the headcage and has to be checked frequently). Both the Abbs' headcage and Optotrack are relatively cheap and easy to use. However, overheads are associated with assembly and calibration. It is also possible to go a step beyond the multisensory Optotrack system and video the movements of the entire face (and other parts of the body involved in speech activity). Hill (in press) has provided a useful summary of the articulatory features available from views of the face. The overall length of the vocal tract, position of maximum constriction of the tongue (when the lips are open) as well as lip aperture may be obtained from a static image. Dynamic images provide additional information (particularly regarding the place of articulation of consonants). Image analysis procedures can be applied to video images to identify regions of movement associated with articulation. These are computationally expensive but may be justified in terms of the additional information they supply.

Ultrasound is another measure that is particularly useful for examining tongue movements for clinical (Stone, 2005) and basic research (Davidson, 2005; Gick, 2002). These systems are easy to use, produce relatively good images and currently are being developed for use in speech movement measurements. A drawback is that ultrasound does not provide images of other structures in the vocal tract that need to be coordinated with tongue movement. For example, the position of the tongue relative to the hard palate cannot be determined, and it cannot provide information about the velum.

MRI also is starting to be used to measure articulatory activity. The articulators and their movement are imaged and provide all information necessary for determining variability and coordination. The application of these techniques is still in its research phase though and costs are likely to continue to be high, prohibiting their routine use for the foreseeable future.

Direct Internal Measurements

Several procedures are available to measure activity within the vocal tract. One example is the electromagnetic articulograph (EMA) system. This system tracks the movement of pellets attached to particular articulators of interest to the experimenter. This could include lips and different parts of the tongue. The markers are relatively easy to track, but the problem for clinical applications is that they are invasive and use expensive equipment.

Electropalatographs (EPGs) provide a record of the contact pattern of the tongue against the palate. These provide detailed information about contact patterns, which then can be compared across repetitions of the same speech item. However, a special palate has to be made for each speaker that may preclude immediate examination, and costs might not justify the production of such a palate for variability testing alone.

Indirect Measurements

The internal activity of the vocal tract also can be estimated indirectly. For instance, measures of laryngeal activity can be obtained from the audio signal in terms of fundamental frequency, intensity, voice quality measures, etc. Similarly, formant frequencies provide information on the position of the tongue; spectrographic information can indicate how individual articulators work and how well different speech systems coordinate through timing measures such as segment duration or voice onset time, indications of nasality and voicing, etc.

Studies employing the STI measure historically have employed direct measures of lip movement (Smith & Goffman, 2004), hence the standard test sentence "Buy Bobby a puppy." However, Howell et al. (2009) have shown that indirect measures such as speech energy variation over time obtained directly from audio recordings (signal rectified and low-pass filtered) also can be used to provide a suitable signal for estimating STI. This opens up new avenues for the use of variability measures, particularly in disordered populations. First of all, the fact that no specialized equipment beyond a high quality sound recorder and microphone is necessary reduces costs significantly and paves the way for clinical application of the technique. In addition, acoustic data capture can be combined with fMRI (recordings made during silent scan phases), which is precluded by approaches dependent on metal components. Finally, audio recordings are noninvasive and, thus, easier to obtain from the participants' point of view, particularly when these come from disordered populations who might experience hypersensitivity of oral structures, etc. The reduced time required in setting up the experiment contributes further to this advantage.

Measurement of Coordination

Before leaving this section, a brief word is necessary about measuring concurrent activity in different articulators that is necessary to examine coordinated movements in speech (and in swallowing). The headcage and Optotrack systems can measure only externally visible components of speech. Audio measures (laryngeal and vocal tract indirect measures) could be used on their own in some cases, or in conjunction with the preceding systems (this also applies to EPG and EMA). EMA and MRI represent marker and markerless schemes, respectively, for assessing articulators that need to be coordinated.

Quantifying Variability and Coordination

Clock and Motor Variance

The Wing and Kristofferson (1973) technique uses isochronous (finger and speech tapping) data and decomposes the total variance into clock and motor components. Variance associated with time-keeping processes (clock variance, Cv) can be estimated separately from that associated with motor (motor variance, Mv) components. To do this, Wing and Kristofferson (1973) assumed that when a motor response deviated from its required position, two intervals were affected: If the response was ahead of its required position, the preceding interval would be short, and the following interval would be long. In contrast, time-keeper variability would be independent of the previous tap. Based on this, an estimate of Mv was obtained from the negative covariance between adjacent response intervals (lag one autocovariance). Cv and other residual components then were obtained by subtracting 2Mv from the total variance (Tv). In further work, Wing (1980) validated that the residual provided an estimate of Cv by showing that Cv increased in line with the length of the interval that subjects were required to repeat (repetition interval). This would be expected if keeping the time of long intervals is more difficult than keeping the time of short intervals and if difficulty is reflected in more variable responses. Mv, on the other hand, remained constant across the repetition interval.

More complicated models have been developed by Wing and other authors (Vorberg and Wing, 1996; Williamson 1998; Beek, Peper, & Daffertshofer, 2002). All trace their origins back, to some extent, to the Wing-Kristofferson model. This model endures because it is robust and simple to use relative to the other related methods. Results from such analysis paradigms have been used to make assumptions about the nature of motor timing, both in healthy subjects as well as in those with neurological disorders such as cerebellar damage, Parkinson's Disease, or Huntington's Disease (e.g., Ivry, 1997; Ivry & Richardson, 2002). These are based largely on finger tapping or other repetitive manual tasks. In addition, other authors have used the speech version of the Wing-Kristofferson technique for the investigation of motor timing in people who stutter with tasks in which iso-chronous repetition of a syllable was required (Howell, Au-Yeung, & Rustin, 1997; Hulstijn, Summers, van Lieshout, & Peters, 1992; Max & Yudman, 2003). The technique also has been used to show that delayed auditory feedback of speech (DAF) selectively affects the time-keeping process (Howell & Sackin, 2002). This is of interest here because DAF has been reported to improve the fluency of speakers who stutter. Thus, the effect of DAF on Cv may provide a clue about why DAF improves speech control in individuals with speech motor disorders and may throw light on the etiology of specific disorders.

One major disadvantage of the Wing-Kristofferson technique is the fact that it is restricted to short speech episodes (such as single syllable repetitions). There is some argument in the literature that this is not reflective of connected speech processes (e.g., Ziegler, 2003). This is not to say that such tasks are not useful in the diagnosis of the presence or subtype of a motor speech disorder (Kent & Kent 2000); however, it will be difficult to generalize any claims made on motor impairment to connected speech performance.

Linear and Nonlinear Estimators

The techniques discussed in the remainder of this section use exact phrase repetition data. There are two approaches for preparing repetition data to estimate variability and coordination—linear and nonlinear. The difference in philosophy behind these approaches has implications about what can be done subsequently with the data.

Linear Methods

Currently, the most popular technique for estimating variability is Smith's spatio-temporal index, STI (Smith et al., 1995). The STI is a statistic that reflects joint temporal and amplitude variation. To calculate an STI for lower lip displacement, 10 or more recordings of an utterance that involves lip closures are obtained. The first step in the procedure is to adjust the time base linearly (proportional stretching or squeezing to give all records a common length).

Changes in average speech rate, or average magnitude of articulator displacement, therefore are discounted from the analysis. The individual lip-movement records then are amplitude-normalized using a z transformation. The standard deviation (*sd*) across all records then is obtained at 2% intervals on the normalized time axis, and the computed quantities are summed to give the single STI score (Figure 13–1). The STI can be applied to estimate interarticulator coordination by combining information from concurrently

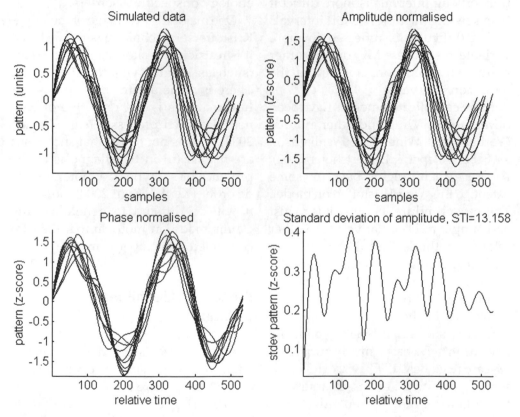

Figure 13–1. Steps in calculation of the STI illustrated using simulated data with randomly generated spatial and temporal variation. The *top right* plot is the data amplitude normalized. The *bottom left* plot is each amplitude normalized record fit to the same relative time line. The *bottom right* plot is the standard deviation of amplitudes from the bottom left plot. The STI is the sum of standard deviations taken at 50 equally spaced sample points on the relative time line.

recorded articulator trajectories, for example, computing the STI on the difference between two articulator signals. However, as described in the following paragraph this estimate of coordination is muddied by a confound in the source of error.

As stated previously, STI has provided extensive data on variability over the course of speech development and has been applied to discriminate disordered and healthy speakers. A limitation of the STI is that it confounds error in timing with error in articulator displacement. It is often the case that speech rate is modulated within an utterance and the pattern of rate modulation changes across repetitions of that utterance. In this case, linearly scaling records to the same time line will result in similar features between records being offset in relative time. The average displacement pattern will be blurred by event offsets, and it is not possible to attribute deviations from the average pattern to mistimings, or misplacements. From the perspective of motor disorders, it may be beneficial to estimate whether a deficit is localized to timing as opposed to displacement, but the STI does not allow this to be done. This observation also applies to the analysis of coordination. The nonlinear methods described in the next section address this issue.

Nonlinear Methods

As discussed in the previous section, differences in within-utterance timing between speech repetitions mean that similar events will occur at different relative times. To get a good estimate of the average speech pattern (and deviations from the average pattern), it is

necessary to pair up similar events between records—that is, to estimate the average displacement at a peak opening, all peak opening events must be put in line with each other (and likewise for all other instants in the utterance). There are different ways that this may be approached. Conceptually, the simplest is to mark landmarks manually (Ward & Armfield, 2001). Records then are adjusted linearly (as with the STI) between features (referred to as piecewise linear). The technique is nonlinear because the amount of adjustment required between the landmark features will vary typically. The disadvantage is that the procedure is manual. This makes the process slow and subjective and requires features to be predefined. This can pose problems in the analysis of motor speech disorders as such landmarks might not be sufficiently clear or altered in some way due to mispronunciations. Irrespective of the quality of the signal, there also may not be enough or too many landmarks in the data, and elicitation materials, thus, have to be chosen with care if this method is to be applied.

Nonlinear Time Warping

A detailed description of dynamic time warping is beyond the scope of this chapter and is provided in other texts (e.g., Lucero et al., 1997; Ramsay, Munhall, Gracco, & Ostry, 1996; Sakoe & Chiba, 1978). A brief overview is helpful, though. The essence of dynamic time warping is to undo between record differences in timing, by distorting (or warping) the time line of each record to best line up features in the entire set. Finding appropriate time warps can be approached in different ways. The dynamic programming approach firstly involves differencing every combination of pairs of points between records. If two records consisted of 10 points, this would give a square grid of 10*10 differences. A new time line best aligning the records is found by stepping back in time from the end point of both records in the grid: [10,10] to the start point [0,0]. Each step is chosen to move to the neighboring grid point with the minimum value.

Several advantages of Functional Data Analysis exist over the earlier dynamic programming approach (discussed in Lucero, 2005), predominantly that the new time lines are continuous and differentiable, potentially facilitating more detailed follow-up analyses of warp characteristics.

In addition, FDA makes it possible to extract information about amplitude (pattern) variability separately from timing variability. This would not be possible if an arbitrary linear scaling were performed. Thus, pattern and timing variability that cannot be separated using the linear STI method are distinguishable with the FDA method as follows:

Because FDA manipulates the time lines of records nonlinearly so as to bring their features into alignment across the set, variation in the degree of adjustment necessary to bring the records into alignment provides an estimate of temporal variability over the course of the records. After the set of records has been aligned, differences on the amplitude axis provide an estimate of amplitude variability over time. This allows separate statistics to be formulated indexing temporal and amplitude variability in an analogous way to that in Smith's STI (Smith et al., 1995). Timing variability can be indexed by estimat-

ing the standard deviation (*sd*) in phase adjustments over the normalized time axis and averaging across the extract. The *sd* of the amplitudes can be processed in a similar way to index amplitude variability (see also Lucero, 2005).

An illustrative application of Functional Data Analysis to patients with Parkinson's Disease and Friedreich's ataxia is described in Anderson, Lowit, and Howell (2008). Howell et al., (2010) have advanced this technique further by developing a method to assess the degree of coordination between two articulatory signals (such as upper and lower lip). This technique involves obtaining the time deformations for each signal independently, prior to differencing them. The amplitudes of the aligned signals can be obtained and processed in a similar way to estimate the amount of pattern variability.

Software Tools

Software to support the majority of analyses discussed in this chapter is freely available on the Web. Praat (http://www.fon.hum.uva.nl/praat/) and SFS (http://www.phon.ucl.ac.uk/resource/sfs/) may be used for digitizing speech, estimating conventional speech properties such as energy, formants, and pitch, and manually segmenting items of interest. MATTAP (Elliot, Welchman, & Wing, 2009), is a MATLAB toolbox to support high fidelity Wing-Kristofferson style tapping experiments. Note that the toolbox is reliant on a data acquisition toolbox and specialized (but relatively inexpensive) hardware.

The authors of this chapter provide MATLAB software to calculate the PVI,

Wing-Kristofferson variance decomposition, and the STI, as well as code to synthesis experimental data and components of variability (at http://www.speech.psychol.ucl.ac.uk/ under "Shared Resources").

A suite of Functional Data Analysis software for R, S-PLUS and MATLAB is provided by Gordon Ramsay at ftp://ego.psych.mcgill.ca/pub/ramsay/FDAfuns. In due course, the present authors will be releasing an integrated time series analysis package interfacing with SFS and the Functional Data Analysis tools described previously.

Clinical Applicability of Variability and Coordination Indices

Single Articulator Variability

Most of the research into speech movement variability has been based on the Spatio-Temporal Index (STI) originally developed by Smith et al. (1995). Research with unimpaired adult speakers has so far been able to suggest a normal range of variability, and to identify conditions under which the stability of speech production can be reduced. Smith et al. noted that adult speakers tended to be the most stable at their habitual rate and became more variable when rate was slowed or increased. Wohlert and Smith (1998) additionally observed that the slow condition resulted in greater variability than the fast condition, and that older speakers were more variable than younger adults. Dromey and Benson (2003) and Dromey and Bates (2005) observed higher degrees of variability when speakers were performing in con-

current task paradigms. Furthermore, evidence for the influence of linguistic planning on motor stability was presented by Kleinow and Smith (2000), who observed that variability increased along with the complexity of the carrier phrase for the test utterance.

Variability measures also have been applied to speakers with a range of disorders. Kleinow and Smith (2000) and Smith and Kleinow (2000) investigated people who stutter (PWS). This group showed the same effects as the unimpaired participants in relation to speech rate changes—that is, elevated variability levels in fast and slow compared to habitual tempo. However, PWS also showed greater variability across all conditions and were affected more by the linguistic complexity of the speech task. In addition, a number of authors report subtle rate control problems in PWS, which could not be identified by gross speech rate measures (Howell, Au-Yeung, & Pilgrim, 1999; Howell & Sackin, 2001; Max & Caruso, 1997; van Lieshout, & Namasivayam, 2010).

A small number of studies also have looked at speakers with dysarthria. Kleinow, Smith, and Ramig (2001) investigated the motor performance of speakers with Parkinson's Disease (PD) in different rate (habitual, slow, and fast) and loudness conditions (loud and soft voice). Similar to previous studies all participant groups showed elevated STI levels in the slow rate condition. The speakers with PD did not differ significantly from the age-matched control group, but they were of very mild severity. The STI also was able to show that the loud voice condition resulted in more stable articulation in all groups, which was interpreted as evidence for the benefits of LSVT®

(Ramig, Countryman, Thompson, & Horii, 1995) treatment. In another study, McHenry (2003) compared participants with different severity of dysarthria across speech rate conditions. STI values were able to highlight differences in severity as well differentiated effects of rate reduction strategies—that is, stretched speech versus pausing. McHenry (2003) thus argued that the STI has an important role to play diagnostically, as well as in establishing optimum treatment strategies. Although the participant groups included different types of dysarthria, she was unable to comment on such differences due to small speaker numbers. McHenry (2003) did, however, hypothesize that the type of disorder might have an influence on the STI in addition to severity.

A study by Anderson et al (2008) also provided some evidence for the potential benefits of an FDA over an STI analysis of speech disorders. Based on the general symptom complex reported for hypokinetic and ataxic dysarthria (e.g., Duffy, 2005), the authors hypothesized that these disorders would differ at the levels of spatial and temporal variability, a fact that could not be picked up by the STI. Although the study included only a few participants, there were tentative signs that PD speakers differed from healthy control speakers in spatial variability, whereas ataxic speakers were distinguishable in terms of temporal variability. Figure 13–2 illustrates such differences between an ataxic and a control speaker. The authors concluded that the nonlinear analysis technique was worth investigating further for its potential in revealing the differences underlying motor speech pathologies. In addition to demonstrating the benefits of FDA over STI, they also support McHenry's (2003) assumption that variability measures can be applied diagnostically to distinguish different types of disorders. The study furthermore lends weight to the argument of using acoustic instead of instrumental data to gain variability data, the benefits of which were already discussed earlier (Measures of Articulatory Movement).

Coordination Measures

At the same time as looking at the variability of single articulators, researchers also have investigated issues of coordination of movement. In their study on children with cleft palate, van Lieshout, Rutjens, and Spauwen (2002) noted that although children with a repaired cleft had a reduced range and greater movement variability in the upper than lower lip, the coordination of the two articulators was not affected. The authors, therefore, stress the importance of investigating speech as a system of coordinated rather than individual movements. Similar arguments have been made in the study of PWS (Howell et al., 2010) who had a poorer ability to coordinate articulatory movements than their healthy counterparts. Problems with co-articulation and the general coordination of speech movements have long been identified as a significant factor in motor speech disorders (see van Lieshout & Namasivayam 2010, for a review). A more refined measure of coordination that can be combined with measures of variability for single articulators would, thus, be helpful in order to further inves-

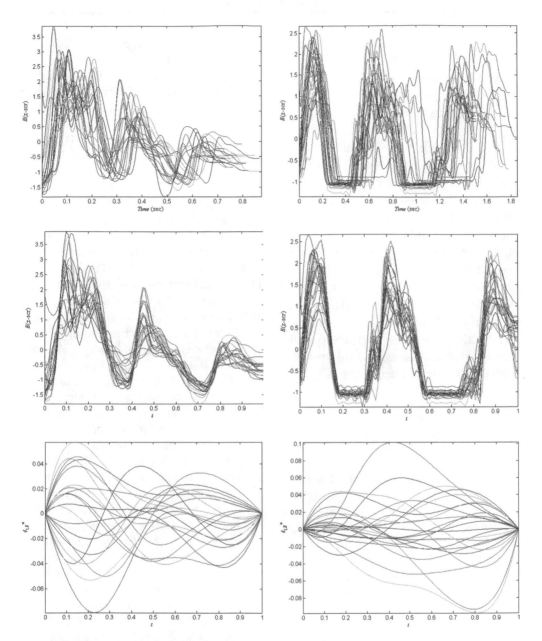

Figure 13–2. Example results comparing variability in a healthy speaker (*left column*) and an ataxic speaker (*right column*) for repetitions of "Well we'll will." The *first row* is low pass filtered speech energy (20Hz cut-off) transformed to z-scores. The *second row* shows the data registered using Functional Data Analysis. The *bottom row* plots the phase error, i.e. the distortion to the relative time line used to bring the records into alignment (as seen in the *middle row*). Negative values correspond to relatively early occurrences of speech events and vice versa. Variability in relative timing can be indexed by averaging the standard deviation of phase errors in a similar manner to the STI. For further examples of these data see Anderson et al. (2008) (See Color Plate 4).

tigate the motor control characteristics for disordered speakers.

The preceding studies suggest that variability measures are a valid and reliable indicator of pathologies affecting the speech production mechanism. Different levels and presentations of problems with movement stability as well as coordination might be able to differentiate underlying physiological changes. They also can inform about more general motor control processes, such as which speaking conditions are more taxing for individuals and what changes might help speakers to exert more control over their articulatory maneuvers. They, thus, have the potential to aid diagnosis, identify populations at risk and assess the suitability of different treatment approaches.

References

Anderson, A., Lowit, A., & Howell, P. (2008). Temporal and spatial variability in speakers with Parkinson's Disease and Friedreich's ataxia. *Journal of Medical Speech Language Pathology, 16*, 173–180.

Barlow, S. M., Cole, K. J., & Abbs, J. H. (1983). A new head-mounted lip-jaw movement transduction system for the study of motor speech disorders. *Journal of Speech and Hearing Research, 26*, 283–288.

Beek, P. J., Peper, C. E., & Daffertshofer, A. (2002). Modeling rhythmic interlimb coordination: Beyond the Haken-Kelso-Bunz model. *Brain and Cognition, 48*, 149–165.

Davidson, L. (2005) Addressing phonological questions with ultrasound. *Clinical Linguistics & Phonetics, 19*, 619–633.

Elliot, M., T., Welchman, A. E., & Wing, A. M. (2009). MatTap: A MATLAB toolbox for the control and analysis of movement synchronisation experiments. *Journal of Neuroscience Methods, 177*, 250–257.

Gick, B. (2002). The use of ultrasound for linguistic phonetic fieldwork. *Journal of the International Phonetic Association, 32*, 113–121.

Gracco, V. L., & Löfqvist, A. (1994). Speech motor coordination and control: Evidence from lip, jaw, and laryngeal movements. *Journal of Neuroscience, 14*, 6585–6597.

Hill, H. (in press). Dynamic facial speech: What, who and how? In M. Giese, C. Curio, & H. H. Bülthoff (Eds.), *Dynamic faces: Insights from experiments and computation*. Boston, MA: MIT Press.

Howell, P., Anderson, A. J., Bartrip, J., & Bailey, E. (2009). Comparison of acoustic and kinematic approaches to measuring utterance-level speech variability. *Journal of Speech, Language and Hearing Research, 52*, 1088–1096.

Howell, P., Anderson, A., & Lucero, J. (2010). Motor timing and fluency. In B. Maasen & P. H. H. M. van Lieshout (Eds.), *Speech motor control: New developments in basic and applied research* (pp. 215–225). Oxford, UK: Oxford University Press.

Howell, P., Au-Yeung, J., & Pilgrim, L. (1999). Utterance rate and linguistic properties as determinants of speech dysfluency in children who stutter. *Journal of the Acoustical Society of America, 105*, 481–490.

Howell, P., Au-Yeung, J., & Rustin, L. (1997). Clock and motor variance in lip tracking: A comparison between children who stutter and those who do not. In W. Hulstijn, H. F. M. Peters, & P. H. H. M. van Lieshout (Eds.), *Speech production: Motor control, brain research and fluency disorders* (pp. 573–578). Amsterdam, The Netherlands: Elsevier.

Howell, P., & Sackin, S. (2000). Speech rate manipulation and its effects on fluency reversal in children who stutter. *Journal of Developmental and Physical Disabilities, 12*, 291–315.

Howell, P., & Sackin, S. (2002). Timing interference to speech in altered listening conditions. *Journal of the Acoustical Society of America, 111,* 2842–2852.

Hulstijn W., Summers J. J., van Lieshout, P. H. M., & Peters, H. F. M. (1992). Timing in finger tapping and speech: A comparison between stutterers and fluent speakers. *Human Movement Sciences, 11,* 113–124.

Ivry, R. (1997). Cerebellar timing systems. *International Review of Neurobiology, 41,* 555–573.

Ivry, R. B., & Richardson, T. (2002). Temporal control and coordination: The multiple timer model. *Brain & Cognition, 48,* 117–132.

Kleinow, J., & Smith, A. (2000). Influence of length and syntactic complexity on the speech motor stability of the fluent speech of adults who stutter. *Journal of Speech, Language, and Hearing Research, 43,* 548–559.

Kleinow, J., Smith, A., & Ramig, L. O. (2001). Speech motor stability in IPD: Effects of rate and loudness manipulations. *Journal of Speech, Language, and Hearing Research, 44,* 1041–1051.

Lucero, J. C. (2005). Comparison of measures of variability of speech movement trajectories using synthetic records. *Journal of Speech, Language and Hearing Research, 48,* 336–344.

Lucero, J. C., Munhall, K. G., Gracco, V. L., & Ramsay, J. O. (1997). On the registration of time and the patterning of speech movements. *Journal of Speech, Language and Hearing Research, 40,* 1111–1117.

Max, L., & Caruso, A. J. (1997). Acoustic measures of temporal intervals across speaking rates: Variability of syllable- and phrase-level relative timing. *Journal of Speech, Language and Hearing Research, 40,* 1097–1110.

Max L., & Yudman, E. A. (2003). Accuracy and variability of isochronous rhythmic timing across motor systems in stuttering versus nonstuttering individuals. *Journal of Speech, Language, and Hearing Research, 46,* 146–163.

McHenry, M. A. (2003). The effect of pacing strategies on the variability of speech movement sequences in dysarthria. *Journal of Speech, Language, and Hearing Research, 46,* 702–710.

Ramig, L. O., Countryman, S., Thompson, L. L., & Horii, Y. (1995). Comparison of two forms of intensive speech treatment for Parkinson disease. *Journal of Speech and Hearing Research, 38,* 1232–1251.

Ramsay, J. O., Munhall, K. G., Gracco, V. L., & Ostry D. J. (1996). Functional data analyses of lip motion. *Journal of the Acoustical Society of America, 99,* 3718–3727.

Ramsay, J. O., & Silverman, B. W. (1997). *Functional data analysis.* New York, NY: Springer-Verlag.

Riley, G. D. (1994). *Stuttering severity instrument for children and adults, Third Edition.* Austin, TX: Pro-Ed.

Sakoe, H., & Chiba, S. (1978). Dynamic programming algorithm optimization for spoken word recognition. *IEEE Transactions on Acoustics, Speech, and Signal Processing, 26,* 43–49.

Smith, A., & Goffman, L. (2004). Interaction of motor and language factors in the development of speech production. In B. Maasen, R. Kent, H. Peters, P. van Lieshout, & W. Hulstijn (Eds.), *Speech motor control in normal and disordered speech* (pp. 227–252). Oxford, UK: Oxford University Press.

Smith, A., Goffman, L., Zelaznik, H. N., Ying, G., & McGillem, C. (1995). Spatiotemporal stability and the patterning of speech movement sequences. *Experimental Brain Research, 104,* 493–501.

Smith, A., & Kleinow, J. (2000). Kinematic correlates of speaking rate changes in stuttering and normally fluent adults. *Journal of Speech, Language, and Hearing Research, 43,* 521–536.

Smith, A., & Zelaznik, H. N. (2004). Development of functional synergies for speech motor coordination in childhood and adolescence. *Developmental Psychobiology, 45,* 22–33.

Stone, M. (2005). A guide to analyzing tongue motion from ultrasound images. *Clinical Linguistics & Phonetics, 19,* 455–501.

van Lieshout, P. H. H. M., & Namasivayam, A. K. (2010). Speech motor variability in people who stutter. In B. Maassen & P. H. H. M. van Lieshout (Eds.), *Speech motor control: New developments in basic and applied research* (pp. 171–188). Oxford, UK: Oxford University Press.

van Lieshout, P. H. H. M., Rutjens, C. A. W., & Spauwen, P. H. M. (2002). The dynamics of interlip coupling in speakers with a repaired unilateral cleft-lip history. *Journal of Speech Language and Hearing Research, 45,* 5–19.

Vorberg, D., & Wing, A. (1996). Modeling variability and dependence in timing. In S. Keele & H. Heuer (Eds.), *Handbook of perception and action* (Vol. 2, pp. 181–262). New York, NY: Academic Press.

Ward, D., & Arnfield, S. (2001). Linear and nonlinear analysis of the stability of gestural organization in speech movement sequences. *Journal of Speech, Language, and Hearing Research, 44,* 108–117.

Wing, A. M., & Kristofferson, A. B. (1973). Response delays and the timing of discrete motor responses. *Perception & Psychophysics, 14,* 5–12.

Williamson, M. M. (1998). Neural control of rhythmic arm movements. *Neural Networks, 11,* 1379–1394.

Wohlert, A. B., & Smith, A. (1998). Spatiotemporal stability of lip movements in older adult speakers. *Journal of Speech, Language, and Hearing Research, 41,* 41–50.

Ziegler, W. (2003). Speech motor control is task-specific: Evidence from dysarthria and apraxia of speech. *Aphasiology, 17,* 3–36.

14

Functional Neuroimaging for the Investigation of Motor Speech Disorders

SERGE PINTO, PH.D.

Introduction

Recent years have seen significant developments in our ability to study the structure and functioning of the brain, furthering our understanding of normal motor and cognitive processes as well as specifying structures underlying disturbances in these processes. There are two principal ways of imaging the brain. The first relies on the structural description of the organ, as part of an anatomical approach delineating specific areas and highlighting brain lesions or tumours. Computed tomography (CT, using X-rays), optical imaging (using near-infrared light) and magnetic resonance imaging (MRI, using magnetic fields) represent some examples of methods of structural neuroimaging. The second imaging possibility investigates the correlation between anatomical locations and brain functioning, linking brain areas with the degree of activation during experimental tasks. Such investigations are referred to as

functional neuroimaging, which encompasses a range of methodologies such as single photon emission computed tomography (SPECT), positron emission tomography (PET), near-infrared spectroscopy (NIRS), functional magnetic resonance imaging (fMRI), electroencephalography (EEG), and magnetoencephalography (MEG). This chapter reviews these functional imaging techniques in relation to their suitability for use in patients with motor speech disorders, providing a description of the procedure as well as summarizing pertinent findings from these investigations.

Functional Neuroimaging Techniques: A Brief Overview

Direct Measurement of Brain Activity

Brain functioning can be assessed by two different means, either directly by measuring the global electrical field at the scalp surface or indirectly by estimating cerebral blood flow. EEG and MEG are techniques that monitor electrical brain activity. EEG and evoked potentials (EPs) globally estimate the electrical activity whose modulations represent physiological markers of brain functioning; MEG assesses brain activity by regionally measuring the associated magnetic emanations (Babiloni, Pizzella, Gratta, Ferretti, & Romani, 2009). EEG and MEG are noninvasive and of great interest for studying the cortical implications of the function considered. However, subcortical structures cannot be easily assessed with these techniques.

Electrical activity also can be measured directly within the brain. Presurgical explorations of cortical areas surrounding epileptic centers or tumors often include the implantation of electrodes deep within the cortex for stereo-EEG (SEEG), which allows the detection of altered brain areas (Wieser, 1991). Deep brain stimulation (DBS) also uses electrodes that have been implanted permanently within subcortical structures for chronic treatment. During implantation surgery, measurements of cell activity and electrical local field potentials (LFPs) are possible, mainly to explore dysfunction at the level of the brain cells within a pathological context (Hutchison et al., 1998; Eusebio et al., 2009). Although these techniques can provide information on subcortical structures, they are not as suitable as an experimental method to assess brain activity as EEG and MEG. Direct measures of brain activity, thus, are restricted largely to cortical activity.

Neurovascular Coupling and Cerebral Blood Flow: The Principles of Indirect Assessment of Brain Functioning

Most neuroimaging techniques are based on brain metabolism estimations. Basically, the more the neurons are recruited for the accomplishment of a function, the more they require glucose and oxygen to support such an increment in activity. This increase in metabolic needs is accounted for by specifically located modulations of regional cerebral blood flow (rCBF). The coupling between neuronal activity and vascular modulation has been extensively studied (Choi, Chen, Hamel, & Jenkins, 2006; Enager et al., 2009) and, thus, represents the basis of the haemodynamic approach for the measurement of brain functioning.

The SPECT and PET techniques involve the use of the injection of a radioactive tracer into the blood stream. Radioactive emissions then are measured by the tomograph scanner, computerized and transformed into images associated with the explored function. The final average image is a static representation of the overall brain areas activated during the completion of the function and within the time window of image acquisition (e.g., around 60–90 seconds for a PET acquisition with labelled [^{15}O]-H$_2$O). Several radioactive products can be used; they must be constructed within a cyclotron located near the scanner since the half-lives of the products used for the blood flow estimation are quite short. Injections of labelled-water ([^{15}O]-H$_2$O; half-life = 2 min.) or labelled-glucose ([^{18}F]-

fluorodesoxyglucose or $[^{18}F]$-FDG); half-life = 109 min.) are, for example, two main strategies for assessing rCBFs by PET. SPECT offers the same information as PET, but it also uses radio-tracers with longer half-lives (like the 99^m-technetium). SPECT and PET can contribute to differentiating disease diagnoses by using adequate radio-markers—that is, the use of a dopamine receptor binder can contribute diagnosing idiopathic Parkinson's Disease (PD) among Parkinsonian syndromes.

Functional magnetic resonance imaging (fMRI) is based upon the para magnetic properties of the hemoglobin, which can be oxygenated (diamagnetic) or deoxygenated (paramagnetic). During the explored experimental condition, the activated neurons need more oxygen, which reaches the cells via an increase of blood flow. Thus, the oxygenated hemoglobin quantity increases within the brain areas functionnally implicated in the condition performance. The ratio between the two hemoglobin states refers to the Blood Oxygenation Level Dependent (BOLD) effect. As a consequence, this ratio differs during a rest condition and an activation paradigm within which cerebral blood flow is increased to supply for the increment of oxygen need for activated neurons. A control condition (which often is called "rest") and an experimental condition usually are alternated in a fMRI block design, and the comparison between the two conditions provides information about the signal, which then can be reconstructed as a functional image. The control condition is not necessarily a proper "rest" as in no activity taking place, instead, it is a condition that contrasts the activation

paradigm used in the experimental condition. The same set up also would be used in an event-related fMRI.

Specificities and Constraints of Direct and Indirect Methods

Each of the previously described techniques has advantages and constraints, and their choice depends heavily on the aims and the experimental design of the investigation (Figure 14–1; inspired by Matthews, 2001). For example, the spatial resolution of PET/SPECT (around 5 millimetres) and fMRI (1–2 millimetres) images is better than that of MEG/EEG; however, the PET/SPECT temporal resolution of around one minute is much lower compared to fMRI (around 500 milliseconds) and MEG/EEG (1 millisecond).

As Figure 14–1 indicates, fMRI represents a compromise between achieving good spatial as well as temporal resolution, and it has, therefore, been preferred over the other techniques as a research tool. However, other methods such as PET still have important assets as a functional neuroimaging technique. For example, only PET retains the possibility of using specific labelled molecules that are able to bind brain receptors or transporters. Participants are scanned in a quiet and undisturbed environment, opposed to the noisy setting of the MRI scanner. This allows for the possibility of subsequent speech/voice analysis and provides less interference for certain speech and language experiments. Physical and visual contact with the participant can be almost constant, thus decreasing stress and anxiety caused by the camera tube and

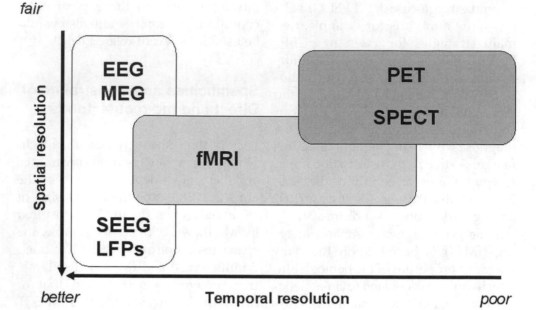

Figure 14–1. Temporal and spatial resolutions of functional neuroimaging techniques: a simple and global overview.

the potentially claustrophobic feeling in the scanner. It is also possible to run studies with participants carrying implanted material (pacemaker, neurostimulator, prostheses, etc.), which is not possible with fMRI scanning, due to the potential diathermy and/or burning effects.

The main disadvantage of PET and SPECT imaging lies in exposure to ionizing radiation. Even if the dose is controlled, it remains an instinctive barrier for some participants. Each injection of [^{15}O]-H$_2$O, for example, requires a waiting time of about 10 minutes before the next injection and the performance of the next experimental task. This time is necessary to allow the radioactivity of the previous injection to decay. As a consequence, the total duration of the experiment can be rather long (between 2 and 3 hours on average) compared to an fMRI experiment (1 hour or less).

Neuroimaging techniques that provide the most relevant information in terms of local brain areas (fMRI and PET) thus have some technical constraints (long duration, possible claustrophic environment, noisy setting, etc.). Although EEG and MEG present fewer constraints of this type, they offer less access to spatial data. As a consequence, an increasing number of studies combine different imaging techniques in order to exploit their advantages as much as possible. For example, combined EEG/fMRI studies may benefit from both the fine-grained temporal (EEG) and spatial (fMRI) resolutions (Grouiller et al., 2010; Ortigue, Thompson, Parasuraman, & Grafton, 2009).

Functional Neuroimaging Investigations of Motor Speech Control

Historically, SPECT and PET were the first techniques used for functional neuroimaging experiments. The 1970s marked the development and advent of PET (Phelps et al., 1976; Yamamoto, Thompson, Meyer, Little, & Feindel, 1977). The first international symposium on PET took place in 1978 in Montreal, Canada. From there, multiple studies aimed at measuring the cerebral blood flow at rest by using different radioligands (Raichle et al., 1978; Ackermann, Subramanyam, Correia, Alpert, & Taveras, 1980; Frackowiak, Lenzi, Jones, & Heather, 1980). The interest continued with the possibility of measuring this same blood flow during various task performances (Phelps et al., 1980).

Heritage of the Princeps Studies

At the end of the 1980s, a series of publications from Petersen and collaborators posed the basis of what would represent for the following decades a reference for cerebral activation profiles associated with speech and language (Petersen et al., 1988, 1989, 1990). As an example, one of the experimental designs used the four following paradigms (Petersen et al., 1988; 1989): (1) attentional fixation of nonverbal symbols; (2) passive presentation (e.g., visual) of words; (3) reading and production of these words; and (4) verbal generation task correlated with these words. The PET subtractive method made it possible to identify cerebral activations associated with, among others, the motor aspects of speech production by using the contrast (3 – 2): in this contrast, activations associated with reading words presented visually (paradigm 2) were "withdrawn" from those of the profile corresponding to the reading and production of the same words (paradigm 3); thus, only the cerebral areas associated with speech production were revealed, since the cerebral profile of reading has been masked. Bilateral hemodynamic modifications on the sensorimotor cortex and antero-superior parts of the cerebellum were displayed. Moreover, activation of the supplementary motor area (SMA), particularly localized in the interhemispherical space between the frontal lobes also could have been observed. A deeply localized activation within the Sylvian fissure in the left insula also was noticed, whereas activation of Broca's area and the basal ganglia (BG) did not reach any significant threshold.

Lower-Order Speech Processes

One of the most unexpected results of these studies was the quasi-absence of the activation of Broca's area during the motor realization of speech production, suggesting that this region plays a crucial role in motor planning and coordination. Since then, its importance for higher-order speech processes has been widely accepted. In time, multiple PET studies along with other studies using different neuroimaging techniques, confirmed and extended Petersen's results (Figure 14–2).

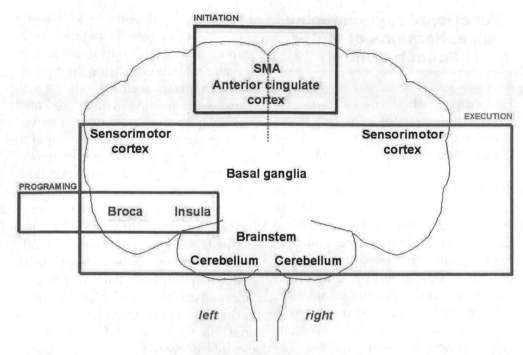

Figure 14–2. Regions specifically implicated in the motor execution of speech: a summary.

These neuroimaging studies commonly revealed that regions specifically implicated in the motor execution of speech were the inferior part of the primary sensorimotor cortex bilaterally, the left and right cerebellum and the right thalamus and caudate nucleus (Blank, Scott, Murphy, Warburton, & Wise, 2002; Bookheimer, Zeffiro, Blaxton, Gaillard, & Theodore, 2000; Dogil et al., 2002; Murphy et al., 1997; Lotze, Seggewies, Erb, Grodd, & Birbaumer, 2000; Ternovoi, Sinitsyn, Evzikov, Morozov, & Kholodov, 2004; Tzourio-Mazoyer, Josse, Crivello, & Mazoyer, 2004; Vigneau, Jobard, Mazoyer, & Tzourio-Mazoyer, 2005; Wise, Greene, Buchel, & Scott, 1999). Moreover, an increase in cerebral blood flow also was observed in the dorsal part of the cerebral trunk, the anterior cingular cortex, and the poste-

rior left pallidum. Particularly, Wise et al. (1999) stressed that the activated regions associated with articulation involved the left anterior insula, lateral premotor cortex, and basal ganglia.

Higher-Order Speech Processes

Speech articulation in stroke patients specifically affected by apraxia of speech was studied by magnetic resonance imaging (MRI) and computerized tomography scans (Dronkers, 1996). All participants had brain lesions that included a discrete region of the left precentral gyrus of the insula, which suggests a role of this area in the motor planning of speech (Donnan, Darby, & Saling, 1997). However, the implication of this area in speech motor tasks revealed by fMRI has been a source of debate (Riecker, Ackermann, Wildgruber, Dogil, & Grodd, 2000; Shuster and Lemieux, 2005), principally highlighting the fact that activation of the insula is dependent on the syllabic structure, including their length and complexity. Moreover, production of pseudo-words produced greater activation in much of the speech production network, which includes the anterior insula (Shuster, 2009). In such experimental paradigms, covert and overt speech did not display the same BOLD activation profiles. During overt speech, activation was larger in the areas associated with speech production, including the left insula (Shuster, 2009).

An up-to-date review of the implications of insula on speech production is provided by Ackermann and Riecker (2010).

Speech Motor Control Theories

Perkell's Theory (1980)

The Moll and Daniloff (1971), Daniloff (1973), and Hammarberg (1976) models, presented by Levelt (1989), considered that temporal adjustments of each motor speech sequence represent tardive events in the process of speech execution. In this vision, auditory targets corresponded to representations that should be reached for proper articulation. Perkell (1980) further introduced the concept of an early coarticulation process, based on orosensitive articulatory representations whose purpose would be to provide the locutor with the sensory information emerging from the speech organs and representing some spatio-temporal

goals to be achieved in order to ensure speech motor execution. This sort of target would be the beginning of a motor cascade, whose second step would represent the temporal planification and adjustment of the programmed muscular contractions. This command would not depend exclusively on the articulatory aim, but also on feedback coming from the articulators (proprioception, orosensitive representations) or other structures (auditory feedback). Coarticulation thus would be defined as abstract preparatory activities, occuring prior to the final step of the motor cascade, which is motor execution.

Levelt's Model (1989)

Levelt's point of view (1989) went further than the previously described concepts based on articulatory representations. It suggested that during speech production, each speaker accesses a mental syllabary. According to this model, the most frequently used syllables are sufficient for the production of the major part of the verbal productions of a language. These syllables are associated by nature with the most frequently used motor activities. These frequent syllables would not be sequenced in real time, but rather would be recovered as complete, prelearned motor programs, stored in the mental syllabary. In other words, the motor programs of the high-frequency syllables are already precompiled and ready for retrieval, in contrast to the motor plans of new or low-frequency syllables, which have to be assembled online segment by segment. Levelt, Roelofs, and Meyer (1999) do not exclude that the stored motor plans also might correspond to units that are greater than syllables. Retrieval of these frequent motor performances could reduce the processing time necessary for speech production. Levelt et al. (1999) proposed the presence of this mental lexicon in the premotor cortex.

Riecker and Colleagues' Contribution (2000–2008)

Levelt and coworkers assume that for silent/inner speech, the same processes take place as in overt speech with the exception of the actual motor action; however, this hypothesis is not yet fully confirmed. Recent fMRI studies showed that silent speech production was associated with a hemodynamic response in a lower left frontal precentral gyrus area (gathering premotor surfaces), in addition to the primary motor cortex (Riecker et al., 2000). This activation could reflect the recruitment of the mental syllabary. Silent internal speech production would induce the need for a temporal organization of the syllables similar to that of the effective production of these syllables. Associated with the left premotor cortex activation, a controlateral cerebellar activation also was observed during internal speech production. In a syllable synchronization task, a separation between two networks of speech motor control has been reported in the basis of functional connectivity (Riecker et al., 2005). The first network seems to support motor preparation (SMA, dorsolateral prefrontal cortex including Broca's area, anterior insula, superior cerebellum), whereas the second is linked to motor execution processes (sensorimotor cortex, basal ganglia, thalamus, inferior cerebellum). A recent fMRI study (Riecker, Brendel, Ziegler, Erb, & Ackermann, 2008) could not find a neuroanatomical correlate of the hypothesized mental syllabary. However, as stated in this study report (Riecker et al., 2008, page 110), "a rejection of the mental syllabary concept still must be considered premature, since a preceding study reported enhanced activation of the left insula in association with low-frequency as compared to high-frequency syllables, irrespective of word frequency, during reading of lexical items." (Carreiras, Mechelli, & Price, 2006)

Guenther and Colleagues' Neurocomputational DIVA Model (1994–2010)

The DIVA (Directions Into Velocities of Articulators) neural network model of speech production represents an attempt to link speech processes both computationally and neurophysiologically (Guenther, Ghosh, & Tourville, 2006; Golfinopoulos, Tourville, & Guenther, 2009). In a certain point of view, this model synthesizes and goes beyond all the previous works, which principally used covert (or silent) speech as a predominant experimental task. The DIVA model is based on the learning of the required movements inducing overt speech production from a computerized-simulation vocal tract, modified from the synthesizer described by Maeda (1990). Feedforward and feedback control subsystems compound the main frame of this model. The former is dedicated to the elaboration of a speech motor program, emerging from the generation of an Articulator Velocity and Position Map and the activation of a Speech Sound Map. This motor program also is projected within an Initiation Map that aims to release it. The auditory and somatosensory feedback control subsystems represent the ability, within the DIVA model, to detect and correct the errors occuring during speech production. Functional neuroimaging studies have contributed to construct this model. A particularity, and strength, of the DIVA model is to localize the neural networks for each of the speech production steps (Figure 14–3). As an example, a "minimal network for overt speech production" can be described as including mesiofrontal areas, intrasylvian cortex, pre- and postcentral gyri, left inferior posterior frontal cortex, basal ganglia, cerebellum, and thalamus. This neural network has been addressed based upon syllable repetitions, production of pseudo-words or even isolated vowels. More recently, fMRI investiga-

tions also focused on neural substrates predominantly engaged in phonemic, syllabic, and supra-syllabic levels of speech (Ghosh, Tourville, & Guenther, 2008; Peeva et al., 2010). The idea was to further the DIVA model with a first approach to define a brain map for language output.

Functional Neuroimaging Investigations of Motor Speech Disorders

Disordered speech, and particularly motor speech disorders, implicates cerebral activation dysfunctions that must be interpreted as part of altered cerebral speech networks. This would be the case for dysarthrias whose

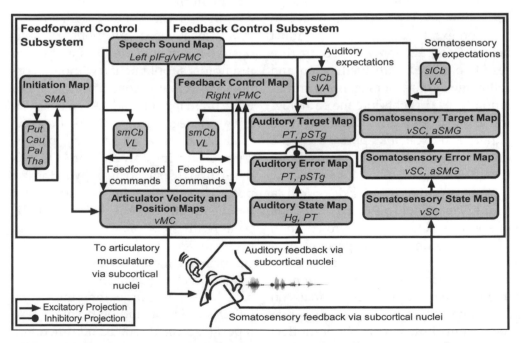

Figure 14–3. The DIVA model schematic representation (Courtesy of Golfinopoulos and colleagues, 2009, Neuroimage, Elsevier).

lesion would be located within the central nervous system (hypokinetic, hyperkinetic, ataxic), but not necessarily for dysarthrias with peripheral origin of the dysfunction (flaccid, spastic, mixed). The previously reported studies represent a relevant context to understand the functional changes identified in disordered speech investigation.

The use of functional neuroimaging methods in the assessment of motor speech disorders, or any other motor or cognitive dysfunction, is highly dependent on the pathophysiological substrate and the therapeutic state of the patients. As a consequence, brain dysfunction assessed via functional imaging will depend on the progression of the disease, associated with a specific severity or degree of the disease. Additionally, some treatments may have significant effects on brain functioning and can change activation levels in cerebral areas. In this context, particular attention must be paid to functional neuroimaging results obtained with medication and following surgery or deep brain stimulation. These insights into the pathological brain during altered speech have paralleled the scientific approach focused on understanding the speaking brain (Dogil et al., 2002).

Among motor speech disorders, a simple vision could differentiate apraxia of speech (AOS) as the representation of higher-order speech process dysfunction, and the group of dysarthrias as lower-order speech process impairments. The following sections focus on functional neuroimaging studies that have contributed to a better understanding of the pathophysiologies of these disorders.

Apraxia of Speech

Speech articulation in stroke patients specifically affected by a motor planning dysfunction of articulatory movements, so-called apraxia of speech (AOS), was studied by magnetic resonance imaging (MRI) and computerized tomography scans. All participants had brain lesions that included a discrete region of the left precentral gyrus of the insula (Dronkers, 1996), thus confirming previous findings about lesion sites associated with AOS (Shuren, 1993), whereas no lesion in the inferior frontal gyrus was noted. However, other studies have since questioned these findings by providing evidence of no association between AOS and lesions of the left insula, anterior insula, or superior border of the precentral gyrus of the insula. Instead, a link with speech impairment and the left posterior inferior frontal gyrus dysfunction was evident (Hillis et al., 2004). Voxel-based morphometry demonstrated a grey matter loss within the premotor/supplementary motor cortices, reflecting a connection between these brain regions and AOS whose origin was a degenerative disease (Josephs et al., 2006). In another study, participants presenting only AOS or AOS plus dysarthria displayed atrophy in the left posterior frontal, anterior insular, and basal ganglia regions, while participants with AOS plus dysarthria also presented greater damage in the orofacial primary motor cortex and the left caudate nucleus (Ogar, Dronkers, Brambati, Miller, & Gorno-Tempini, 2007). Other studies, including a single case report (Ricci et al., 2008) and functional neuroimaging in unimpaired speakers (Moser et al., 2009), have contributed further to the understanding of the neuranatomical substrates of AOS.

Dysarthrias

According to the classification of Darley and colleagues, dysarthria refers to a specific motor speech disorder associated with a particular pathological lesion (Darley, Aronson, & Brown, 1969a, 1969b, 1975). Among the dysarthrias, the hypokinetic and ataxic types have benefited particularly from functional neuroimaging investigation.

Hypokinetic Dysarthria

Liotti et al. (2003) studied the cerebral haemodynamic response to various speech tasks in five PD speakers extensively by PET. The participants were assessed twice, once before and once after voice therapy. In addition to highlighting the neural correlates of treatment efficacy, a bilateral overactivation of cortical motor/premotor regions, including the SMA and inferior lateral premotor cortex was revealed prior to the therapy. Another study also confirmed these pretreatment overactivations in 10 PD speakers (Narayana et al., 2010). PD dysarthria also has been associated with (1) a decreased activation in the right orofacial motor cortex and bilateral cerebellar hemispheres; (2) an abnormal increase of rCBF in the right superior premotor cortex and bilateral dorsolateral prefrontal cortex (DLPFC); and (3) an overactivation of the SMA (Pinto et al., 2004). Parkinsonian dysarthria may result from an altered recruitment of the main cerebral motor regions (orofacial motor cortex, cerebellum) and an increased involvement of premotor and prefrontal cortices (DLPFC, SMA, superior premotor cortex). An SMA overactivation also has been observed by PET in a recent single case study, in which a primary motor cortex overactivation also was reported in an off state (subthalamic stimulation turned off) as compared with the on state (Narayana et al., 2009). Cerebral activation changes, such as the recruitment of additional temporal regions during phonation and phoneme repetition, seem to be an emerging issue of speech in PD (Sachin et al., 2008). They might represent a compensatory phenomenon underlying the reorganized activation pattern associated with PD dysarthria. Another fMRI investigation reported data obtained in a group of nine medicated PD speakers (Rektorova, Barrett, Mikl, Rektor, & Paus, 2007). A significantly higher regional cerebral blood flow in the right orofacial sensorimotor cortex in PD participants as compared to controls was interpreted by the authors as a compensatory phenomenon for reduced brain activations, in order to preserve speech production in PD.

PD speakers also can present with higher order language difficulties (Berg, Björnram, Hartelius, Laakso, & Johnels, 2003). The literature reports significant deficits in verb generation (Bertella et al., 2002; Castner et al., 2008; Péran et al., 2003), aspects of lexical-semantic inhibitory mechanisms (Castner et al., 2007a), semantic and affective priming (Castner et al., 2007b), as well as sentence comprehension (Angwin, Chenery, Copland, Murdoch, & Silburn, 2005, 2007; Angwin, Copland, Chenery, Murdoch, & Silburn, 2006) and processing

(Grossman, Lee, Morris, Stern, & Hurtig, 2002). Such difficulties rely on basal ganglia nonmotor circuit dysfunction (Castner et al., 2007a, 2007b). Notably, impairment of a fronto-temporal network associated with word production has been suggested (Castner et al., 2008), as well as overaction of the right inferior frontal and left posterior-lateral temporal and parietal areas during sentence comprehension (Grossman et al., 2003).

Ataxic Dysarthria

Ischaemic lesions in the superior and inferior cerebellar arteries are known to be associated with dysarthric speech (Ackermann, Vogel, Petersen, & Poremba, 1992; Urban, Wicht, Hopf, Fleischer, & Nickel, 1999; Urban et al., 2001). These lesion studies have suggested a predominant lateralization of motor speech control within the right cerebellum. As expected, functional neuroimaging studies performed with ataxic participants have revealed some changes in brain activations, as compared to control subjects, within the cerebellar hemispheres, vermis, and brainstem (Kluin et al., 1988; Honjo et al., 2004), but also in other regions including posterior temporal and inferior frontal regions, and the supplementary motor area (Moeller, Strother, Sidtis, & Rottenberg., 1987; Anderson et al., 1988). However, as mentioned by Sidtis, Gomez, Groshong, Strother, and Rottenberg (2006, page 247), "some of the reported associations between brain activity and dysarthria likely reflect disease severity rather than specific abnormalities related to motor speech control." Dysarthric speech following cerebellar dysfunction also has been described in some case studies by neuroimaging techniques (Urban et al., 1999;

Okuda, Kawabata, Tachibana, & Sugita, 1999; Gasparini et al., 1999). Apart from the consistent cerebellar metabolism, other cerebral areas such as frontal, temporal, and sensorimotor cortices also have displayed a reduction in rCBF.

Recent fMRI (Riecker, Kassubek, Gröschel, Grodd, & Ackermann, 2006) and PET (Sidtis et al., 2006) studies investigated larger participant groups and largely confirmed some previous findings. As an example, Sidtis et al. (2006, page 252) reported "significant reductions in cerebellar but not cerebral blood flow in a group of hereditary ataxic subjects (...) Cerebellar disease may well amplify the normal role of the cerebellum in motor speech control, as it is identifiable in the ataxic but not the normal subjects." These studies particularly highlight the key role played by the predominant projection from the right cerebellum to the left motor cortex in speech motor control (Ackermann, Wildgruber, Daum, & Grodd, 1998). Cerebellar dysfunction has furthermore contributed to questioning the connection between the cerebellum and some cognitive processes of speech (Ackermann et al., 1998; Ackermann, 2008).

Other Speech Manifestations

SPECT was used in some individual cases presenting with speech deterioration, such as speakers with Foix-Chavany-Marie syndrome (Lang, Reichwein, Iro, & Treig, 1989) or foreign-accent syndrome (Fridriksson et al., 2005; Mariën et al., 2006) to confirm diagnosis and highlighted the lack of implication of the basal ganglia or cerebellum as substrates of altered speech. Another example illustrates the use of PET to follow disease progression and anarthria development in a case of multiple neuro-degenerations (Tebartz van Elst et al., 2002). Functional neuroimaging also has been used sporadically, mainly in single case studies or small populations, to investigate hyperkinetic speech disorders as present in Huntington's disease (Metter, Riege, Hanson, Phelps, & Kuhl, 1984) as well as spasmodic dysphonia (Takahashi, Oki, Miyamoto, & Okuno, 1998; Hirano et al., 2001; Haslinger et al., 2005). In these studies, a SMA underactivation and the basal ganglia dysfunction appeared to play an important role in the pathophysiology of the associated speech impairment.

The evaluation of a single family across three generations, known as the KE family, and presenting with a severe verbal dyspraxia, gave the opportunity to link this syndrome with a specific abnormal gene at the origin of structural brain abnormalities in the caudate nucleus and frontal areas (Fisher, Vargha-Khadem, Watkins, Monaco, & Pembrey, 1998). The functional neuro-imaging investigation of speech in this family revealed "abnormalities in both cortical and sub-cortical motor-related areas of the frontal lobe" (Vargha-Khadem et al., 1998, page 12695), questioning the implication of the basal ganglia circuit in this particular speech deterioration.

The Remaining Challenges for Functional Neuroimaging of Motor Speech Disorders

Motor speech disorders result from dysfunctions in specific brain areas. Lesion location within the central and/ or peripheral nervous systems can help us to understand the pathophysiology of speech disorders, as can the alteration of cerebral blood flow assessed by functional neuroimaging. Logically, lesion sites can be associated with specific speech dysfunctions, thus also arguing for the implication of such brain areas in normal speech. However, it is still difficult to understand the proper involvement of other areas that present dysfunctional activity, without any lesion or degeneration. For this reason, functional neuroimaging is needed to elucidate such implications and to test for hypotheses that rely on models of speech production.

These models are updated permanently, corrected, confirmed, or even rejected. So far, the DIVA model developed by Guenther and colleagues (Guenther et al., 2006; Golfinopoulos et al., 2009) represents an interesting point of view that integrates most of the neurophysiological constraints inherent to the actual processes of speech motor control (Bohland, Bullock, & Guenther, 2010).

One challenge for such a model is to document the role of the basal ganglia in speech, which is still not yet fully understood (Radanovic & Scaff, 2003). Development of fMRI investigations of motor speech disorders presents a crucial opportunity for the better understanding of the impact of basal ganglia deficits on speech. In this context, dysarthric speech is one of the pathological models of choice and justifies the need for further investigations involving various speech tasks using functional neuroimaging.

The nature of the speech task used for the experimental paradigm is extremely important. Cerebral activations are highly dependent on such variables; they can be very different depending on whether the speech task is externally or internally cued, overtly or covertly produced, visually or auditory guided, cognitively demanding or not, automatic, complex, and so on. Experimenters must be aware of such issues, since data interpretation will depend on them. Motor speech disorders deserve further investigations in order to elucidate the pathophysiological neural substrate of speech deficits in specific diseases and to afford the possibility of predicting treatment effects on speech production.

References

Ackermann, H. (2008). Cerebellar contributions to speech production and speech perception: psycholinguistic and neurobiological perspectives. *Trends in Neuroscience, 31*, 265–272.

Ackermann, H., & Riecker, A. (2010). The contribution(s) of the insula to speech production: a review of the clinical and functional imaging literature. *Brain Structure and Function.* [Epub ahead of print]

Ackermann, H., Vogel, M., Petersen, D., & Poremba, M. (1992). Speech deficits in ischaemic cerebellar lesions. *Journal of Neurology, 239*, 223–227.

Ackermann, H., Wildgruber, D., Daum, I., & Grodd, W. (1998). Does the cerebellum contribute to cognitive aspects of speech production? A functional magnetic resonance imaging (fMRI) study in humans. *Neuroscience Letters, 247*(2–3), 187–190.

Ackerman, R. H., Subramanyam, R., Correia, J. A., Alpert, N. M., & Taveras, J. M. (1980). Positron imaging of cerebral blood flow during continuous inhalation of C15O2. *Stroke, 11*(1), 45–49.

Anderson, N. E., Posner, J. B., Sidtis, J. J., Moeller, J. R., Strother, S. C., Dhawan, V., & Rottenberg, D. A. (1988). The metabolic anatomy of paraneoplastic cerebellar degeneration. *Annals of Neurology, 23*, 533–540.

Angwin, A. J., Chenery, H. J., Copland, D. A., Murdoch, B. E., & Silburn, P. A. (2005). Summation of semantic priming and complex sentence comprehension in Parkinson's disease. *Cognitive Brain Research, 25*, 78–89.

Angwin, A. J., Chenery, H. J., Copland, D. A., Murdoch, B. E., & Silburn, P. A. (2007). The speed of lexical activation is altered in Parkinson's disease. *Journal of Clinical Experimental Neuropsychology, 29*, 73–85.

Angwin, A. J., Copland, D. A., Chenery, H. J., Murdoch, B. E., & Silburn, P. A. (2006). The influence of dopamine on semantic activation in Parkinson's disease: Evidence from a multipriming task. *Neuropsychology, 20*, 299–306.

Babiloni, C., Pizzella, V., Gratta, C. D., Ferretti, A., & Romani, G. L. (2009). Fundamentals of electroencefalography, magnetoencefalography, and functional magnetic resonance imaging. *International Review of Neurobiology, 86*, 67–80.

Berg, E., Björnram, C., Hartelius, L., Laakso, K., & Johnels, B. (2003). High-level language difficulties in Parkinson's disease. *Clinical Linguistics & Phonetics, 17*, 63–80.

Bertella, L., Albani, G., Greco, E., Priano, L., Mauro, A., Marchi, S., . . . Semenza, C. (2002). Noun-verb dissociation in Parkinson's disease. *Brain & Cognition, 48*, 277–280.

Blank, S. C., Scott, S. K., Murphy, K., Warburton, E., & Wise, R. J. (2002). Speech production: Wernicke, Broca, and beyond. *Brain, 125*(Pt 8), 1829–1838.

Bohland, J. W., Bullock, D., & Guenther, F. H. (2010). Neural representations and mechanisms for the performance of simple speech sequences. *Journal of Cognitive Neuroscience, 22*(7), 1504–1529.

Bookheimer, S. Y., Zeffiro, T. A., Blaxton, T. A., Gaillard, P. W., & Theodore, W. H. (2000). Activation of language cortex with automatic speech tasks. *Neurology, 55*, 1151–1157.

Carreiras, M., Mechelli, A., & Price, C. J. (2006). Effect of word and syllable frequency on activation during lexical decision and reading aloud. *Human Brain Mapping, 27*, 963–972.

Castner, J. E., Copland, D. A., Silburn, P. A., Coyne, T. J., Sinclair, F., & Chenery, H. J. (2007a). Lexical-semantic inhibitory mechanisms in Parkinson's disease as a function of subthalamic stimulation. *Neuropsychologia, 45*, 3167–3177.

Castner, J. E., Chenery, H. J., Copland, D. A., Coyne, T. J., Sinclair, F., & Silburn, P. A. (2007b). Semantic and affective priming as a function of stimulation of the subthalamic nucleus in Parkinson's disease. *Brain, 130*, 1395–1407.

Castner, J. E., Chenery, H. J., Silburn, P. A., Smith, E. R., Coyne, T. J., Sinclair, F., & Copland, D. A. (2008). The effects of subthalamic deep brain stimulation on noun/verb generation and selection from competing alternatives in Parkinson's disease. *Journal of Neurology, Neurosurgery and Psychiatry, 79*(6), 700–705.

Choi, J. K., Chen, Y .I., Hamel, E., & Jenkins, B. G. (2006) Brain hemodynamic changes mediated by dopamine receptors: Role of the cerebral microvasculature in dopamine-mediated neurovascular coupling. *Neuroimage, 30*(3), 700–712.

Daniloff, R. G. (1973). Normal articulation processes. In F. D. Minifie, T. J. Hixon, & F. Williams (Eds.), *Normal aspects of speech, hearing and language* (pp. 169–209). Englewood Cliffs, NJ: Prentice-Hall

Darley, F. L., Aronson, A. E. & Brown, J. R. (1969a). Differential diagnostic patterns of dysarthria. *Journal of Speech and Hearing Research, 12*, 246–269.

Darley, F. L., Aronson, A. E. & Brown, J. R. (1969b). Clusters of deviant speech dimensions in the dysarthrias. *Journal of Speech and Hearing Research, 12*, 462–496.

Darley, F. L., Aronson, A. E. & Brown, J. R. (1975). *Motor speech disorders.* Philadelphia, PA: Saunders.

Dogil, G., Ackermann, H., Grodd, W., Haider, H., Kamp, H., Mayer, J. . . . Wildgruber, D. (2002). The speaking brain: A tutorial introduction to fMRI experiments in the production of speech, prosody and syntax. *Journal of Neurolinguistics, 15*, 59–90.

Donnan, G. A., Darby, D. G., & Saling, M. M. (1997). Identification of brain region for coordinating speech articulation. *Lancet, 349*, 221–222.

Dronkers, N. F. (1996). A new brain region for coordinating speech articulation. *Nature, 384*(6605), 159–161.

Enager, P., Piilgaard, H., Offenhauser, N., Kocharyan, A., Fernandes, P., Hamel, E., & Lauritzen, M. (2009). Pathway-specific variations in neurovascular and neurometabolic coupling in rat primary somatosensory cortex. *Journal of Cerebral Blood Flow and Metabolism, 29*(5), 976–986.

Eusebio, A., Pogosyan, A., Wang, S., Averbeck, B., Gaynor, L. D., Cantiniaux, S., . . . Brown, P. (2009). Resonance in subthalamocortical circuits in Parkinson's disease. *Brain, 132*(Pt 8), 2139–2150.

Fisher S. E., Vargha-Khadem, F., Watkins, K.E., Monaco, A.P., & Pembrey, M.E. (1998). Localization of a gene implicated in a severe speech and language disorder. *Nature Genetics, 18*(2), 168–170. Erratum in *Nature Genetics 18*(3), 298.

Frackowiak, R., Lenzi, G., Jones, T., & Heather, J. D. (1980). Quantitative measurement of regional cerebral blood flow and oxygen metabolism in man using 15O and positron emission tomography: Theory, procedure, and normal values. *Journal of Computer Assisted Tomography, 4*, 727–736.

Fridriksson, J., Ryalls, J., Rorden, C., Morgan, P. S., George, M. S., & Baylis, G. C. (2005.) Brain damage and cortical compensation in foreign accent syndrome. *Neurocase, 11*(5), 319–324.

Gasparini, M., Di Piero, V., Ciccarelli, O., Cacioppo, M. M., Pantano, P., & Lenzi, G. L. (1999). Linguistic impairment after right cerebellar stroke: A case report. *European Journal of Neurology, 6*(3), 353–356.

Ghosh, S. S., Tourville, J. A., & Guenther, F. H. (2008). A neuroimaging study of premotor lateralization and cerebellar involvement in the production of phonemes and syllables. *Journal of Speech Language Hearing Research, 51*(5), 1183–1202.

Golfinopoulos, E., Tourville, J. A., & Guenther, F.H. (2009). The integration of large-scale neural network modeling and functional brain imaging in speech motor control. *Neuroimage*. [Epub ahead of print].

Grossman, M., Cooke, A., DeVita, C., Lee, C., Alsop, D., Detre, J., . . . Hurtig, H. I. (2003). Grammatical and resource components of sentence processing in Parkinson's disease: An fMRI study. *Neurology, 60*, 775–781.

Grossman, M., Lee, C., Morris, J., Stern, M. B. & Hurtig, H. I. (2002). Assessing resource demands during sentence processing in Parkinson's disease. *Brain & Language, 80*, 603–616.

Grouiller, F., Vercueil, L., Krainik, A., Segebarth, C., Kahane, P., & David, O. (2010). Characterization of the hemodynamic modes associated with interictal epileptic activity using a deformable model-based analysis of combined EEG and functional MRI recordings. *Human Brain Mapping*. [Epub ahead of print].

Guenther, F. H., Ghosh, S. S., & Tourville, J. A. (2006). Neural modelling and imaging of the cortical interactions underlying syllable production. *Brain & Language, 96*, 280–301.

Hammarberg, R. E. (1976). The metaphysics of coarticulation. *Journal of Phonetics, 4*, 353–363.

Haslinger, B., Erhard, P., Dresel, C., Castrop, F., Roettinger, M., & Ceballos-Baumann, A. O. (2005). "Silent event-related" fMRI reveals reduced sensorimotor activation in laryngeal dystonia. *Neurology, 65*(10), 1562–1569.

Hillis, A. E., Work, M., Barker, P. B., Jacobs, M. A., Breese, E. L., & Maurer, K. (2004). Re-examining the brain regions crucial for orchestrating speech articulation. *Brain, 127*(Pt 7), 1479–1487.

Hirano, S., Kojima, H., Naito, Y., Tateya, I., Shoji, K., Kaneko, K., . . . Konishi J. (2001). Cortical dysfunction of the supplementary motor area in a spasmodic dysphonia patient. *American Journal of Otolaryngology, 22*(3), 219–222.

Honjo, K., Ohshita, T., Kawakami, H., Naka, H., Imon, Y., Maruyama, H., . . . Matsumoto, M. (2004). Quantitative assessment of cerebral blood flow in genetically confirmed spinocerebellar ataxia type 6. *Archives of Neurology, 61*, 933–937.

Hutchison, W. D., Allan, R. J., Opitz, H., Levy, R., Dostrovsky, J. O., Lang, A. E., & Lozano A. M. (1998). Neurophysiological identification of the subthalamic nucleus in surgery for Parkinson's disease. *Annals of Neurology, 44*(4), 622–628.

Josephs, K. A., Duffy, J. R., Strand, E. A., Whitwell, J. L., Layton, K. F., Parisi, J. E., . . . Petersen, R.C. (2006). Clinicopathological and imaging correlates of progressive aphasia and apraxia of speech. *Brain, 129*(Pt 6), 1385–1398.

Kluin, K. J., Gilman, S., Markel, D. S., Koeppe, R. A., Rosenthal, G., & Junck, L. (1988). Speech disorders in olivopontocerebellar atrophy correlate with positron emission tomography findings. *Annals of Neurology, 23*, 547–554.

Lang, C., Reichwein, J., Iro, H., & Treig, T. (1989). Foix-Chavany-Marie-syndrome —neurological, neuropsychological, CT, MRI, and SPECT findings in a case progressive for more than 10 years. *European Archives of Psychiatry and Clinical Neuroscience, 239*(3), 188–193.

Levelt, W. J. M. (1989). *Speaking: From intention to articulation.* Cambridge, MA: MIT Press.

Levelt, W. J. M., Roelofs, A., & Meyer, A. (1999). A theory of lexical access in speech production. *Behavioral and Brain Sciences*, 22, 1–75.

Liotti, M., Ramig, L. O., Vogel, D., New, P., Cook, C. I., Ingham, R. J., . . . Fox, P.T. (2003). Hypophonia in Parkinson's disease: neural correlates of voice treatment revealed by PET. *Neurology*, *60*(3), 432–440.

Lotze, M., Seggewies, G., Erb, M., Grodd, W., & Birbaumer, N. (2000). The representation of articulation in the primary sensorimotor cortex. *Neuroreport*, *11*(13), 2985–2989.

Maeda, S. (1990). Compensatory articulation during speech: Evidence from the analysis and synthesis of vocal tract shapes using an articulatory model. In W. J. Hardcastle & A.Marchal (Eds.), *Speech production and speech modelling* (pp. 131–149). Boston, MA: Kluwer Academic.

Mariën, P., Verhoeven, J., Engelborghs, S., Rooker, S., Pickut, B. A., & De Deyn, P. P. (2006). A role for the cerebellum in motor speech planning: Evidence from foreign accent syndrome. *Clinical Neurology and Neurosurgery, 108*(5), 518–522.

Matthews, P. M. (2001). An introduction to functional magnetic resonance imaging of the brain. In P. Jezzard, P. M. Matthews, S. M. Smith (Eds.), *Functional MRI: An introduction to methods* (pp. 3–34). Oxford, UK: Oxford University Press.

Metter, E. J., Riege, W. H., Hanson, W. R., Phelps, M. E., & Kuhl, D. E. (1984). Local cerebral metabolic rates of glucose in movement and language disorders from positron tomography. *American Journal of Physiology, 246*(6 Pt 2), R897–R900.

Moeller, J. R., Strother, S. C., Sidtis, J. J., & Rottenberg, D. A. (1987). The scaled subprofile model: A statistical approach to the analysis of functional patterns of brain metabolism in positron emission tomographic/fluorodeoxyglucose data. *Journal of Cerebral Blood Flow and Metabolism, 7*, 649–658.

Moll, K. L., & Daniloff, R. G. (1971). An investigation of the timing of velar movements during speech. *Journal of the Acoustical Society of America, 50*, 678–684.

Moser, D., Fridriksson, J., Bonilha, L., Healy, E. W., Baylis, G., Baker, J. M., & Rorden, C. (2009). Neural recruitment for the production of native and novel speech sounds. *Neuroimage, 46*(2), 549–557.

Murphy, K., Corfield, D. R., Guz, A., Fink, G. R., Wise, R. J., Harrison, J., & Adams, L. (1997). Cerebral areas associated with motor control of speech in humans. *Journal of Applied Physiology, 83*, 1438–1447.

Narayana, S., Fox, P. T., Zhang, W., Franklin, C., Robin, D. A., Vogel, D., & Ramig, L. O. (2010). Neural correlates of efficacy of voice therapy in Parkinson's disease identified by performance-correlation analysis. *Human Brain Mapping*. [Epub ahead of print].

Narayana, S., Jacks, A., Robin, D. A., Poizner, H., Zhang, W., Franklin, C., . . . Fox, P. T. (2009). A noninvasive imaging approach to understanding speech changes following deep brain stimulation in Parkinson's disease. *American Journal of Speech and Language Pathology, 18*(2), 146–161.

Ogar, J. M., Dronkers, N. F., Brambati, S. M., Miller, B. L., & Gorno-Tempini, M. L. (2007). Progressive nonfluent aphasia and its characteristic motor speech deficits. *Alzheimer Disease and Associated Disorders, 21*(4): S23–S30.

Okuda, B., Kawabata, K., Tachibana, H., & Sugita, M. (1999). Cerebral blood flow in pure dysarthria: Role of frontal cortical hypoperfusion. *Stroke, 30*, 109–113.

Ortigue, S., Thompson, J. C., Parasuraman, R., & Grafton, S. T. (2009). Spatio-temporal dynamics of human intention understanding in temporo-parietal cortex: A combined EEG/fMRI repetition suppression paradigm. *PLoS One, 4*(9): e6962.

Peeva, M. G., Guenther, F. H., Tourville, J. A., Nieto-Castanon, A., Anton, J. L., Nazarian, B., & Alario, F. X. (2010). Distinct representations of phonemes, syllables, and supra-syllabic sequences in the speech production network. *Neuroimage, 50*(2), 626–638.

Péran, P., Rascol, O., Démonet, J. F., Celsis, P., Nespoulous, J. L., Dubois, B., & Cardebat, D. (2003). Deficit of verb generation in nondemented patients with Parkinson's disease. *Movement Disorders, 18,* 150–156.

Perkell, J. S. (1980). Phonetic features and the physiology of speech production. In B. Butterworth (Ed.), *Language production, volume 1: Speech and talk* (pp. 337–372). New York, NY: Academic Press.

Petersen, S. E., Fox, P. T., Posner, M. I., & Raichle, M. E. (1988). Positron emission tomographic studies of the cortical anatomy of single-word processing. *Nature, 331,* 585–589.

Petersen, S. E., Fox, P. T., Posner, M. I., & Raichle, M. E. (1989). Positron emission tomographic studies of the processing of single words. *Journal of Cognitive Neuroscience, 1,* 153–170.

Petersen, S. E., Fox, P. T., Snyder, A. Z., & Raichle, M. E. (1990). Activation of extrastriate and frontal cortical areas by visual words and word-like stimuli. *Science, 249,* 1041–1044.

Phelps, M. E., Hoffman, E. J., Coleman, R. E., Welch, M. J., Raichle, M. E., Weiss, E. S., . . . Ter-Pogossian, M. M. (1976). Tomographic images of blood pool and perfusion in brain and heart. *Journal of Nuclear Medecine, 17,* 603–612.

Phelps, M. E., Mazziotta, J. C., Kuhl, D. E., Nuwer, M., Packwood, J., Metter, J., & Engel, J. Jr. (1980). Tomographic mapping of human cerebral metabolism visual stimulation and deprivation. *Journal of Computer Assisted Tomography, 4,* 727–736.

Pinto, S., Thobois, S., Costes, N., Le Bars, D., Benabid, A. L., Broussolle, E., . . . Gentil, M. (2004). Subthalamic nucleus stimulation and dysarthria in Parkinson's disease: A PET study. *Brain, 127*(Pt 3), 602–615.

Radanovic, M., & Scaff, M. (2003). Speech and language disturbances due to sub-cortical lesions. *Brain & Language, 84*(3), 337–352.

Raichle, M. E., Welch, M. J., Grubb, R. L. Jr., Larson, K. B., Laux, B. E., & Ter-Pogossian, M.M. (1978). Regional cerebral oxygen utilization with positron emission tomography. *Journal of Computer Assisted Tomography, 2,* 637–664.

Rektorova, I., Barrett, J., Mikl, M., Rektor, I. & Paus, T. (2007). Functional abnormalities in the primary orofacial sensorimotor cortex during speech in Parkinson's disease. *Movement Disorders, 22,* 2043–2051.

Ricci, M., Magarelli, M., Todino, V., Bianchini, A., Calandriello, E., & Tramutoli, R. (2008). Progressive apraxia of speech presenting as isolated disorder of speech articulation and prosody: a case report. *Neurocase, 14*(2), 162–168.

Riecker, A., Ackermann, H., Wildgruber, D., Dogil, G., & Grodd, W. (2000). Opposite hemispheric lateralization effects during speaking and singing at motor cortex, insula and cerebellum. *Neuroreport, 11,* 1997–2000.

Riecker, A., Brendel, B., Ziegler, W., Erb, M., & Ackermann, H. (2008). The influence of syllable onset complexity and syllable frequency on speech motor control. *Brain & Language, 107*(2), 102–113.

Riecker, A., Kassubek, J., Gröschel, K., Grodd, W., & Ackermann, H. (2006). The cerebral control of speech tempo: Opposite relationship between speaking rate and BOLD signal changes at striatal and cerebellar structures. *Neuroimage, 29*(1), 46–53.

Riecker, A., Mathiak, K., Wildgruber, D., Erb, M., Hertrich, I., Grodd, W., & Ackermann, H. (2005). fMRI reveals two distinct cerebral networks subserving speech motor control. *Neurology, 64*(4), 700–706.

Sachin, S., Senthil Kumaran, S., Singh, S., Goyal, V., Shukla, G., Mahajan, H., & Behari, M. (2008). Functional mapping in PD and PSP for sustained phonation and phoneme tasks. *Journal of Neurological Sciences, 273,* 51–56.

Shuren, J. (1993). Insula and aphasia. *Journal of Neurology, 240*(4), 216–218.

Shuster, L. I. (2009). The effect of sublexical and lexical frequency on speech production: An fMRI investigation. *Brain & Language, 111*(1), 66–72.

Shuster, L. I., & Lemieux, S. K. (2005). An fMRI investigation of covertly and overtly produced mono- and multisyllabic words. *Brain & Language, 93*(1), 20–31.

Sidtis, J. J., Gomez, C., Groshong, A., Strother, S. C., & Rottenberg, D. A. (2006). Mapping cerebral blood flow during speech production in hereditary ataxia. *Neuroimage, 31*(1), 246–254.

Takahashi, S., Oki, J., Miyamoto, A., & Okuno, A. (1998). Hemidystonia, hemichorea, and motor aphasia associated with bilateral ischemic lesions in the striatum: Regional cerebral blood flow studies to clarify the pathophysiology. *Journal of Child Neurology, 13*(8), 408–411.

Tebartz van Elst, L. H., Juengling, F. D., Kassubek, J., Schmidtke, K., Thiel, T., Ebert, D., Dykierek, P., & Hüll, M. (2002). On the role of quantitative brain imaging in the differential diagnosis of speech disorders. *Psychiatry and Clinical Neurosciences, 56*(1), 111–115.

Ternovoi, S. K., Sinitsyn, V. E., Evzikov, G. Y., Morozov, S. P., & Kholodov, B. V. (2004). Localization of the motor and speech zones of the cerebral cortex by functional magnetic resonance tomography. *Neuroscience and Behavioral Physiology, 34*(5), 431–437.

Tzourio-Mazoyer, N., Josse, G., Crivello, F., & Mazoyer, B. (2004). Interindividual variability in the hemispheric organization for speech. *Neuroimage, 21*, 422–435.

Urban, P. P., Wicht, S., Hopf, H. C., Fleischer, S., & Nickel, O. (1999). Isolated dysarthria due to extracerebellar lacunar stroke: A central monoparesis of the tongue. *Journal of Neurology, Neurosurgery and Psychiatry, 66*, 495–501.

Urban, P. P., Wicht, S., Vukurevic, G., Fitzek, C., Fitzek, S., Stoeter, P., . . . Hopf, H. C. (2001). Dysarthria in acute ischemic stroke: Lesion topography, clinicoradiologic correlation, and etiology. *Neurology, 56*, 1021–1027.

Vargha-Khadem, F., Watkins, K. E., Price, C. J., Ashburner, J., Alcock, K. J., Connelly, A., . . . Passingham, R. E. (1998). Neural basis of an inherited speech and language disorder. *Proceedings of the National Academy of Sciences of the United States of America, 95*(21), 12695–12700.

Vigneau, M., Jobard, G., Mazoyer, B., & Tzourio-Mazoyer, N. (2005). Word and non-word reading: What role for the visual word form area? *Neuroimage, 27*, 694–705.

Wieser, H. G. (1991). Temporal lobe epilepsy, sleep and arousal: stereo-EEG findings. *Epilepsy Research (Suppl.), 2*, 97–119.

Wise, R. J., Greene, J., Buchel, C., & Scott, S. K. (1999). Brain regions involved in articulation. *Lancet, 353*, 1057–1061.

Yamamoto, Y. L., Thompson, C. J., Meyer, E., Little, J., & Feindel, W. (1977). Krypton-77 positron emission tomography for measurement of regional cerebral blood flow in a cross section of the head. *Acta Neurologica Scandinavica (Suppl.), 64*, 448–449.

15

Apraxic Failure and the Hierarchical Structure of Speech Motor Plans

A Nonlinear Probabilistic Model

WOLFRAM ZIEGLER, PH.D.

Apraxia of Speech and Learned Speech Motor Behavior

Apraxia of speech (AOS) is considered as an impairment affecting the acquired, overlearned aspects of the motor skill of spoken language production.[1] This stance is taken in most of the historical and the modern perspectives of this disorder. The French neurologist Paul Broca, for instance, who speculated about patients who had lost the "faculty of articulate language" after lesions to the posterior part of the left inferior frontal gyrus, claimed that these patients (whom he called "aphemic") have lost the "memory of the procedures for the production of words"[2] (Broca, 1861). In

modern terms, they have lost the implicit, acquired, procedural knowledge underlying their motor skill of spoken word production. Lichtheim and Wernicke later used the term "speech motor images" (german: *Sprechbewegungsbilder*) to characterize normal adult speakers' capacity of coordinating their vocal tract movements for the generation of words (Lichtheim, 1885). In the associationist thinking of this time, Lichtheim's speech motor images, like Broca's motor memories, were not inborn; they were rather considered as emerging during the maturation of an individual's linguistic and motor abilities. Later, Liepmann (1907) coined the term "apraxia of the speech musculature" (*Apraxie der Sprechmuskulatur*), basing on his view that the faculty of performing

---

[1]See the appendix of this chapter for a list of diagnostic criteria for AOS.
[2]. . . le souvenir du procédé qu'il faut suivre pour articuler les mots." (Broca, 1861, p. 333)

skilled actions relies on an "image of the intended action" and a capability of translating these images into movement patterns (Liepmann, 1907). In his perspective, apraxia (of the limbs or the speech muscles) resulted from a disconnection of the motor images from their associated motor commands. Liepmann considered the left hemisphere to be specialized for the performance of motor actions "freely from memory," i.e., in a feedforward manner, without support from sensory input or from a manipulated object, and in his view, articulation was a prototypical exemplar of an action without an object (Goldenberg, 2003). Therefore, Liepmann implicitly postulated the existence of stored, acquired knowledge about specific motor actions, such as speaking, and their transformation into movement.

Much later, in the 1960s, Darley took up Liepmann's term "apraxia" and the idea of a translation of abstract motor goals into tangible movements when he characterized apraxia of speech as an impairment of the capacity to *program* the movements of the articulators for the purpose of speaking (Darley, 1968). Darley used the *motor program* metaphor to describe the link between the phonological idea of a speech movement and the motor commands that guide the articulations. In the 1960s the notion of the *motor program* had been elaborated most explicitly by Keele (1968), who made the assumption that the muscular specifications of a movement to be performed are stored as units in motor memory, enabling us to access pre-assembled motor patterns and implement them in an automated, error-safe manner. Similar to Liepmann's ideo-kinetic translation pro-

cess, a motor program in Keele's early understanding orchestrates the motor organs in a feedforward-manner—that is, without requiring any sensory input or feedback. Therefore, an implicit assumption of the motor program theory, again, was that these stored representations must have been acquired through a motor learning process.

An obvious drawback of the motor program concept developed by Keele (1968) was that it could not explain the adaptivity of skilled motor actions; if movements were guided by stored, static algorithms, there would be little room for flexible adaptations of a motor activity to changing environments. Therefore, Schmidt (1988) elaborated on a modified motor program theory by introducing the concept of a generalized motor program (GMP), which until today influences some approaches to AOS (e.g., Robin, Jacks, Hageman, Clark, & Woodworth, 2008). Unlike Keele's "open-loop" view of motor programs specifying all details of a movement, the GMP is viewed as a more abstract representation (a schema) of an action to be performed, which is unspecified for parametric details of the action, such as speed or amplitude of performance. GMPs are considered to contain knowledge about the invariants of an action; for example, the relative timing of the components that are part of a more complex motor act. Based on evidence from nonspeech motor performance of patients with apraxia of speech (see the following section), Maas, Robin, Wright, and Ballard (2008) speculated that the neuropathology underlying AOS interferes with GMPs in a universal sense; that is, independent of the type of movement to be performed (e.g., speech or non-speech) and independent of the movement effector implicated in a movement (i.e., vocal tract muscles, fingers, feet, etc.).

What Is the Content of Learned Speech Motor Representations?

The theories sketched previously and several others not mentioned here are —explicitly or implicitly—based on the view that apraxia of speech interferes with learned motor behavior, which, in some unknown manner, is stored in an adult speaker's brain. However, these theories differ strongly in their thinking about what exactly we acquire through speech motor learning and what the contents of our procedural knowledge about the art of speaking are.

Speech-Specific Motor Perspectives

Neurologists of the 19th century were strongly bound to *lexical* theories of language, hence Broca's idea was that speakers dispose of memories of the movements for the production of *words* (Figure 15–1a). Similarly, the speech motor images of the Wernicke-Lichtheim model were of the size of words. However, the view that a separate motor representation exists for each word lacks any generative and adaptive power. If words were the motor primitives of spoken language production, we would have to incur the pain of acquiring a new motor program every time we encounter a new word and for any inflected or cliticized form of a word. Modern perspectives, therefore, usually acknowledge the principle of a *particulation* of word forms as the basis of our ability to create a potentially infinite

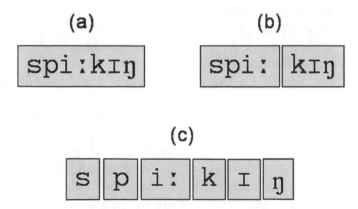

Figure 15–1. Linear accounts of phonetic planning. **(a)** Holistic motor plans for words (e.g., Broca, 1861). **(b)** Syllable-based phonetic planning (e.g., Aichert & Ziegler, 2004; Levelt, 1999). **(c)** Motor programs for phonemes (e.g., Darley, 1968).

number of verbal messages from a small number of primitives (Levelt, 1998), that is, from *sublexical* units. Since these smaller units occur over and over again when we speak, their motor patterns become more and more entrained during speech acquisition and thereby acquire the status of a stored, automated, and error-safe prescription of the corresponding motor pattern. This idea was expressed by Darley when he defined AOS as an impairment of the capacity to program the movements "for the volitional production of *phonemes*" (cited after Wertz, Lapointe, & Rosenbek, 1984, p. 48). On this account, a store of some 50 phoneme programs would be sufficient to generate any verbal message whatsoever, meaning that phoneme-theories of speech planning have an enormous generative power (Figure 15–1c). However, this option obviously suffers from the disadvantage that a large amount of work still remains to be done to adapt the phoneme-sized motor programs to their environment. Therefore, phoneme-based models of phonetic planning shift the whole load of interphonemic coarticulation and supra-segmental integration to subsequent motor execution processes, without further explaining these mechanisms.

Levelt's theory of phonetic encoding partly circumvents this problem by postulating that the major phonetic planning unit is the *syllable* (Levelt, Roelofs, & Meyer, 1999; Cholin, Levelt, & Schiller, 2006; cf., Figure 15–1b). In this view, the syllables that occur most frequently in a language are stored as holistic motor plans in a "mental syllabary." Since a relatively small number of syllables covers a large proportion of our daily spoken output, this organization prin-

ciple would be highly efficient. The importance of the syllable also is substantiated by its key role in mediating between gestural and rhythmical aspects of speech motor control. Furthermore, according to Levelt et al. (1999) only little coarticulation occurs *between* syllables, which reduces the unexplained amount of speech motor organization that needs to be shifted from the planning to the execution stage of the speech production process. The footprints of syllabic mechanisms in speech planning also were found in investigations of syllable structure and frequency effects on apraxic speech errors (Aichert & Ziegler, 2004; Staiger & Ziegler, 2008).

A common assumption implicit to the lexical, the segmental, and the syllabic view is that the phonetic plan of an utterance consists of a linear string of phonetic plans (or motor programs) for the motor primitives that constitute the utterance (see Figure 15–1). Later in this chapter, we refer to these approaches as *linear* theories of phonetic encoding.

Universal Motor Perspectives

The theories reviewed in the preceding section are all based on the idea that we dispose of motor plans that are specific to the motor act of *speaking*. Their implicit assumption is that speech motor learning and practice creates motor representations that are useful for the purpose of producing the sounds of words and phrases, but not for other purposes (Ziegler, 2006). Yet, as mentioned in the preceding paragraph, other theories neglect that goal-specific organization principles of speaking are relevant for explaining the patho-mechanism underlying apraxia of speech (Ballard, Granier, & Robin, 2000; Maas et al., 2008; Robin et al., 2008). To the contrary, they claim that apraxia of speech is merely an epiphenomenon of a more general inability to create a generalized motor program for whatever type of movement, of either the vocal tract muscles or even any other motor system, such as the fingers. This assumption was based on experimental observations in patients with apraxia of speech who demonstrated problems of tracking predictable movements of a cursor on a computer screen by their lip or jaw movements (Robin et al., 2008) or had delayed reactions in producing rhythmical vocal or finger tapping patterns in choice reaction tasks (Maas et al., 2008). From these data the authors inferred that brain lesions causing apraxia of speech in effect destroy our general ability to generate a program for any motor activity that is within the range of our physical potentials and that speaking is simply one of an arbitrary number of action domains of a universal and pluripotent GMP-capacity of humans.

However, this view is incompatible with the fact that adult speakers do not possess an unconstrained potential of generating motor programs for any physiologically possible combination of vocal tract gestures. To the contrary, the range of feasible vocal tract configurations during speaking is strongly limited by the patterns that occur in an adult speaker's native language. For instance, most English speakers have severe problems producing front-rounded vowels ([y] and [ø]), although they are able to round their lips (e.g., for [u] or [o]) and to advance their tongue (e.g., for [i] or [e]), as long as these gestures do not co-occur. Likewise, German speakers have a notorious problem of keeping their vocal folds adducted when a syllable ends with an obstructed vocal tract configuration, like in [lʌv] (love) or [ʀuːʒ] (*French:* red), although glottal adduction *per se* is no problem for them. Similarly, adult French speakers are unable to approach their vocal folds for the production of a voiceless breathy noise (i.e., the consonant [h]) as soon as it comes to speaking, although they have this gesture within their motor repertoire in other circumstances; for example, when they breathe upon their sunglasses to clean them.[3] Many more examples could be generated to demonstrate that speech motor acquisition is not describable as a virtually limitless expansion of gestural potentials. To the contrary, the increase in motor proficiency during speech acquisition is associated with a concomitant limitation of the speaker's gestural repertoire by the constraints of the sound system of her/his native language (e.g., Levitt & Utman, 1992). Universal theories of motor programming cannot account for these language-specific motor constraints.

How, then, can we explain the results of Maas et al. (2008) and Robin et al. (2008)? The observation that patients with lesions to the left posterior inferior frontal region may, in addition to their apraxia of speech, also have problems with choice reaction paradigms or with

---

[3]French infants seem to be able to produce this gesture when they use [h] in their babbling (Vihman, 1992), but lose this ability later during speech acquisition.

the tracking of predictable cursor movements may be ascribable to the fact that this brain region houses a wealth of motor, perceptual or conceptual capabilities, in both the linguistic and the nonlinguistic domain (cf., Schubotz & Fiebach, 2006, and the special issue of Cortex 42, 2006). Therefore, statistical relationships between AOS, on the one hand, and impairments of artificial nonlinguistic tasks like finger tapping or visuomotor tracking, on the other, may tell us something about the proximity of articulate language relative to many other cognitive or motor capacities in left inferior frontal cortex, but they do not explain the mechanisms underlying apraxic speaking.

A Nonlinear Probabilistic Model of Motor Plans for Speaking

If, as it appears, our motor skill of producing words and phrases is based on the acquisition of motor routines that are specific to our native idiom, what is the content of this acquired proficiency? In the preceding section, *linear* theories proposing a sequencing of phoneme- or syllable-sized motor programs were mentioned. However, neither of these approaches provides a satisfactory account of the patterns of impairment seen in apraxic speakers. For instance, a series of model calculations performed recently (Ziegler, Thelen, Staiger, & Liepold, 2008) demonstrated that nei-

ther phonemes nor syllables nor other sublexical units, such as syllable constituents (e.g., rhymes) or metrical feet, are likely to function as the building blocks of motor plans for utterances. This suggests that speech motor plans for words or phrases should not be considered as linear strings of phonetic primitives, as illustrated in Figure 15–1, but rather as hierarchically organized structures, similar to the structures proposed, for instance, in nonlinear phonologies (e.g., Liberman & Prince, 1977).

The model sketched here, therefore, embarks on a nonlinear account of the architecture of motor plans for speaking.[4] It is based on probabilistic considerations of the likelihood of an apraxic speaker to produce a given utterance accurately. Assuming that a patient's likelihood of accurately producing a given speech unit U (e.g., a phonetic gesture, a phoneme, a syllable, etc.) is of the magnitude p $(0 < p < 1)$, one may, in a first approximation, calculate the probability that a combination, V, of two of these units is accurate as

(1a) $\quad p(V) = p(U) * p(U) = p^2.$

However, this approach is only valid if the two subunits of V are independent of each other, as suggested by linear string theories. If, for instance, the two subunits of V are integrated into some higher order motor plan, the probability that V is accurate will be greater than p^2. To the contrary, if the concatenation of the two segments to a larger unit V requires additional motor plan-

---

[4]For a more exhaustive explanation of the architecture of the model presented here, see (Ziegler, 2005, 2009).

ning effort, the probability that V is accurate will decrease, because the process of combining them is also vulnerable to apraxic failure. Generally, therefore,

(1b) $p(V) = p(U) * p(U) * c_V = p^2 * c_V,$

where the coefficient c_V corrects for interdependencies between the two subunits of V. As an example, if the likelihood of a patient to produce a syllable accurately is $p = .8$, then probability that a bisyllabic trochaic word is accurate is $.64 * c_{troc}$. In case the composition of a trochaic word from two syllables creates extra programming expenses, c_{troc} will assume a value < 1. On the contrary, if the two combined syllables form a natural motor unit, for example as parts of a metrical foot, c_{troc} will turn out greater than 1. If, as a third option, the two syllables are encoded independently of each other, as assumed in Levelt's model, the coefficient will not be different from 1. In this sense, the coefficient here represents the strength of the "glue" between the two syllables of a trochee, or the relative stability of motor plans for trochees.

We may apply this combinatorial principle in a recursive manner to construct increasingly larger phonological structures from smaller ones. The approach described here borrows from Articulatory Phonology (AP) (Goldstein, Byrd, & Saltzman, 2006), on the one hand, and from Metrical Phonology (Liberman & Prince, 1977), on the

other. The recursion starts at a basic level of phonetic gestures, as conceptualized by the proponents of Articulatory Phonology and extends to the level at which two or more metrical feet are combined to form a complex utterance. Figure 15–2 explains the principle, using the word *speaking* as an example.

In this word, two syllables combine to form a trochaic foot. The gestures that constitute the word's phonetic plan are arranged around the vocalic nuclei of the two syllables, which are considered to be produced through gross vocal tract gestures.[5] Within each syllable, consonantal gestures can be attached at the end of the syllabic nucleus to form a coda, as for example the consonant [ŋ] in the unstressed syllable of *speaking*. The resulting syllabic rhyme can, in a further step, be expanded by attaching one or more consonantal gestures at the beginning of the syllable's vocalic gesture to form a syllable onset, like the [sp]-related gestures of *spea* or the [k]-related gestures of *king*. Consonantal gestures can be lip (LP), tongue-tip (TT), or tongue-back (TB) gestures, with varying degrees of constriction for plosives, fricatives, and so on. Furthermore, glottal aperture (GA) or velar aperture (VA) gestures can occur in synchrony with these gestures to form voiceless or nasal consonants, respectively (see Figure 15–2).

As a starting point of the computational model, the probability of a vocalic gesture being produced accurately is set to $p \in \,]0, 1[$. When a consonantal

---

[5]For the sake of simplicity, vowel gestures in the present model are considered as holistic vocal tract gestures, without specifying the involved articulator(s). That is, no distinction is made between, for instance, rounded and unrounded vowels. In AP, vowel gestures usually are represented as tongue body gestures (cf., Goldstein et al., 2006).

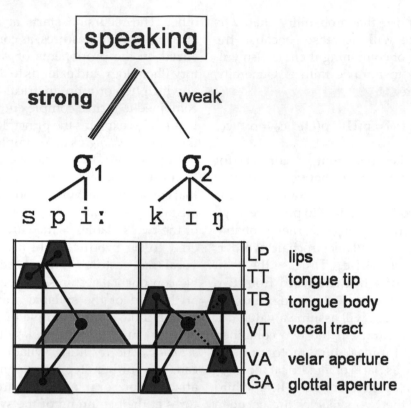

Figure 15–2. A nonlinear gestural model of the phonetic plan for the word *speaking*, inspired by the frameworks of Articulatory Phonology (AP; e.g., Goldstein et al., 2006) and Metrical Phonology (e.g., Liberman & Prince, 1977). Vocal tract gestures for vowels are represented by large trapezoids at the VT-tier (light grey), consonantal gestures by smaller trapezoids (dark grey), arranged at five different articulatory tiers. Consonant gestures of the coda and the onset of each syllable are connected to their vowel nucleus gesture at different phase angles (solid connections for onset, dashed connections for coda). Gestures for consonant clusters are deflected from their CC-centers by a smaller phase angle (see text). Synchronization of velar and glottal aperture gestures with lip, tongue tip or tongue body gestures is represented by vertical connections. The gestural scores of the two syllables are connected under the metrical domain of a trochaic foot, with a strong first and a weak second syllable.

gesture is attached to a vocalic gesture in the coda position, the likelihood that the combination of the two gestures is accurate is, according to (1),

$$(2) \quad p' = p^2 * c_{cod},$$

where c_{cod} is a real number such that $p' \in \,]0, 1[$. The coefficient c_{cod} accounts for the specific phase relationship between the two involved gestures[6] and represents the strength of the "glue" by which the two gestures are interlinked in the motor plan of the syllable rhyme.

Likewise, when a consonantal gesture is attached to the onset of a vowel nucleus gesture, the likelihood that the resulting gestural sequence is accurate is

$$(3) \quad p'' = p^2 * c_{ons},$$

where c_{ons} is a real number such that $p'' \in]0, 1[$. Again the coefficient c_{ons} accounts for the specific phase relationship between onset and nucleus gestures.[7]

In a further step, the model has to account for consonant clusters. If two consecutive labial, tongue tip, or tongue back gestures occur in a sequence within the coda or the onset position of a syllable (i.e., in a consonant cluster), it is assumed that these two gestures have a specific inter-gestural phase relation, irrespective of their position relative to the vowel gesture (i.e., onset or coda). For the likelihood of two sequential gestures in a consonant cluster to be accurate we set, analogous to (2) and (3),

$$(4) \quad p''' = p^2 * c_{clu}.$$

The coefficient c_{clu} here accounts for the phase relationship between two primary articulations in a consonant cluster, as for instance the tongue tip gesture and the lip gesture in [sp]

of *speaking* (see Figure 15–2). Hence, relative to the vowel gesture, these two gestures are specified, first, by their onset phase relation, and, second, by a small phase-shift relative to their "CC-centre" due to the clustering. In Figure 15–2, this is illustrated by the lines connecting the vowel nucleus gesture of *spea* with the TT-LP-sequence of *sp* for the onset phase relation, and between the two *sp*-gestures for the cluster phase relation.

Regarding the VA- and GA-layers in Figure 15–2, the consonant gestures in these layers also are specified for their phase-relation to the syllable nucleus gesture, hence their attachment to the vowel gesture is weighted by the coefficients c_{cod}, c_{ons}, and c_{clu}, respectively. At the same time, the model also accounts for the fact that the VA- and GA-gestures need to be synchronized with one or more of the primary articulations of the LP-, TT-, or TB-layers (see Figure 15–1). To account for this, each VA- or GA- attachment also is weighted by a synchronization coefficient c_{sync}. Note that only a single GA gesture is assumed to occur in the onset of *spea*, which is weighted for its onset position (c_{ons}) and for its synchronization with the TT- and LP- gestures (c_{sync}), but not for clustering.

So far, only within-syllable structural relationships were explained. However, the model also accounts for supra-syllabic, that is, metrical properties.

---

[6]Recall that AP postulates that gestures for coda consonants are in a 180° phase relationship with their vowel nucleus gestures (cf., Goldstein et al., 2006). For the purpose of the present model this assumption is not substantial.

[7]AP postulates that gestures for onset consonants are in a 0° phase relationship with their vowel nucleus gestures (cf., Goldstein et al., 2006). Again, for the purpose of the present model this assumption is not substantial.

Regarding the example of Figure 15–2, the fact that *king* constitutes the weak syllable of a trochaic foot is accounted for by weighting each of its gestures by a specific coefficient, c_{tail}, which accounts for the alternatives that planning a gesture in the position of the tail of a metrical foot may cause supra-exponential programming costs ($c_{tail} < 1$) or may be facilitated by some super-ordinate motor integration process at the foot level ($c_{tail} > 1$). In metrical feet containing two weak syllables, like in the word *CAnada*, the gestures of the second weak syllable are weighted likewise.

Finally, a word may contain more than one foot, for instance a trochaic foot with an upbeat (e.g., *aPRAxic*) or two metrical feet (e.g., *CORresPONdence*). In these cases, there is always a prominent foot (e.g., *praxic*, *pondence*) and a subordinate metrical component, that is, an anacrusis (e.g., *a* in *apraxia*) or a subordinate foot (e.g., *corres* in *correspondence*). In the probabilistic model sketched here, metrical structure above the foot level is accounted for by weighting each gesture that is part of the subordinate appendage to a full metrical foot by a further model coefficient, c_{sft}. Again, this coefficient stands for the amount of motor planning costs for gestures in a metrically subordinate position, yet this time at a higher metrical level.

Summing up, in the computational architecture of phonetic planning described here a word is modeled by analyzing its gestural and metrical structure, as in the example of Figure 15–2, and calculating weighted probabilities of correct production in a hierarchically nested way, based on a total of seven coefficients. For the example depicted in Figure 15–2, the resulting equation is

$$(5) \quad p_{speaking} = p_{spea} * (p_{king} * c^5_{tail})$$
$$= p^4 * c^3_{ons} * c^2_{clu} * c_{sync} *$$
$$(p^5 * c^2_{cod} * c^2_{ons} * c^2_{sync} * c^5_{tail}).$$

Since the word *speaking* consists of only a single metrical foot, the coefficient c_{sft} does not occur in its parametric modeling.

Calculating the Model Coefficients

In order to determine numerically the coefficients of the model, equations of type (5) shown previously must be resolved. For this purpose, estimates of the likelihood of correct articulation are needed for a sufficiently large number of words with different structures, to be filled in on the left of these equations. These estimates need to have a fairly high resolution, in order to be able to predict small differences between the phonetic planning efforts required for words with different shapes.

Participants and Materials

We used accuracy data from a large pool of speech samples obtained from 40 carefully selected patients with apraxia of speech who had undergone a total of 120 examinations with a word repetition test (Liepold, Ziegler, & Brendel, 2003). The data were collected over a period of more than 10 years, during the course of the evaluation of the *Hierarchical Word Lists* (Liepold et al., 2003) and during several research projects on apraxia of speech (Aichert, 2009; Brendel & Ziegler, 2008; Staiger, 2009). The patients were based in the

Clinic for Neuropsychology of the *Munich City Hospital* or were referred from private practices and clinical centers in different parts of the country. All of them had apraxia of speech as their major clinical impairment, according to the criteria reported in Ziegler (2008) (cf., the appendix). Yet, most of them also had additional aphasic symptoms, such as agrammatism or impaired word retrieval (for a more comprehensive description of the patient sample, see Ziegler, 2009). The materials were composed of a selection of 72-word and nonword items drawn from the *Hierarchical Word Lists* (Liepold et al., 2003). The items varied in length (1–4 syllables) and syllable complexity (empty or filled onsets or codas, with single consonants or consonant clusters) and were controlled for a number of variables (cf., Ziegler, 2005).

Accuracy Scores

Each word was rated for accurate production on a pass-fail-basis. An error was notified if at least one of the phonemes of a word was affected by a phonemic error (substitution, omission, or addition), a phonetic distortion, or both. Ratings were performed by experienced clinicians who were not familiar with the hypotheses of this study.[8] A reliability analysis revealed that listener agreement on these ratings was good (Kendall's tau = 0.80; Liepold et al., 2003). For each word, an accuracy index was calculated as the proportion of correct productions among the 120 samples of the population studied here. This index was considered as an estimate of the likelihood that a particular word is produced accurately by an "ideal average apraxic speaker." A rather low index was, for instance, obtained for the word "Mikroskop," (Engl. *microscope*) ($p_{mikroskop} = 0.260$), meaning that this word is highly vulnerable to apraxic failure, hence it presumably requires a high phonetic encoding effort. On the contrary, a much higher index was obtained for the disyllabic word "blume," (Engl. *flower*) ($p_{blume} = 0.531$), indicating that considerably fewer apraxic speakers made errors on blume, which suggests that much less motor planning effort is required to produce it.

Each word's accuracy index was inserted in the corresponding model equation, as in (5), yielding a total of 72 nonlinear equations of different complexities, with seven unknown coefficients.[9] A nonlinear regression analysis was calculated to obtain statistical estimates for the model coefficients.

Shape and Properties of the Nonlinear Model

Goodness-of-Fit

The regression model converged to a stable solution, with a goodness-of-fit that was similarly high as in the two

---

[8]Michaela Liepold, Bettina Brendel, and Marco Mebus are acknowledged for their evaluation of most of these materials. Further contributions were made by Anja Staiger and Ingrid Aichert.
[9]Effectively, one additional coefficient was needed to account for the difference between words and nonwords. Each gesture of a nonword was weighted for nonlexicality, analogous to the procedure described in Ziegler (2009).

earlier approaches (Ziegler, 2005, 2009), namely 0.83. It is remarkable that a gestural and metrical parametric description of the 72 words and nonwords was obviously sufficient to explain, with a high mathematical stability, more than 80% of the variation in the average accuracy scores of these words.

Given the high simulation accuracy of the nonlinear model, it is most interesting to see what the numerical values of the seven coefficients tell us about the shape of the model.

The base value obtained for the estimated likelihood of accurate gesture production was .972, which appears considerably high, given that the average proportion of accurate word production in the whole sample was .39. An obvious explanation is that accurate word production requires correct production of a larger number of gestures at the same time, which may cause an exponential decay of the accuracy scores with increasing numbers of gestures.

The remaining model coefficients yield a description of the relative strength of the glue by which the gestures of a word are coupled at different levels. To illustrate this, Figure 15–3 presents the coupling graph (Goldstein, Pouplier, Chen, Saltzman, & Byrd, 2007) of the gestural model of the word "speaking," as depicted in Figure 15–2, with the numerical values of the model coefficients for each of the connections. Asterisks indicate where a coefficient was significantly different from 1 at a significance level of .05.

Coda versus Onset Gestures

The weightings obtained for the combination of a vowel gesture with a coda

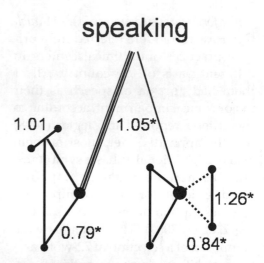

Figure 15–3. Coupling graph of the word *speaking* (see Figure 15–2), labeled by empirically determined weights for the coupling of gestures at different hierarchical levels (see text). The base value describing the probability of accurate gesture production is p = .97. Not indicated in this graph is the weighting of gestures above the foot level (c_{sft} = 1.002).

or onset gesture were .84 and .79, respectively. The fact that these gestural combinations include a supra-exponential decay in accuracy is probably ascribable to the fact that consonantal gestures generally impose higher demands than vowel gestures. More importantly, however, c_{ons} (= .79) was remarkably lower than c_{coda} (= .84), which is consistent with the view that onsets are more vulnerable to apraxic errors than coda consonants (Aichert & Ziegler, 2004). As an example, simulation of two syllables containing the same consonant in either the coda or the onset position, such as [al] versus [la], yields markedly different accuracy scores, i.e., $p_{[la]}$ = .75 vs. $p_{[al]}$ = .79.

Consonant Clusters

The encoding of two consonantal gestures within the onset or the coda position, that is, in a consonant cluster, turned out to be neither more nor less expensive than one would predict on purely combinatorial grounds (c_{clu} = 1.005; p > .05). This result is compatible with what we found in a first, phoneme-based version of this model (Ziegler, 2005) but is at variance with the feature-based account of Ziegler (2009), in which a weak but significant cluster effect was obtained. It generally is accepted that clusters are particularly error-prone in apraxic speech, but this may simply be due to the almost trivial fact that they involve more gestures than single consonants. Given the inconsistent results of our different nonlinear modeling approaches, it is still an open question if the increase of phonetic encoding expenses involved in consonant clusters is disproportionately large and, therefore, requires for some additional explanation, for example, by specifically challenging timing demands. Alternatively, cluster effects simply may be explained by the higher number of gestures involved in a cluster, as evident from the current results. Simulation of the onsets of [ka] versus [kla], for instance, yields considerably different accuracy values, that is, $p_{[ka]}$ = 0.72 vs. $p_{[kla]}$ = 0.56, but this effect is ascribable solely to the additional TT onset gesture that is present in [kla], but not in [ka].

Synchronous Articulations

As a further result, the combination of primary articulations with synchronous gestures of the larynx or the velum was weighted by a rather high value of the coefficient c_{sync} (= 1.26), meaning that parallel velar or laryngeal articulations pose no specific synchronization problem. To the contrary, they are much less expensive than one would predict from the fact that an additional gesture has to be produced, which is consistent with the results obtained for an earlier, feature-based version of the nonlinear model (Ziegler, 2009). It should be noted that the model still forecasts a lower accuracy for an onset like [kna] ($p_{[kna]}$ = 0.54), which involves a velar aperture gesture, as opposed to [kla] ($p_{[kla]}$ = 0.56), where no such gesture is involved. However, the difference is smaller than the presence of an additional velar gesture would predict. One explanation of this outcome could be that there is no real need to synchronize laryngeal and velar gestures with lip or tongue gestures, because the timing of any consonantal gesture is determined uniquely by its phase relation relative to the vowel gesture. Since this would only imply that c_{sync} is not significantly smaller than 1, a further argument is needed to explain why c_{sync} was indeed much larger than 1. One might speculate that many of the gestural combinations with velar or laryngeal abductions considered here occur with a high frequency. For instance, in German glottal abduction in the coda position occurs as a rule if the primary articulation is obstruent. Furthermore, velar lowering occurs very frequently in combination with alveolar closure, because [n] is the most frequent consonant in German. More generally, the high value of c_{sync} may be indexical of language-specific frequency properties at the gestural level.

Metrical Influences

At the supra-syllabic level, the combination of a strong syllable with one or two weak syllables to form a metrical foot was weighted by $c_{tail} = 1.05$, which was significantly larger than 1 (p<.05). Therefore, production of a trochaic or dactylic foot turned out less expensive than the independent production of two or three syllables in a row, suggesting that metrical feet represent a natural unit of phonetic integration. Again, this is a replication of earlier results (Ziegler, 2005, 2009). The fact that trochaic feet are particularly stable units in apraxia of speech may result from this metrical pattern occurring with a very high frequency among German content words, which implies that the corresponding motor rhythm is exercised to a particularly high degree. It is also consistent with the finding of a preference for trochaic feet very early during speech acquisition in infants who grow up in a German speaking environment (Fischer, 2009).

A final coefficient, which is not represented in Figure 15–3, accounts for the combination of units at the level of metrical feet. The numerical value of the corresponding coefficient turned out to be very close to 1 (and not significantly different from 1), that is, $c_{sft} = 1.002$. As an interpretation, the likelihood that two feet or an upbeat and a foot are produced accurately is strictly *multiplicative*, that is, the phonetic codes of these units appear to be generated independently of each other. This may mean that with each new metrical foot in an utterance, speakers with apraxia open a new motor planning window. As we had found in an earlier study, there may be differences between patients with mild and severe apraxia of speech, to the extent that patients with a less severe impairment may tend to generate overarching phonetic plans for more than one foot and thereby increase their likelihood of making errors to a disproportionate extent on these longer utterances (Ziegler, 2009).

Nonlinear versus Linear Modeling

Figure 15–4 illustrates some of the properties of the nonlinear probabilistic model of apraxic speech production as compared to linear accounts. In Figure 15–4a, the observed proportions of accurate word production are plotted against syllabic length (filled symbols). The left panel of Figure 15–4a also depicts estimates of production accuracy based on a linear, syllable-by-syllable view of word production, starting from the observed proportion of .51 correct productions of monosyllables (open symbols). A linear string model as postulated in Levelt et al. (1999) would for instance predict that two-syllabic words have an estimated accuracy score of $.51 \times .51 = .26$, but it becomes obvious from the observed data that the proportion of accurate disyllabic word productions was considerably higher. Considering that the underlying word list contained only regular (trochaic) metrical forms among the disyllabic words, this difference suggests that the two syllables in a trochee are integrated at the phonetic encoding level. Most of the three-syllabic words of the underlying word list included more than a single metrical foot, hence the decay of accurate word productions was slightly steeper from the two- to the

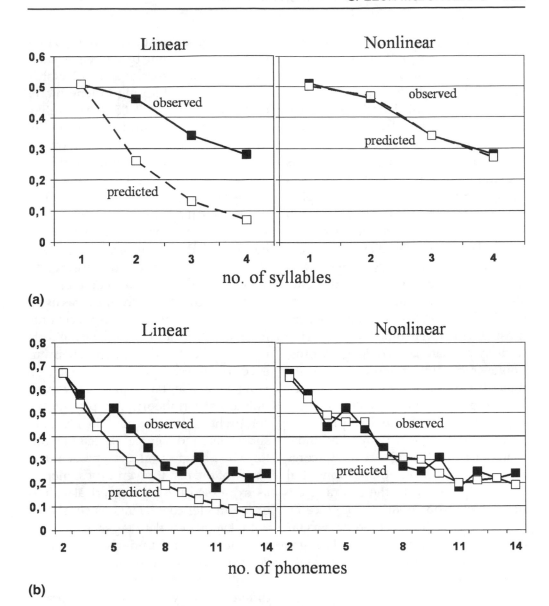

Figure 15–4. Linear versus nonlinear models of phonetic planning for accuracy scores across word length **(a)** in syllables (*top*) and **(b)** in phonemes (*bottom*). The linear models (*left panels*) are based on the assumption that phonetic plans for words are linear strings of motor programs for smaller units, that is, syllables or phonemes, respectively. Model calculations for the linear models are based on empirical accuracy scores for monosyllabic (*top*) or biphonemic words (*bottom*). The panels on the right illustrate the simulation of accuracy scores by the nonlinear probabilistic model presented in this chapter.

three-syllabic words as compared to mono- versus disyllables. However, overall the observed data by no means followed the exponential decay that would be predicted by a syllable-by-syllable theory of phonetic encoding.

On the right of Figure 15–4a, the observed data are plotted together with the accuracy estimates simulated by the nonlinear model, demonstrating that the effect of syllabic length was almost perfectly described by the nonlinear approach sketched here.

Figure 15–4b provides an analogous illustration of how the nonlinear model fitted the observed data across phoneme lengths. Again, a linear approach to phonetic encoding would, on combinatorial grounds—predict an exponential decay of accuracy scores with increasing word length. The actual data show that this account makes good predictions for 2- to 4-phoneme words, most of which were monosyllabic in the underlying materials. For longer words, however, the linear model underestimates the empirical accuracy scores (see Figure 15–4b, left panel, open symbols). Because many of the five-phoneme words and all longer words had more than one syllable, their accuracy scores no longer followed the exponential decay hypothesis. To the contrary, the nonlinear probabilistic model came rather close to the observed data as far as the influence of segmental length is concerned (see Figure 15–4b, right panel, open symbols).

Conclusions

In the first instance, the model presented here was developed to explain the variation of apraxic failure as a function of word structure. The nonlinear approach sketched in this chapter resembles the approach taken in two earlier studies, in that it used metrical tree analyses of word structure and a statistical model based on probabilistic reasoning to predict the errors made by a large population of apraxic speakers on 72 words and nonwords differing in length and complexity (Ziegler, 2005, 2009). Unlike these earlier two studies, the model presented here was largely built on the theoretical and terminological framework of Articulatory Phonology (e.g., Goldstein, Byrd, & Saltzman, 2006). It turned out that more than 80% of the variability between the 72 items could be explained on the basis of skeletal structure alone, and no information about the location and degree of constriction of consonant gestures was used.

The theory elaborated here accounts for the length and complexity effects that often have been described to influence accuracy in apraxic speakers (e.g., Staiger & Ziegler, 2008). However, unlike earlier theories, it provides a comprehensive account of the gestural, subsyllabic and metrical aspects of word form by a single, unitary approach. The shape of the resulting empirical model, as expressed by the numerical values of the model coefficients, is consistent with several prevalent hypotheses about the mechanisms underlying apraxic speech errors. For instance, it simulates the often-described vowel-consonant differences in vulnerability to apraxic failure; it provides explanations for onset and cluster effects (e.g., Aichert & Ziegler, 2004; Staiger & Ziegler, 2008), and it gives a new account of the timing problem of velar and laryngeal gestures (e.g., Ziegler & von Cramon, 1986). The nonlinear model also offers a solution to the problem of whether length effects on apraxic speech errors reflect phoneme or syllable number, or the presence of consonant clusters (Nickels & Howard, 2004), by conceiving motor plans for words as nonlinear objects. On the whole, the model conceptualizes apraxia of speech as an impairment that interferes with the language-specific aspects of the gestural, syllabic, and metrical organization of articulation.

It should be pointed out that the fact that this theory borrows from metrical phonology must not be mistaken as suggesting a linguistic-symbolic understanding of the patho-mechanism underlying apraxia of speech. To the contrary, the approach taken here considers the nonlinear phonological framework as a blueprint of the architecture of speech motor plans. Under the assumption that apraxia of speech interferes with phonetic planning processes, therefore, the present model provides clues to a better understanding of the cognitive processes involved in the planning of articulation in unimpaired speakers. In this sense, the model coefficients obtained here may be taken as a description of the relative temporal and spatial stability of gestural coalitions and of the local coherence of motor planning components at different levels, from phonetic gestures to rhythmical units of the size of metrical feet. Relatively strong bindings were found to exist (1) between gestures of the primary articulators, on the one hand, and concomitant synchronized velar and laryngeal gestures, on the other; (2) between vowel and coda as opposed to onset consonant gestures; and (3) between the syllables within a metrical foot. This architecture is claimed to emerge as a result of speech motor learning, through repeated exercises of the recurring gestural and metrical patterns of the speaker's language. The patho-mechanism underlying apraxia of speech is considered to disintegrate these structures, with weaker connections being more vulnerable to apraxic failure than stronger connections.

The nonlinear approach proposed here describes the motor hierarchies of speech production in an entirely new way. This thinking may, in the future, influence our way of designing hierarchically organized materials for the assessment of apraxia of speech. It also may provide clues about how motor requirements can be manipulated more systematically in the treatment of patients with this disorder.

Acknowledgment. The development of this model was supported by DFG-grants Zi469 / 6–1 / 6–2 / 8–1 / 9–1 / 10–2 and by ReHa-Hilfe e.V. Ingrid Aichert and Anja Staiger are acknowledged for continuing valuable discussions of theoretical and clinical issues; Michaela Liepold, Marko Mebus, and Bettina Brendel are thanked for their contributions to the design and evaluation of the materials. I also am indebted to numerous colleagues from the Bogenhausen Hospital, Clinic of Neuropsychology, and from other clinical centers for their collaboration and to the many patients with apraxia of speech who were enrolled in these investigations.

References

Aichert, I. (2009). *Die Bausteine der phonetischen Enkodierung: Untersuchungen zum sprechmotorischen Lernen bei Sprechapraxie.* Tönning, Germany: Der Andere Verlag.

Aichert, I., & Ziegler, W. (2004). Syllable frequency and syllable structure in apraxia of speech. *Brain & Language, 88,* 148–159.

Ballard, K. J., Granier, J. P., & Robin, D. A. (2000). Understanding the nature of apraxia of speech: Theory, analysis, and treatment. *Aphasiology, 14,* 969–995.

Brendel, B., & Ziegler, W. (2008). Effectiveness of metrical pacing in the treatment of apraxia of speech. *Aphasiology, 22,* 77–102.

Broca, P. (1861). Remarques sur le siège de la faculté du langage articulé; suives d'une observation d'aphémie. *Bull. Soc. Anat., 6,* 330–357.

Cholin, J., Levelt, W. J., & Schiller, N. O. (2006). Effects of syllable frequency in speech production. *Cognition, 99,* 205–235.

Darley, F. L. (1968). *Apraxia of speech: 107 years of terminological confusion.* Paper presented at the Annual Convention of the ASHA.

Fischer, A. (2009). *Prosodic organization in the babbling of German-learning infants between the age of six and twelve months.* Humboldt-Universität Berlin.

Goldenberg, G. (2003). Apraxia and beyond: Life and work of Hugo Liepmann. *Cortex, 39,* 509–524.

Goldstein, L., Byrd, D., & Saltzman, E. (2006). The role of vocal tract gestural action units in understanding the evolution of phonology. In M. A. Arbib (Ed.), *Action to language via the mirror neuron system* (pp. 215). Cambridge, UK: University Press.

Goldstein, L., Pouplier, M., Chen, L., Saltzman, E., & Byrd, D. (2007). Dynamic action units slip in speech production errors. *Cognition, 103,* 386–412.

Keele, S. W. (1968). Movement control in skilled motor performance. *Psychological Bulletin, 70,* 387–403.

Levelt, W. J. M. (1998). The genetic perspective in psycholinguistics or where do spoken words come from. *Journal of Psycholinguistic Research, 27,* 167–180.

Levelt, W. J. M., Roelofs, A., & Meyer, A. S. (1999). A theory of lexical access in speech production. *Behavioral and Brain Sciences, 22,* 1–38.

Liberman, A. M., & Prince, A. (1977). On stress and linguistic rhythm. *Linguistic Inquiry, 8,* 249–336.

Lichtheim, L. (1885). Ueber Aphasie. Aus der medicinischen Klinik in Bern. *Deutsches Archiv für klinische Medicin, 36,* 204–268.

Liepmann, H. (1907). Zwei Fälle von Zerstörung der unteren linken Stirnwindung. *Journal für Psychologie und Neurologie, IX,* 279–289.

Liepold, M., Ziegler, W., & Brendel, B. (2003). Hierarchische Wortlisten. Ein Nachsprechtest für die Sprechapraxiediagnostik. Dortmund, Borgmann.

Maas, E., Robin, D. A., Wright, D. L., & Ballard, K. J. (2008). Motor programming in apraxia of speech. *Brain & Language, 106,* 107–118.

Nickels, L., & Howard, D. (2004). Dissociating effects of number of phonemes, number of syllables, and syllabic complexity on word production in aphasia: It's the number of phonemes that counts. *Cognitive Neuropsychology, 21,* 57–78.

Robin, D. A., Jacks, A., Hageman, C., Clark, H. M., & Woodworth, G. (2008). Visuomotor tracking abilities of speakers with apraxia of speech or conduction aphasia. *Brain & Language, 106,* 98–106.

Schmidt, R. A. (1988). *Motor control and learning* (2nd ed.). Champaign, IL: Human Kinetics.

Schubotz, R. I., & Fiebach, C. J. (2006). Integrative models of Broca's area and the ventral premotor cortex. *Cortex, 42,* 461–463.

Staiger, A. (2009). *Frequenz und Struktur sublexikalischer Einheiten in der Spontansprache bei Sprechapraxie.* Tönning, Germany: Der Andere Verlag.

Staiger, A., & Ziegler, W. (2008). Syllable frequency and syllable structure in the spontaneous speech production of patients with apraxia of speech. *Aphasiology, 22,* 1201–1215.

Wertz, R. T., Lapointe, L. L., & Rosenbek, J. C. (1984). *Apraxia of speech in adults. The disorder and its management.* Orlando, FL: Grune & Stratton.

Ziegler, W. (2005). A nonlinear model of word length effects in apraxia of speech. *Cognitive Neuropsychology, 22,* 603–623.

Ziegler, W. (2006). Distinctions between speech and nonspeech motor control. A neurophonetic view. In M. Tabain & J. Harrington (Eds.), *Speech production: Models, phonetic processes, and techniques* (pp. 41–54). New York, NY: Psychology Press.

Ziegler, W. (2008). Apraxia of speech. In G. Goldenberg & B. L. Miller (Eds.), *Neuropsychology and behavioral neurology* (3rd ed., pp. 269–286). Edinburgh, UK: Elsevier.

Ziegler, W. (2009). Modeling the architecture of phonetic plans: Evidence from apraxia of speech. *Language and Cognitive Processes, 24,* 631–661

Ziegler, W., & Cramon, D. Y. V. (1986). Timing deficits in apraxia of speech. *European Archives of Psychiatry and Neurological Sciences, 236,* 44–49.

Ziegler, W., Thelen, A.-K., Staiger, A., & Liepold, M. (2008). The domain of phonetic encoding in apraxia of speech: Which sub-lexical units count? *Aphasiology, 22,* 1230–1247.

Appendix:
Diagnostic Criteria for Apraxia of Speech

(cf., Ziegler, 2008).

(1) Patients with AOS produce *segmental errors*.
   (a) Unlike patients with aphasic phonological impairment, they produce a substantial amount of phonetic distortions in addition to (perceived) phonemic errors.
   (b) Unlike the uniformly aberrant articulatory settings encountered in dysarthric speakers, the distortions of patients with AOS often can be allocated to individual phonemes or phoneme transitions and are highly variable.
   (c) At times, even moderately impaired patients may produce entirely error-free words or phrases.

(2) Patients with AOS present with prosodic abnormalities.
   (a) Their speech is dysfluent due to frequent sound prolongations and frequent within- or between-syllable pauses.
   (b) They often produce false-starts and self-corrections, causing additional dysfluency.
   (c) The dysfluent and hesitant nature of their speech often entails destruction of natural stress and intonation patterns.

(3) Patients with AOS are conspicuous for their speaking behavior.
   (a) Their speaking appears effortful and laborious.
   (b) They often demonstrate visible and/or audible groping.
   (c) They are aware of their articulation problems and often express frustration about their incapacity.

16

Defective Neural Motor Speech Mappings As a Source for Apraxia of Speech

Evidence from a Quantitative Neural Model of Speech Processing

BERND J. KRÖGER, PH.D., NICK MILLER, PH.D., ANJA LOWIT, PH.D., AND CHRISTIANE NEUSCHÄFER-RUBE, PH.D.

Introduction

Since apraxia of speech (AOS) emerged as a focus of attention in the 1960s (Darley, Aronson, & Brown, 1975) the design and interpretation of studies has been dogged by variations in definitions used and consequent characteristics of cases investigated. The plethora of psycholinguistic, neurological, and speech motor control models employed to derive or justify diagnostic markers has led to sets of clinical criteria that are not all universally accepted. A major obstacle to investigations is the rarity with which AOS occurs in isolation from other disorders. Nevertheless, it generally is accepted that AOS represents some kind of distinct motor speech disorder (Ogar, Slama, Dronkers, Amici, & Gorno-Tempini, 2005) or a form of a phonetic-motoric disorder (McNeil, 2008), separating it from other neurological disorders of speech and language, most notably aphasia and dysarthria (Jordan & Hillis 2006). From a cognitive or functional point of view, AOS has been labeled or defined as "inefficiencies in the translation of well-formed and -filled phonological frames into previously learned kinematic information used for carrying out intended movements" (McNeil, 2008, p. 264), or more generally "impairment in the translation of phonological representations into specifications for articulation" (Croot, 2002). On the one hand, these cognitive definitions of AOS separate it from aphasia since linguistic processing (comprising conceptual, lexical, and grammatical processing) is not deemed to be impaired. On the other hand, they separate AOS from the dysarthrias since it is the specification of articulations but not the basic neuromuscular articulatory system *per se*, that is believed to be impaired. Following these definitions, both the linguistic processing system as well as the entire speech production apparatus (lungs, larynx, pharynx, nasal and oral cavity, lower jaw, lips, tongue, and velum) and its muscular system, including (peripheral) neuromuscular activation, are seen as separate and unimpaired. Furthermore, most definitions cite primary peripheral sensory (auditory and somatosensory, i.e., tactile and proprioceptive) processing as unimpaired in AOS (see McNeil, 2008).

Behavioral definitions of AOS rely on descriptions of typical symptoms such as "intra- and inter-articulator temporal and spatial segmental and prosodic distortions, (. . .) distortions of segments and intersegment transitionalization," with errors being "relatively consistent in location within the utterance and invariable in type" (McNeil, Robin, & Schmidt, 1997, p. 329). Earlier summaries pointed to "(1) effortful, trial and error groping articulatory movements and attempts at self-correction, (2) dysprosody unrelieved by extended periods of normal rhythm, stress, and intonation, (3) articulatory inconsistency on repeated productions of the same utterance, (4) obvious difficulty initiating utterances" (Wertz, LaPointe, & Rosenbeck, 1984, p. 81).

A major drawback of behavioral definitions of AOS is that none of these symptoms can be accepted as unambiguous or strong indicators for the disorder (Croot, 2002). Numerous signs, such as inconsistency in production errors, remain highly controversial, and debate continues as to how far many of the perceived segmental errors (insertions, elisions, segmental changes, for example, from voiced to voiceless, etc.) are not actually segmental in nature but are associated with deficits in the overall coordination of articulatory movements.

Furthermore, a lack of a comprehensive definition provides transparency between functional, behavioral, and psycholinguistic conceptualizations, motoric characterizations, and neurophysiological and anatomical specifications of AOS. One barrier to this is that the brain networks associated with translating phonological representations into specifications for articulation are distributed widely over cortical and subcortical regions (Hickok and Poeppel, 2004; Hillis et al. 2004; Miller, 2002; Riecker, Brendel, Ziegler, Erb, & Ackermann, 2008) and distinct brain regions can be active during very different tasks (speech and nonspeech). Nevertheless several writers have called for a definition of AOS based on a detailed and quantitative model of speech processing comprising cognitive as well as sensorimotor aspects of speech production (Croot, 2002; Miller, 2000; Miller, 2002) as the only way to proceed to a full understanding of AOS.

The aim of this chapter is to demonstrate how a quantitative neural model of speech processing, comprising both cognitive and sensorimotor aspects of speech production, works toward a more comprehensive understanding of AOS. Such a model could lead to insights into possible underlying neural functional processes of speech production and, particularly, the relations between neural dysfunctions in the process of speech production and the resulting articulatory misbehavior. We will proceed by highlighting the main features of the model and then illustrate how so-called "typical symptoms" of apraxia of speech arise from lesions at different points in the model. Through this, we hope to throw more light onto the nature of the mechanisms in speech

apraxic break down and the relationship between perceived and underlying disturbance in AOS.

An Action-Based Quantitative Neurocomputational Model of Speech Processing

The neurocomputational action-based model (ACT, Figure 16–1) is described in detail in Kröger, Kannampuzha, and Neuschaefer-Rube (2009) and Kröger, Kannampuzha, Lowit, and Neuschaefer-Rube (2009). As these papers have

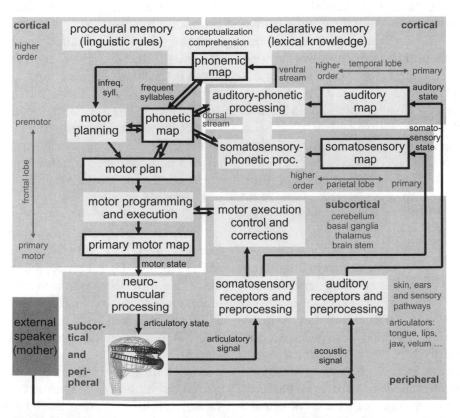

Figure 16–1. Organization of the neural model. Boxes with black outline represent neural maps. Arrows indicate processing paths or neural mappings. Boxes without outline indicate processing modules.

shown, this model is capable of producing real articulatory and acoustic signals and simulating the normal speech acquisition process. The model introduced here is computer-implemented and, thus, strongly quantitative. Mappings co-activate neural states in those maps, which are connected by a mapping. Thus, the mappings between phonetic map, motor plan map, and sensory maps (see Figure 16–1) co-activate neural representations of phonemic states, auditory states, somatosensory states, and motor plan states of speech items under production. Thus, we assume that the phonetic map comprises mirror neurons capable of closely linking sensory and motor states. We further assume that the appropriate mappings are distributed widely within frontal, temporal, and parietal cortical regions. It is beyond the scope of this chapter to give a comprehensive discussion of anatomical location of brain functions for speech processing, but it should be noted that many of our neural processing stages are comparable to those defined by Guenther (2006) and Guenther, Ghosh, and Tourville (2006). These authors offer a comprehensive discussion of the anatomical cortical and subcortical location of functional modules, maps, and mappings for speech processing.

ACT is capable of producing articulatory movement patterns and acoustic signals by controlling a 3-D articulatory-acoustic model. In parallel to the quantitative neural model of speech production introduced by Guenther (2006) and Guenther et al. (2006) (DIVA), our model separates feed-forward and feedback control. A major difference of our approach compared to DIVA is the separation of motor planning and motor execution. This separation results from the assumption that speech movements (similar to limb movements) are controlled by action units. Using this concept (Goldstein, Byrd, & Saltzman, 2006; Goldstein, Pouplier, Chen, Saltzman, & Byrd, 2007), a motor plan (also termed vocal tract action score or gestural score) specified for a speech item under production is the result of action planning. On the motor plan level, all gestures forming an utterance are selected, and their intergestural temporal coordination is specified. Subsequently, these gestures or vocal tract action units are executed; that is, gestures or vocal tract actions are the relevant control units for programming and executing articulatory movements. A differentiation of motor planning, programming, and execution also was introduced in the detailed model of speech production given by van der Merwe (2008). A shortcoming of her approach, however, is that it is not strongly quantitative, and the model cannot be tested by producing or perceiving speech items. Furthermore, it should be noted that van der Merwe's approach is not strongly action based but segment oriented.

The importance of the concept of action (action planning, programming, and execution) in AOS is argued by Miller (2000, 2002). Likewise, the importance of models of speech production embracing cognitive linguistic as well as sensorimotor aspects of speech production has been advocated (Miller, 2002; Croot, 2002). For example, the production of a labial closure or of a glottal opening is a "speech action" or "speech gesture." A complete language-specific system of speech actions is introduced by Kröger and Birkholz (2007) for standard German. Criticism concerning the action concept, at least in its formulation as articulatory phonology (Browman & Goldstein, 1989, 1992), focused mainly on the lack of integration of the auditory domain into the gestural theory (Kohler, 1992). In our modeling approach, the concept of vocal tract action units or gestures is introduced as a concept for sensorimotor control of speech production. Thus gestures are not interpreted primarily as phonological or linguistic units. Rather, in our modeling approach, no linguistic unit is favored. Different linguistic units (i.e., features, phonological gestures, segments, syllable constituents such as onset, rhyme or coda, syllables, words, and larger prosodic units) are seen as potential and co-existing units of linguistic speech processing. These different units are ordered hierarchically: prosodic units can be subdivided into one or more words, words into one or more syllables and so on. Thus, phonological gestures have an intermediate status between segments and features. A bundle of features determines a gesture (e.g., manner and place features determine the labial closing gesture), and one or more gestures determine a segment (e.g., labial closing and glottal opening gesture determine the phoneme /p/). These linguistic units lead to specifications of sensorimotor action units (i.e., sensorimotor gestures). Moreover, in contrast to Browman and Goldstein (1992), gestural targets or goals are not seen primarily as articulatory targets in our approach but as functional goals that can be specified in a functional manner in the sensory (somatosensory and auditory) domain in our model. It should be emphasized that the phonetic map—that is, the core

of the "mental syllabary" in our model (Kröger et al., 2009)—is organized on a syllabic level.

A further feature of our model is the assumption that a disruption of the phonetic to motor plan network (or mapping) can occur separately for different types of syllables (e.g., V, CV, and CCV) since the neural self-organization of the phonetic maps always leads to topologically connected or continuous subregions for these syllable types (see experiment 1). In addition, we assume that particular neural defects always occur in spatially connected subregions of the phonetic map. This allows the modeling of different degrees of severity when disturbances are introduced into the model, for example, defective mapping of V, CV, and CCV items as opposed to CCV items only (see Experiment 2).

ACT also assumes the existence of a motor planning module (Kröger et al., 2009). The motor planning module forms a neural processing pathway (or route) for infrequent syllables. This arises from the fact that the storage of motor plans and sensory states of syllables as whole patterns within a mental syllabary implies practicing this syllable frequently until the motor pattern is "overlearned" (Levelt, Roelofs, & Meyer, 1999). This cannot be achieved for infrequent syllables. Therefore, a module for the generation of motor plans for infrequent or novel syllables must exist, and by extension, two neural pathways for motor planning are needed (Levelt et al., 1999).

A final feature of our model relevant to the current discussion is the postulation of four processing levels within the motor planning module (Table 16–1). Level 1 of the motor planning module is a generator for proto-gestures, which are

Table 16–1. Knowledge Stored on Different Levels of the Motor Planning Module

Level of Motor Planning Module	Knowledge Stored per Level for the Production of . . .
1	proto-gestures, for example, mouth opening for producing a proto-vowel, tongue elevation for producing a proto-consonant
2	fine-tuned language-specific gestures (see language-specific gesture system in Kröger and Birkholz, 2007)
3	language-specific temporal coordination of gestures for syllables
4	words and sentences, that is, knowledge concerning connecting syllables to words and sentences and modification of gestures and gesture timing with respect to stress and intonation

gestures defined before any language-specific fine-tuning of targets has taken place (proto-gestures are explained in Kröger, Birkholz, Kannampuzha, & Neuschaefer-Rube, 2006). Levels 2 and 3 reflect the organization of (language-specific) motor plans. In order to produce a language-specific speech item, proto-gestures have to be fine-tuned, and intergestural temporal coordination must be fixed. A set of language-specific gestures and its temporal coordination within syllables is established after language-specific imitation training (Kröger et al., 2006, Kröger and Birkholz, 2007). The resulting knowledge concerning the set of language-specific gestures is stored on level 2 of the motor planning module while the knowledge concerning the language specific temporal coordination of gestures within syllables is stored on level 3. Level 4 is involved mainly in modifying gestures and gestural coordination with respect to connecting syllables into words and words into sentences. It, thus, involves specific prosodic categories such as differ-ent levels of stress (e.g., unstressed vs. stressed) or types of intonation.

Experiment 1: Learning a Model Language— The Unimpaired Speaker

In order to simulate different types of lesions with our model, it first had to be trained for normal speech production (and perception) as a "model speaker before stroke." The model language consisted of a five vowel system in which Vs were /i/, /e/, /a/, /o/, or /u/ along with nine consonants in which Cs were voiced and voiceless plosives /b/, /d/, /g/, /p/, /t/, and /k/, the nasals /m/ and /n/ as well as the lateral /l/. Consonants could be combined with all vowels and C_1C_2V syllables were trained in which C_1 is /b/, /p/, /g/, or /k/ and in which C_2 was always the lateral /l/, again in combination with all five vowels. The model language thus comprised 5 vowels, 15 CV syllables with voiced plosives, 15 CV syllables with voiceless plosives, 10 CV syllables with nasal consonants, and 20 CCV syllables (/plV/, /blV/, /klV/, and /glV/). Furthermore, the model was capable of processing two-syllable words composed from these syllables. All combinations of the 60 syllables occurred as words within the model language and these words were defined as trochee structures (i.e., with stress on the first syllable).

Motor plan states and sensory states of frequent syllables are stored as a whole by the phonetic to motor plan mapping and by the phonetic to sensory mappings (see arrows in Figure 16–1). This results from extensive training of these frequent syllables during speech acquisition (and further during lifetime). Thus, frequent syllables also are called well-practiced, overlearned, or automated syllables in terms of sensorimotor control. Infrequent syllables have to be assembled from subsyllabic parts such as onset, rhyme, or coda, single sound segments, or single vocal tract action units by the motor planning module. The neural pathway, consisting of the motor planning module, may be termed the gestural assembly route, analogous to the idea of a segmental assembly route as introduced by Levelt et al. (1999). In our model language, the production of isolated vowels and most of the CV and CCV syllables was defined as high frequency and these were, therefore, stored in long-term memory—that is in the phonetic to motor plan and phonetic to sensory mappings introduced previously (comparable with the concept of mental syllabary, Levelt & Wheeldon, 1994; Levelt et al., 1999; Indefrey & Levelt, 2004). Only

the syllables /lo/ and /ple/ were defined as infrequent syllables in our model language. Accordingly, the motor plan state for these syllables had to be assembled by the motor planning module. A typical ordering of the automated or well-practiced syllables within a 25×25 neuron self-organizing phonetic map is shown in Figure 16–2. This results from a babbling and imitation training experiment as described in Kröger et al., 2009. One main result of this experiment was that vowels, CV-, and CCV- items were shown to capture different (cortical) regions within the phonetic map.

Experiment 2: Simulations of Different Types of Breakdown—The Virtual Apraxic Speakers

Different instances of the neural model can be trained by starting from (1) several initial settings of link weight values for the mappings, by using (2) different training items resulting from different randomization procedures, and by (3) varying orderings of training items (Kröger et al., 2009). The resulting "trained models" represent different virtual speech processing units—that is, different virtual listeners and virtual speakers.

In the current study, versions of the model comprising different specific neural disruptions were introduced. In addition to the virtual unimpaired speaker described previously, four "impaired" versions were trained that exhibited a variety of dysfunctions of certain neural maps and mappings and

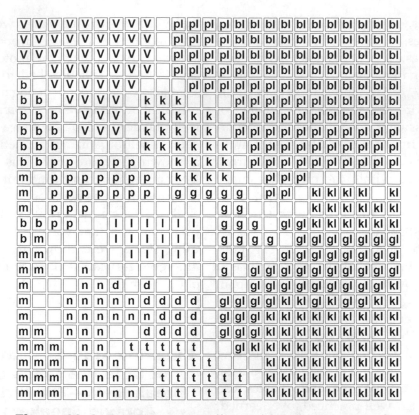

Figure 16–2. 25 × 25 neuron self-organizing phonetic map after babbling and imitation training for the model language (see text). A neuron is marked with a letter V if the neuron represents a vocalic state. Neurons are marked with lower case letters for C or CC if the neuron represents a CV or a CCV state. Clear regions can be found for [V, dV, gV, pV, tV, kV, nV, blV, glV, plV, klV]. A slight mixture of regions occurs for [mV, bV]. Vowels are not broken down to [i, e, a, o, u] in this figure. Unmarked neurons indicate states that cannot be associated clearly with any phonemic state.

varying dysfunctions of particular neural processing modules. The benefit of using a quantitative model of speech processing is that the processing of one speech item (specified on the phonological level) can lead to different anomalous articulation behaviors and different acoustic signals for that speech item due to the specific dysfunction introduced to the model. The resulting phonetic anomalies can be related to the specific neural deficits applied to the model speaker. Table 16–2 subsumes types of combinations of (1) disruptions within the phonetic to motor plan mapping (mental syllabary path for frequent syllables) and (2) disruptions within the motor planning module (gestural assembly path for infrequent syllables). Concerning the phonetic-to-motor plan mapping, we assume that this mapping can be disrupted as a whole or in parts with respect to different groups of speech items such as

Table 16–2. Speech Production Symptoms for Model Instances (Virtual AOS Speakers)

Virtual Speakers	Available (concerning: phonetic-to-motor plan mapping)	Available (concerning: motor planning module)	Symptoms
1 (severe form of AOS)		• Level 1: proto-gestures	• groping for vowels; • no CV, CCV syllables and words; • dysprosody
2	• V	• Level 1: proto-gestures • Level 2: vocalic gestures	• groping for consonants; • gestural timing errors for CV syllables; • no CCV syllables and words; • dysprosody
3a	• V • CV	• Level 1 • Level 2: all language-specific gestures	• gestural timing errors for infrequent CV syllables, • no CCV syllables and words; • dysprosody
3b	• V • CV	• Levels 1 & 2 • Level 3: timing for CV- syllables	• gestural timing errors for CCV- syllables and words; • dysprosody
4a	• V • CV • CCV	• Levels 1 & 2 • Level 3: timing for CV- syllables	• gestural timing errors for infrequent CCV syllables and words; • dysprosody
4b (mild form of AOS)	• V • CV • CCV	• Levels 1, 2 & 3	• gestural timing inaccuracies at syllable boundaries in words (e.g., pauses at syllable boundaries); • dysprosody
normal virtual speaker	• V • CV • CCV	• Level 1, 2, 3 & 4	• none

Note. These symptoms resulted from specific defects of the motor planning module and/or the phonetic to motor plan mapping. It is assumed that all syllables are realized as stressed if the prosodic part of the phonetic-to-motor plan mapping is defective.

CCV syllables, CV syllables, or V-items (vowels) since these groups of speech items form spatially connected regions at the level of the self-organizing phonetic map (see Figure 16–2).

As regards the motor planning module, we assume it may be disrupted in a top-down direction—that is, the motor planning module can be disrupted at higher levels of motor plan specification while lower levels of motor plan specification remain available. The aim of these simulation experiments with contrasting types of "virtual AOS speakers" was to describe the varying speech outcomes from the different lesions and to compare these to features claimed as characteristic of AOS in real speakers. There-by, we aimed to contribute to the debate on possible origins of speech apraxic disruptions within models of speech output in relation to varying types of neural disruption. An overview of virtual speakers exhibiting specific neural defects and of the resulting AOS signs or symptoms is provided in Table 16–2.

Virtual Speaker 1: Lesion at the Level of Phonetic-to-Motor Plan Mapping for Vowels and Consonants

In this version of the model, the phonetic-to-motor plan mapping was cut off entirely, rendering the speaker incapable of executing any language-specific motor plans for vowels or syllables (Experiment 1). However, it is assumed that the phonetic-to-auditory and the phonetic-to-somatosensory mappings remain unaffected. Thus, despite the fact that the virtual speaker is unable to produce language-specific speech items, he still knows what a

vowel or a frequent syllable should sound like and how a vowel or frequent syllable feels during production when he activates this speech item at the level of the phonemic map. It is assumed that for this type of speaker, the motor planning module is disrupted starting at level 2, rendering him incapable of producing language-specific speech items, even via the motor planning module (vocal tract action assembly path). Only proto-actions can be activated from the motor planning module (see Table 16–2).

In order to investigate the effects of this disruption, the production of a simple task was simulated—that is, to produce a realization of the vowel /u/. This leads to the activation of the neuronal representation of the phonemic /u/ state within the phonemic map. Subsequently, this brings about coactivation of the auditory and somatosensory state of the stored /u/ realization via the phonetic map as was trained during speech acquisition (Kröger et al., 2009). Thus, the virtual speaker activates the auditory, tactile, and proprioceptive neural state for /u/ while the motor plan state for a /u/-realization is inaccessible. Despite the fact that speaker 1 is not capable of producing the appropriate motor plan state, he still "feels" (1) the vocal tract state from the prestored proprioceptive activation pattern and (2) the tactile contact pattern from the prestored tactile activation pattern. Since the motor plan state of an /u/ realization is not available to speaker 1, he activates what he is able to—that is, several proto-vocalic actions —and compares the resulting somatosensory (i.e., tactile and proprioceptive) states of his current production trials with the somatosensory target state for a /u/ action. Figure 16–3 gives an

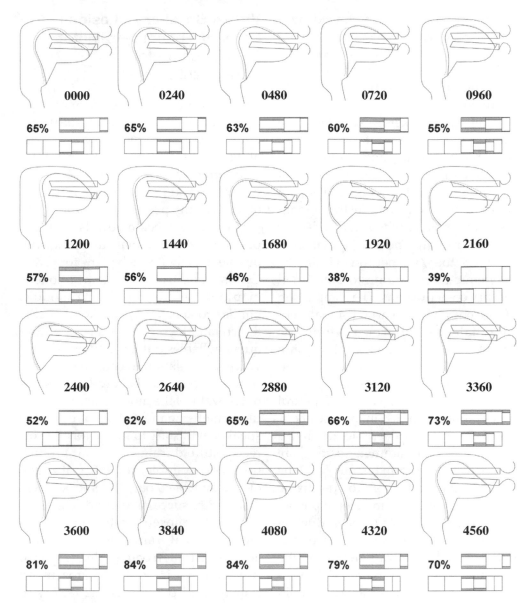

Figure 16–3. Trial and error groping of speaker 1. The speaker tries to articulate a realization of /u/. Time is indicated in ms. Degree of similarity of current somatosensory state with respect to somatosensory state of the /u/ realization is given in percent. The shaded areas in the tactile contact pattern indicate contact of vocal tract organs or articulators (adjacent to the percentage; from left to right: contact area of tongue body, tongue tip, lips) with regions of the vocal tract wall (below; from left to right: lower pharyngeal, upper pharyngeal, velar, palatal, post-alveolar, and alveolar region) (See Color Plate 5).

example for the resulting vocal tract movements. It can be seen that groping behavior occurs for this speaker. He successively produces a number of proto-vocalic actions, first a front-high-unrounded action (from 0 ms to about

960 ms, Figure 16–5), followed by a low-unrounded (from 960 ms to about 1920 ms), a front-high-rounded (from 1920 ms to about 3120 ms) and a back-high-rounded action (from 3120 ms to about 4080 ms).

While the speaker is executing these proto-actions, the somatosensory state is monitored online and compared to the prelearned somatosensory state of a typical /u/ action. This prelearned state is activated in parallel throughout the duration of the whole trial-and-error process since the speaker permanently activates the /u/ neuron within the phonemic map, leading to prelearned sensory co-activations. The comparison of current and prelearned somatosensory states is performed within the somatosensory phonetic processing module. If the current and the prestored somatosensory states are comparable (e.g., degree of similarity of neural states higher than 80% in the case of our simulation) the current proto-action and its intragestural parameter setting are retained in short-term memory, and the speaker now endeavors to co-activate pulmonary initiation and glottal phonation in order to make vowel production audible. A further refinement of the vocalic action realization toward the prestored /u/ can be attempted through comparisons of auditory states. It should be noted that proto-gestures are permitted to vary with respect to all intragestural parameters. Thus, the motor plan state of the vowel /u/ is re-attained by trial-and-error groping. Due to the severe neural defects of this virtual speaker, the production of motor plan items more complex than isolated vowels is assumed to involve too excessive demands and no co-articulation with other phonemes is deemed possible.

Virtual Speaker 2: Lesion at the Level of Phonetic–to-Motor Plan Mapping for Consonants Only

The neural defects modeled for speaker 2 are identical to those of speaker 1 with the exception that the vocalic part of the phonetic-to-motor plan mapping is unaffected (see Table 16–2). This virtual speaker is, therefore, capable of activating prestored motor plans for language-specific vowels from the phonetic-to-motor plan mapping, but unable to activate such plans for CV or CCV syllables, neither via the phonetic map nor the motor planning module. Similar to speaker 1, speaker 2 is able to activate the sensory states of all frequent syllables but in addition, also all vowels. In relation to consonants, only proto-actions can be produced since only level 1 of the motor planning module remains unaffected. As a result, the speaker will start to grope for the correct gesture during consonant production. For example, for the realization of the syllable /pa/, the speaker will start with successive productions of randomly chosen proto-consonantal labial, apical, and dorsal closing actions. Through being able to monitor productions in the somatosensory domain and possessing the facility to compare current productions and a prestored /pa/ realization, the speaker will maintain the proto-labial closing actions in short-term memory. However, to produce an acceptable realization of /pa/, speaker 2 now has to find the correct interaction temporal coordination for all actions of /pa/ (i.e., labial closing action, glottal opening action, and vocalic action) through trial-and-error productions. Typical segmental effects resulting from these trial–and-error productions as generated by the model are provided in Figure 16–4.

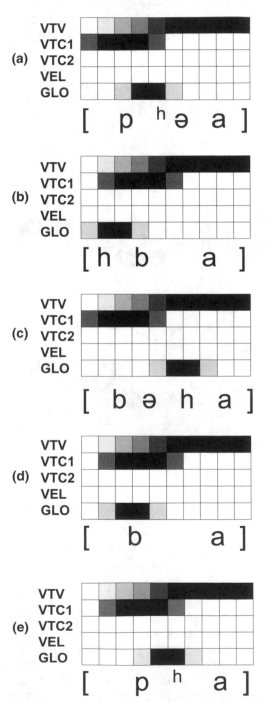

The neural activation pattern of the motor plans for /pa/ and the resulting acoustic signal are listed in Figure 16–4: (a) If the timing of the glottal opening action with respect to the consonantal vocal tract closing action is correct, but if the vocalic tract forming action starts too late with respect to the consonantal closing action, the perceptual impression of an inserted schwa-sound arises. (b) If the timing of the consonantal closing action and of the vocalic action is correct, but the glottal opening action starts too early with respect to the consonantal closing action, pre-aspiration can occur, and the consonant may be perceived as voiceless. (c) If the glottal opening action together with the vocalic action starts too late with respect to the consonantal closing action, schwa-insertion and [h]-insertion are perceived. (d) If the timing of the consonantal closing action and the vocalic action is

Figure 16–4. CV motor plan temporal activation patterns and appropriate phonetic transcriptions of the resulting acoustic speech signal produced by model speaker 2. This model speaker tries to produce an acceptable /pa/ realization. Trial **(a)–(d)**: severe mistiming of gestures resulting in deviating phonetic transcription for /pa/. Trial **(e)**: proper gestural timing for a /pa/ realization. The gestural timing for **(a)–(e)** is illustrated by the motor plan neural activation patterns. These patterns are described in the text. Each box represents a motor plan neuron (white to black: no activation to full activation). The rows indicate gestural activation for actions; from top: vocalic tract forming action as part of V (VTV), consonantal vocal tract closing action as part of C1 and as part of C2 (VTC1, VTC2), velum action (VEL), and glottal action (GLO).

correct, but the glottal opening action is produced temporally synchronous with the consonantal closing action, the perceptual impression of a voiced plosive occurs. (e) The production of an acceptable /pa/ realization is achieved only if the temporal ending of the glottal opening gesture (i.e., time instant of maximum glottal opening) coincides in time with the termination of the consonantal closing action (i.e., time instant of release of consonantal closure). It is assumed that speaker 2 is capable of producing CV syllables after several trials at finding the correct temporal coordination.

Virtual Speakers 3a and 3b: Modeling of Gestural Timing Errors for CCV Syllables

The next progression in the location of neural defects is to have levels 1 and 2 intact, but a breakdown at level 3. That means that phonetic-to-motor plan mapping is functioning for V-items and CV syllables (see Table 16–2). The speaker is, therefore, capable of producing vowels and consonants and combining these to form syllables. The latter ability might be restricted to frequent syllables only (speaker 3a) or can include the production of infrequent syllables as well (speaker 3b). In the case of speaker 3a, infrequent CV syllables are produced by taking the information concerning action timing from phonetically similar frequent CV syllables—that is, by taking the knowledge from the motor part of the intact part of the phonetic map. Irrespective of the ability to produce such CV syllables, neither of the speakers is able to activate motor plans for CCV syllable via the phonetic map, but speaker 3b tries

to produce CCV syllables since he is capable of producing all CV syllables. Typical errors in temporal coordination of actions for the CCV syllable for speaker 3b are illustrated in Figure 16–5 in which the model is instructed to produce /gla/. It is capable of producing

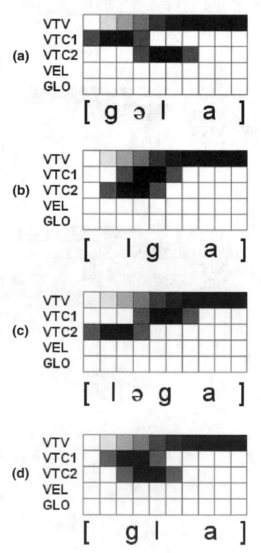

Figure 16–5. (a)–(c): CCV motor plan temporal activation patterns for typical timing errors occurring in realization of /gla/ for model speaker 3b (see text). (d): correct neural activation pattern for the motor plan of /gla/.

the syllables /ga/ or /la/, but as can be seen, the timing errors of actions for /CCV/ syllables lead to segmental effects such as schwa-insertion in the consonant cluster or to metathesis of the two initial consonants with or without schwa-insertion.

Virtual Speakers 4a and 4b: Modeling of Gestural Timing Errors for Infrequent CCV Syllables and Dysprosody

Speakers 4a and 4b present a further decrease in severity of speech problem. Compared to speaker 3b, speaker 4a now has intact motor plans for all (frequent) V, CV, and CCV syllables. However, his knowledge of the correct temporal coordination for infrequent CCV syllables is still unavailable (see Table 16–2). The speech deviations for such syllables thus are comparable to those illustrated for speaker 3b (Figure 16–5). In the case of speaker 4a infrequent CCV syllables are produced by taking the information concerning action timing from phonetically similar frequent CCV syllables—that is, by taking the knowledge from the motor part of the phonetic map.

As a result of disruption of level 4 of the motor planning module, the main defect for speaker 4b, which also occurs as a side defect for all other speakers (1, 2, 3a, 3b, and 4a) in as far as these speakers are capable of producing at least two consecutive syllables, affects the prosodic make up of words. Model speaker 4b is, thus, characteristic of someone with a mild form of AOS. The difference between this speaker and the unimpaired model is that he is not capable of accessing information on how to produce an unstressed version of a syl-

lable (all syllables within the phonetic map are assumed to be stressed versions of syllables) and how to connect two syllables correctly in order to form a word within the model language. Thereby, speaker 4b is capable of producing the syllables of the model language but realizes a bisyllabic word as two equally stressed syllables with an unnatural pause in between.

Discussion

The simulation experiments described in this paper have demonstrated that signs of AOS such as trial-and-error groping or different segmental errors (or effects) resulting from errors in temporal coordination can result from particular neural defects in mappings (here the phonetic-to-motor plan mapping) or processing modules (here, the motor planning module) within our neural model. These findings lend weight to speculations aired by Miller (2000) that within a perspective on speech motor control that integrates cognitive (e.g., attentional, short-term/ working memory, processing capacity), motor as well as neural strands (e.g., interconnectivity), speech derailments would be emergent properties of (disordered) interaction within and across tiers in the speech production system. This is even before one starts to ponder the possibilities for break down that could occur when considering possible interactions between speech processing and broader language processing (e.g., word retrieval; sentence stress assignment). One would not need to posit separate phonological or phonetic ordering, deletion, or insertion processes, and the like to explain perceived speech errors. This is amply illustrated in virtual speaker 2 where schwa-insertion, apparent substitutions, additions, and omissions emerge from disruptions to the timing between gestures. Such a perspective also affords a transparency between perceived speech derailments and understanding them in terms of underlying alterations in neural functioning, such as levels of activation and inhibition, integration of feed-forward and feedback processes and perceptual and output processes. However, the virtual speakers illustrated in Table 16–2 give only a first very broad indication of possible subtypes of AOS speech disruptions. Basic disruption to the phonetic map (V, CV, CCV, prosody) could lead to further subtypes.

It is beyond the scope of this chapter to discuss the different levels of knowledge in specifying the temporal coordination (or intergestural timing) of all gestures forming a specific syllable or speech item. One would need to attend (1) to the detailed knowledge for each syllable attained by looking for the phonetically most similar syllable occurring within the mental syllabary (phonetic-to-motor plan mapping) and by adapting the intra- and intergestural parameters of this specific syllable for the target under production, or (2) to the broader knowledge differentiating types of syllable (e.g., CV with C = nasals; or C = voiced plosives; or C = voiceless plosives; or CCV with C1 = voiced plosives and C2 = /l/; or CCV with C1 = voiceless plosives and C2 = /l/, etc.), which can be generalized from the phonetic-to-motor plan mapping by processing gestural parameters over all CV syllables belonging to a specific syllable type. Although on the one hand the knowledge of how to specify the ges-

tural parameters of a specific syllable in detail needs the online availability of the phonetic-to-motor plan mapping (i.e., needs a nondisrupted phonetic to motor plan mapping) in the current version of ACT; on the other hand, the knowledge for syllable types can be seen as a generalization of motor planning knowledge, and it can be assumed to be available even if phonetic to motor planning mapping is disrupted. This generalization of knowledge for the temporal coordination of gestures is not implemented in our model currently. It would lead to a further separation of the four severity stages suggested in Table 16–2 and is an area for future investigation.

Moreover, it should be noted that due to the speaker's ability to activate the somatosensory state of a syllable during production, groping too could be advantageous in order to prepare the production of a syllable silently. We assume that the somatosensory pattern can be used for selecting proto-gestures as was the case in our silent groping simulations, but we assume that somatosensation does not provide a sufficiently detailed or strong signal to set the correct timing of all gestures of a syllable in advance during silent groping, especially in the case of glottal and velopharyngeal gestures. This offers one explanation of why audible trial and error productions often follow after silent groping and why certain segments may appear more problematic than others.

The Dual Route Paradigm

In agreement with Levelt et al. (1999), we assume a "dual route model" (or as it would be labeled in our approach:

dual neural pathway model) for translating phonological specifications of syllables into articulatory specifications. In agreement with these authors we assume one neural pathway for frequent and another for infrequent syllables. The frequent pathway comprises phonemic-to-motor mapping, which is comparable to the mental syllabary. This neural pathway (also called syllabic encoding route or in terms of our model: syllabic motor plan storage) is implemented in our model by a self organizing (phonetic) map, and its bilateral mappings, which associate phonemic, motor plan, and sensory states. All motor plans and sensory states for frequent syllables are stored within the phonetic to motor plan and phonetic to sensory mappings. For the second neural pathway (also termed subsyllabic encoding route, or in terms of our model motor planning module, generator of motor plans, or generator of gestural scores) we assume that motor plans here are assembled from smaller subsyllabic units (Levelt et al., 1999). These smaller units, though, are basically vocal tract action units (or gestures) in our approach and not necessarily segments as is claimed by other authors. In some cases, one gesture represents one segment (e.g., some vowels such as /i/, /a/; voiced plosives) and so in these cases one might interpret the gesture-by-gesture assembly of motor plans within the motor planning module as segment-by-segment assembly. However, in other cases segments are ensembles or groups of gestures (vowels such as /o/, /u/ comprise lip and tongue gestures; voiceless consonants comprise vocal tract constricting or closing and glottal opening gestures; nasals comprise vocal tract constricting

or closing and velopharyngeal opening gestures). Furthermore, it is possible that the assembly of syllabic motor plans is based on larger subsyllabic units, for example, syllable onset consonantal clusters, since intragestural timing first of all relates all gestures constituting this cluster and then relates the gestures for this cluster with other constituents forming a syllable.

A major difference between our approach and the dual route concepts discussed previously is that a strong neural association between mental syllabary and the gestural assembling module (motor planning module) is assumed in our model (see Figure 16–1). In our approach, it is assumed that the knowledge for assembling infrequent syllables always stems from knowledge stored within the mental syllabary. For example, in the case of the realization of the infrequent syllable /lo/ (designated as low frequency in our model language), the phonemic activation of /lo/ leads to an activation of all frequent /lV/ syllables (i.e., /lu/ as well as /la/, /le/ and /li/). All these syllables are phonetically similar and thus one can assume that the temporal gestural frame of these frequent syllables /lV/, i.e. the specification of all temporal inter- and intra-gestural parameters for the /lV/ syllable type is copied from the syllabary in order to have a prototypical gestural motor plan for /lo/. Thus, only the spatial target information of /l/ and /o/ need be added as "spatial content" to this "temporal gestural frame" (cf., MacNeilage, 1970, for segments) in order to specify completely the motor plan for this infrequent syllable.

Hence, a model of AOS that assumes total impairment of the mentally syllabary and a need to compensate by using an "indirect route" is not compatible with our model. First, knowledge from the mental syllabary is needed to assemble gestural motor plans of infrequent syllables in our approach. Second, the gestural assembly route (i.e., the route using the motor planning module in our approach) cannot be interpreted as an indirect or "second choice" route if the main route, that is, the mental syllabary, is defective. The gestural assembly pathway in our approach (i.e., the motor planning module) is as important as the mental syllabary itself, being, for example, the neural pathway for modifying temporal and spatial gestural parameters in relation to prosody (e.g., speaking rate, emphatic stress).

Moreover, in our approach it is not assumed that one of the motor planning routes can be completely defective. For instance, it is assumed that parts of the mental syllabary (for example, CV syllables or CCV syllables) and in parallel parts (or levels) of the motor planning module are defective. One of the main results of this study, therefore, is that the functional picture of neural defects in terms of our model is not as simplistic as in other approaches (e.g., Varley & Whiteside 2001). Experimental data from speakers with AOS compatible with the assumptions and results given by our model appear for example in Aichert and Ziegler (2004). They conclude that not only the mental syllabary but also the "indirect route must be disturbed as well in AOS patients" (p. 154) and that "a disturbance of the indirect route should not be explained by side-effects . . . of speech motor programming" (p. 154). Moreover, Aichert and Ziegler claim that "patients with AOS do access the mental syllabary . . ." (p. 156). This assumption is again in accordance with the assumptions of our model. Furthermore, Aichert and Ziegler (2004) postulate that AOS speakers retrieve corrupted entries from the mental syllabary. This has not been modeled in our experiments to date, but could lead to more types of segmental errors than were generated in our model so far, for example, by varying the temporal coordination of gestures.

Motor Planning versus Motor Programming

Although motor planning is a central concept in our neural model, motor programming is not addressed here explicitly. It is striking in the literature that the terms motor planning and motor programming currently refer to different control concepts or control models. Thus, Darley et al (1975) claimed a three-step model separating language processing, motor programming, and execution. Van der Merwe (2008) introduced a four-stage sensorimotor model of speech production and separated linguistic processing, motor planning, motor programming, and motor execution. She claimed that motor planning involves (1) activating and organizing the temporal and spatial specifications or the production of sequences of phonemes and (2) adaptation of core motor plans for particular phonemes to specific speech contexts in which they will appear by entering into subroutines that enable movement of the articulatory structures. Further, motor programming means that the motor plan subroutines are fed-forward to the motor programming system in which muscle-specific motor programs for articulatory movements are selected. Following this approach, AOS would be a motor planning disorder while the dysarthrias would be motor programming disorders (cf., Peach, 2004). Kent (2000) separates "the planning and preparation of movements (sometimes called motor programming) and the execution of movement plans to result in muscle contractions and structural displacements" (p. 391). He maintains that "acquired AOS . . . impairs especially the process of planning or programming speech movements . . . " and states that "the dysarthrias affect the execution of movements" (p. 403). Although the model introduced in this paper differentiates only planning and execution, by introducing the motor plan level, it is one of our future tasks to specify the execution module in more detail, for example, in relation to a differentiation of this module with respect to action unit programming and execution (Maas, Robin, Wrigth, & Ballard, 2008; Wright et al., 2009). Currently, we allocate programming between planning and execution, which is in agreement with the model of van der Merve (2008).

Moreover, it should be noted that the model introduced in this paper is a model of speech processing that includes production and perception components. The DIVA model also includes feedback loops, and through this, introduces self-perception. Despite the fact that perception is seldom mentioned in descriptions of AOS, it is assumed in our perspective that peripheral and central sensory speech processing are not affected in AOS. This is important for example in our modeling of groping, since the notion of the auditory and somatosensory target of the speech item is the driving force for groping in our approach.

We set out to introduce the main features of ACT and to examine within this action, gestural- as opposed to segmental-based model, whether lesioning would produce sound derailments compatible with perceptual and instrumental descriptions of apraxic speech derailments that were emergent properties of the system without having to posit a linear, segmental organization of speech output. In as far as the speech "errors" produced in model speakers 1–4 reflected the kinds of disruption reported for people with AOS, we believe we have achieved this. Speech derailments could be seen, for instance, to arise from overall problems in inter- and intragestural timing, in degraded access to computational elements, and so forth. This opens up an avenue of enquiry that can supplement and complement studies of AOS. ACT offers the possibility on the one hand of testing out theoretical predictions concerning the nature of AOS and on the other hand informing the interpretation of apraxic speech output, informing construction of tasks to test out with real AOS speakers and against real lesions. It was seen that predictions and results from ACT were compatible with contemporary models of apraxia of speech in terms of nonlinear dynamics in output and notions of gestural internal versus external breakdown of organization (Maas et al., 2008; Wright et al., 2009; Ziegler, 2005, 2009).

However, it should be noted that the neurocomputational model of speech processing introduced here as well as our modeling of AOS should be interpreted only as an initial endeavor. While the model is among the most detailed quantitative neural models of speech processing currently in existence and is in accordance with very recent results of functional imaging and behavioralistic studies (Eickhoff, Heim, Zilles, & Amunts, 2009; Moser et al., 2009; Martins & Ortiz, 2009), it nevertheless still delivers only a very broad picture of the true complexity of human neural processes in speech processing. Further, the neural deficits introduced here are related strongly to the organization of the model and are highly schematic. In reality, it can be assumed that true neural deficits are far more complex. Thus, this model and the resulting modeling of signs of AOS should be interpreted as only a starting point in understanding AOS. More detailed modeling as well as true clinical studies must focus on this topic in order to gain a better and more detailed understanding of AOS.

Acknowledgment. This work was supported in part by the German Research Council Project Nr. Kr 1439/13-1 and project Nr. Kr 1439/15-1.

References

Aichert, I., & Ziegler, W. (2004). Syllable frequency and syllable structure in apraxia of speech. *Brain & Language, 88*, 148–159.

Browman, C., & Goldstein, L. (1989). Articulatory gestures as phonological units. *Phonology, 6*, 201–251.

Browman, C., & Goldstein, L. (1992). Articulatory phonology: An overview. *Phonetica, 49*, 155–180.

Croot, K. (2002). Diagnosis of AOS: Definition and criteria. *Seminars in Speech and Language, 23*, 267–279.

Darley, F. L., Aronson, A. E., & Brown, J. R. (1975). Motor speech disorders. Philadelphia, PA: Saunders.

Eickhoff, S. G., Heim, S., Zilles, K., & Amunts, K. (2009). A systems perspective on the effective connectivity of overt speech production. *Philosophical transactions of the Royal Society B: Biological Science, 367*, 2399–2421

Goldstein, L., Byrd, D., & Saltzman, E. (2006). The role of vocal tract action units in understanding the evolution of phonology. In M. A. Arbib (Ed.), *Action to language via the mirror neuron system* (pp. 215–249). Cambridge, UK: Cambridge University Press.

Goldstein, L., Pouplier, M., Chen, L., Saltzman, L., & Byrd, D. (2007). Dynamic action units slip in speech production errors. *Cognition, 103*, 386–412.

Guenther, F.H. (2006). Cortical interaction underlying the production of speech sounds. *Journal of Communication Disorders, 39*, 350–365.

Guenther, F. H., Ghosh, S. S., & Tourville, J. A. (2006). Neural modeling and imaging of the cortical interactions underlying syllable production. *Brain & Language, 96*, 280–301.

Hickok, G., & Poeppel, D. (2004). Dorsal and ventral streams: A framework for understanding aspects of the functional anatomy of language. *Cognition, 92*, 67–99.

Hillis, A. E., Work, M., Barker, P. B., Jacobs, M. A., Breese, E. L., & Maurer, K. (2004). Re-examining the brain regions crucial for orchestrating speech articulation. *Brain, 127*, 1479–1487.

Indefrey, P., & Levelt, W. J. M. (2004). The spatial and temporal signatures of word production components. *Cognition, 92*, 101–144.

Jordan, L. C , & Hillis, A. E. (2006). Disorders of speech and language: Aphasia, apraxia and dysarthria. *Current Opinion in Neurology, 19*, 580–585.

Kent, R. (2000). Research on speech motor control and its disorders: a review and prospective. *Journal of Communication Disorders, 33*, 391–428.

Kohler, K. J. (1992). Gestural reorganization in connected speech: A functional viewpoint on "articulatory phonology." *Phonetica, 49,* 205–211.

Kröger, B. J., Birkholz, P., Kannampuzha, J., & Neuschaefer-Rube, C. (2006). Learning to associate speech-like sensory and motor states during babbling. *Proceedings of the 7th International Seminar on Speech Production* (pp. 67–74). Brazil: Belo Horizonte.

Kröger, B. J., & Birkholz, P. (2007). A gesture-based concept for speech movement control in articulatory speech synthesis. In A. Esposito, M. Faundez-Zanuy, E. Keller, & M. Marinaro (Eds.), *Verbal and nonverbal communication behaviours LNAI 4775* (pp. 174–189) Berlin, Heidelberg: Springer.

Kröger, B. J., Kannampuzha, J., Lowit, A., & Neuschaefer-Rube, C. (2009). Phonetotopy within a neurocomputational model of speech production and speech acquisition. In S. Fuchs, H. Loevenbruck, D. Pape, & P. Perrier (Eds.), *Some aspects of speech and the brain* (pp. 59–90). Berlin: Lang.

Kröger, B. J., Kannampuzha, J., & Neuschaefer-Rube, C. (2009). Towards a neurocomputational model of speech production and perception. *Speech Communication 51,* 793–809.

Levelt, W. J. M., Roelofs, A., & Meyer, A. (1999). A theory of lexical access in speech production. *Behavioral and Brain Sciences, 22,* 1–75.

Levelt, W. J. M., & Wheeldon, L. (1994). Do speakers have access to a mental syllabary? *Cognition, 50,* 239–269.

Maas, E., Robin, D. A., Wright, D. L., & Ballard, K. J. (2008). Motor programming in apraxia of speech. *Brain & Language, 106,* 107–118.

Martins, F. C., & Ortiz, K. Z. (2009). The relationship between working memory and apraxia of speech. *Arq Neuropsiquiatr, 67,* 843–848.

MacNeilage, P. F. (1970). Motor control of serial ordering of speech. *Psychological Review, 77,* 182–196.

McNeil, M. R. (Ed.) (2008). *Clinical management of sensorimotor speech disorders.* New York, NY: Thieme.

McNeil, M. R., Robin, D. A., & Schmidt, R. A. (1997). Apraxia of speech: Definition, differentiation, and treatment. In M. R. McNeil (Ed.), *Clinical management of sensorimotor speech disorders* (pp. 311–344). New York, NY: Thieme.

Miller, N. (2000). Changing ideas in apraxia of speech. In I. Papathanasiou (Ed.), *Acquired neurogenic communication disorders* (pp. 173–202). London, UK: Whurr.

Miller, N. (2002). The neurological bases of apraxia of speech. *Seminars in Speech and Language, 23,* 223–230.

Moser, D., Fridriksson, J., Bonila, L., Healy, E. W., Baylis, G., Baker, J. M., & Rorden, C. (2009). Neural recruitment for the production of native and novel speech sounds. *Neuroimage, 46,* 549–557.

Ogar, J., Slama, H., Dronkers, N., Amici, S., & Gorno-Tempini, M. L. (2005). Apraxia of speech: An overview. *Neurocase, 11,* 427–432.

Peach, R. K. (2004). Acquired apraxia of speech: Features, accounts, and treatment. *Topics in Stroke Rehabilitation, 11,* 49–58.

Riecker, A., Brendel, B., Ziegler, W., Erb, M., & Ackermann, H. (2008). The influence of syllable onset complexity and syllable frequency on speech motor control. *Brain & Language, 107,* 102–113.

van der Merwe, A. (2008). Theoretical framework for the characterization of pathological speech sensorimotor control. In M. McNeil (Ed.), *Clinical management of sensorimotor speech disorders* (2nd ed., pp. 3–18). New York, NY: Thieme.

Varley, R., & Whiteside, S. (2001). What is the underlying impairment in acquired apraxia of speech? *Aphasiology, 15,* 39–49.

Wertz, R. T, LaPointe, L. L., & Rosenbeck, J. C. (1984). *Apraxia of speech in adults: The disorder and its management.* Orlando, FL: Grune and Stratton.

Wright, D., Robin, D., Rhee, J., Vaculin, A., Jacks, A., & Guenther, F. (2009). Using the self-select paradigm to delineate the nature of speech motor programming. *Journal of Speech, Language, and Hearing Research, 52*, 755–765.

Ziegler, W, (2005), A nonlinear model of word length effects in apraxia of speech.

Cognitive Neuropsychology, 22, 603–623.

Ziegler, W, (2009), Modelling the architecture of phonetic plans: Evidence from apraxia of speech. *Language and Cognitive Processes, 24*, 631–661.

Index

A